"All of the guidelines in *Nutrition for the Chemotherapy Patient* are practical and realistic; giving short, easy recipes cross-referenced with the diet recommendations and drug descriptions, and emphasizing that individual tolerances to drugs and diet modifications will vary. This book will be very useful for dietitians working with cancer patients, and the friendly, direct and easy writing style will make it a book you'll want to recommend to your patients."

Patricia Booth, MS, RD
Department of Nutritional Sciences
University of California, Berkeley

NUTRITION FOR THE CHEMOTHERAPY PATIENT

Janet L. Ramstack, Dr.P.H.
Ernest H. Rosenbaum, M.D.
Sponsored by Mount Zion Medical Center of U.C. San Francisco

with chapter co-authors
Janine Bernat, R.D. and Carol Stitt, R.D., and Isadora Rosenbaum
(Chapter 3—Useful Recipes and Tables)
Robert J. Ignoffo, Pharm.D.
(Chapter 4—Description of Chemotherapeutic Drugs)
Lawrence W. Margolis, M.D.
(Chapter 5—Nutrition and Radiotherapy)

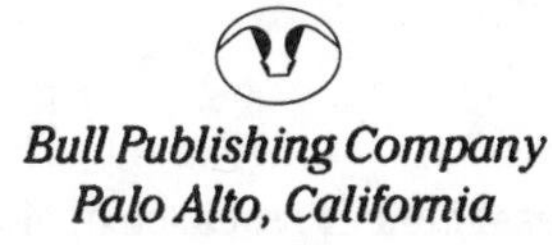

Bull Publishing Company
Palo Alto, California

Bull Publishing Company
P.O. Box 208
Palo Alto, CA 94302-0208
415/322-2855
ISBN 0-915950-99-5

Distributed in the United States by:
Publishers Group West
4065 Hollis Street
Emeryville, California 94608

Library of Congress Cataloging-in-Publication Data
Ramstack, Janet L.
Nutrition for the chemotherapy patient / by Janet L. Ramstack, Ernest H. Rosenbaum.
p. cm.
Includes bibliographical references.
Includes index.
ISBN 0-915950-99-5 : $18.95
1. Cancer—Nutritional aspects. 2. Cancer—Chemotherapy. I. Rosenbaum, Ernest H. II. Title.
(DNLM: 1. Diet. 2. Drug Therapy—adverse effects. 3. Neoplasms—drug therapy. 4. Nutrition. QZ 266 R183n)
RC268.45.R36 1990
616.99'4061—dc20
DNLM/DLC
for Library of Congress 90-1907
CIP

Cover Design: Robb Pawlak
Interior Design: Detta Penna
Production Manager: Helen O'Donnell
Composition by: *The Cowans*
Printer: Bookcrafters, Inc.
Text Face: Cheltenham

All royalties will go to breast cancer research at Mount Zion Medical Center of U.C. San Francisco, San Francisco, California.

This book is dedicated to R. Davilene Carter, M.D.,
whose foresightedness and unmitigated support
are responsible for its genesis.

As a Professor of Surgery at Tulane Medical Center and a surgical oncologist, she recognized the need for nutritional support of the cancer patient long before others in the profession did so.

Acting as a mentor and major academic advisor, she made it possible for the primary author to integrate her knowledge of nutrition with that of cancer chemotherapy treatments to synthesize the concepts set forth here.

Contents

Recipe Table of Contents

About the Authors

Janet L. Ramstack, Dr.PH received her doctorate in Public Health Nutrition from Tulane University in New Orleans. Her primary interests are nutrition and cancer; nutrient-drug interactions; public health nutrition and nutrition education for medical professionals, patients, and the public.

Ernest H. Rosenbaum, MD is Associate Chief of Medicine, Mount Zion Medical Center of U.C. San Francisco; Chief of Oncology, French Hospital, San Francisco; Medical Director of the San Francisco Regional Cancer Foundation; and Clinical Professor of Medicine, University of California, San Francisco.

Nutrition for the Chemotherapy Patient is sponsored by Mount Zion Medical Center of U.C. San Francisco, San Francisco, California.

About the Authors

Acknowledgements

We gratefully acknowledge the following people for their administrative and editorial support: Gay O. Decker, Karen Foreman, Erica Goode, M.D., Julia Homoki, Suzanne Lipset, John Rothberg, Jay Stewart, Mary Anne Stewart, and Jill Wait, R.D. We also wish to credit Elizabeth Silverstein, Charlyn Ignacio-Fotionos, and Paula Chung for typing assistance.

Special thanks for time, effort and editing are due Carmel Finigan, Dwight Starr M.S., and Deborah Hamolsky, R.N. of Mount Zion Hospital and Medical Center.

We wish to thank the Better Health Programs and Jeanine Nesset, M.P.H., R.D. of the Regional Cancer Foundation of San Francisco.

Special thanks is also accorded to the Louisiana Division/American Cancer Society for financial support.

How To Use This Book

This book has two parts. *Part I: Using Nutrition—How Food Can Help* is designed primarily for people with cancer and those helping them at home, while *Part II: Advising the Chemotherapy Patient—The Medical Perspective* is directed primarily at the medical professional. Although many from both groups will naturally be interested in information contained throughout the book, patients and their caregivers will naturally be drawn more to Part I and medical practitioners to Part II.

The first chapter in Part I tells "How to Deal With Specific Problems." Ideally, patients and their caregivers will be advised by their healthcare team, and together they will adopt a nutrition strategy specific for the patient and the particular drug regimen. But the information in this chapter also will enable patients to find immediate help for problems as they arise.

Chapter 2 of Part I contains "General Dietary Guidelines" for sound nutritional management, and Chapter 3 contains "Recipes and Tables," for the actual food planning and preparation that puts the nutrition principles to work.

Chapters 1 and 2 are cross-referenced to the Recipes of Chapter 3, making it easy for the reader to find and prepare the recommended foods.

The Appendix contains a discussion of mouth and dental care, as well as lists of resources for further information and assistance. There is also a Glossary, defining commonly-used technical terms, and an Index for easy reference to specific subjects of interest.

Introduction

This book is a guide for making nutrition choices. The right choices can often prevent, control, and reverse some of the adverse side effects of chemotherapy. They can also help build and maintain general health, and thus improve chances of successful treatment and recovery.

Many factors can interfere with the ability of the patient on chemotherapy to eat well. These include depression, inactivity, pain, digestive and other physical problems, intestinal obstruction, and reactions to the drugs.

Patients who begin treatment well-nourished tolerate treatment better, possibly survive longer, and have a greater sense of well-being than those whose nutrition initially is poor; but even for the well-nourished patient, consuming enough well-chosen foods can become a problem as treatment goes on.

Unless someone—preferably the patient—conscientiously plans a nutritionally-optimal diet and follows through to make sure it is eaten, there is a real danger of malnutrition.

Not only is malnutrition a serious condition in itself, but it greatly increases the difficulty of chemotherapy treatment. The malnourished or marginally-nourished patient experiences more drug side effects. As a result, the treatment is then generally refused or curtailed, which in turn may permit the cancer to progress. It is this vicious cycle that the nutritional plan should be designed to break.

Part I: *Using Nutrition—How Food Can Help*, tells what to do. Patients (and their home caregivers) will use the information here to make nutrition work for them.

Because of what is now known about specific chemotherapy drugs and their nutrition-related characteristics, a nutrition strategy can be developed for each patient, taking into account the particular drugs being administered, as well as the particular circumstances of the patient's health status and treatment. Part I will tell patients what they can do to help themselves.

Written in easy-to-understand language, and laying out simple rules for choosing food and eating, the interrelated sections of Part I will make it easy to adopt a nutritional strategy for each person. If there are changes in treatment or health status, the nutrition prescription (and guidelines for food selection) can be changed accordingly. If the strategy is not as effective as anticipated, further consultation with medical advisors can help pinpoint the reason, utilizing the information in Part II.

Part II: *Advising the Chemotherapy Patient—The Medical Perspective* provides the information base for deciding what sections of Part I are important for a given patient. It is directed more to the physician and other members of the healthcare team; it describes the chemical agents used in chemotherapy treatment, their interactions, side effects, and nutrition-related characteristics.

It assumes some medical background (though the interested lay person can learn a great deal about the particular drugs, and the importance of a nutrition strategy as a part of cancer treatment).

Most patients and those supporting them at home will want to turn directly to the sections of Part I prescribed for them by their medical advisors. These advisors will be able to make copies of and use a "Nutrition Prescription" form, filled in for each patient and designating the sections of Part I of greatest importance for him. This will enable each patient to develop a strategy, using the information in Part I that fits his needs and treatment.

In writing this book, we have drawn both from the scientific literature on the subject and on our own clinical experiences in fashioning dietary applications to reduce drug toxicity. These have proved effective in improving the quality of life of patients on chemotherapy, and in supporting the primary treatment.

It is important to emphasize that this book does not promote diet as a primary therapy for cancer. On the contrary, it approaches nutritional support as an adjunct of standard cancer treatments, with the purpose of increasing patients' comfort, well-being, and tolerance with respect to chemotherapy. Also, to the extent that these factors help enhance general nutritional status, they strengthen the natural powers of the body to help fight the disease.

Besides combating the side effects of drugs, diet and nutrition planning give cancer patients and those who care about them an element of control in circumstances that may well seem beyond control. Once patients find they can mitigate side effects of their chemotherapy through what they choose to eat, they come to feel they are actively participating in their own recovery process. That very participation can only be a positive step in shaping the hopeful optimism that could well be a factor in recovery.

Part I

Using Nutrition—How Food Can Help

Chapter 1

How to Deal with Specific Problems

1. *Loss of Appetite*
2. *Nausea and Vomiting*
3. *Taste Changes*
4. *Sore or Ulcerated Mouth or Throat (Stomatitis/Mucositis)*
5. *Difficulties in Chewing and Swallowing (Dysphagia) and Dry Mouth (Xerostomia)*
6. *Diarrhea*
7. *Protecting the Gastrointestinal Tract (Enteritis)*
8. *Constipation*
9. *Dehydration*

Problem 1

Loss of Appetite

Loss of appetite, called anorexia, is one of the most common side-effects of many of the chemotherapy drugs. Loss of appetite can also occur as a result of stress, depression, or the cancer itself. It may occur as a result of nausea, sore mouth, vomiting, or difficulty swallowing.

It is important for both your general sense of well-being, and your ability to fight the disease, that you eat a nutritious diet and try to maintain your weight. Fortunately, loss of appetite is often temporary, starting around the time of chemotherapy administration.

When appetite no longer motivates you to eat well, you will need a planned approach. You may improve your appetite by experimenting with different ways of preparing and serving food. Here are some hints that other cancer patients have found helpful. **Try to choose foods high in calories so you can get maximum energy and avoid losing weight (which will cause weakness).**

- **Plan your daily menu in advance.**
  Include the recommended number of servings from the Basic Four food groups and the necessary amounts of protein and calories. See General Guideline 1, *Basic Nutrition for the Cancer Patient* (page 30) in Chapter 2: General Dietary Guidelines. Plan precisely what you will eat, and when. Try new or different seasonings to improve your sense of taste—garlic, soy or barbecue sauce, onion, etc. Eat your favorite foods often.

- **Arrange for help in preparing your meals.**
  If you are not feeling well, you may not be up to preparing nutritious meals. A friend or relative may be able to help you by making some main courses for several days ahead of time. In many communities, Meals on Wheels or other meal-delivering services will bring hot meals to your home. Also, home aid in preparing meals is available in many communities. Contact your social worker for more information.

  But even without help with cooking, it is possible to prepare a nutritious diet using canned, packaged, and frozen foods, or to cook and store foods for several days—microwave reheating often simplifies life.

- **Add extra protein and calories to your diet.**
See General Dietary Guideline 2, *A High-Protein/High-Calorie Diet*, (page 38). Use fortified milk—made by adding 1 cup non-fat dry milk to 1 quart whole milk—for drinking and in all recipes calling for milk. If lactose intolerance is a problem, see General Dietary Guideline 6, *A Lactose-Free/Lactose-Restricted Diet* (page 61).
Add protein-rich, chopped hard-boiled eggs to your normal recipes. Add high-calorie foods such as cream or butter to soups, cooked cereals, and vegetables. Use gravies, sauces, and sour cream with vegetables, meat, poultry, and fish. Consider adding a high-protein diet supplement to your menu (see page 40 of General Dietary Guideline 2). (NOTE: Do **NOT** add raw eggs to a milkshake or other beverage. The risk of *Salmonella* poisoning, which can be very serious for a cancer patient, is too great.)

- **Fix small portions of favorite foods and store them.**
Then, when nothing seems appealing, you won't have to think about what to fix—it will already be there. Store food properly in single-meal containers. REMEMBER: To protect against bacterial contamination, which could cause food poisoning, do not leave protein-containing foods at room temperature for long periods of time. *If in doubt, pitch it out!*

- **Hints for eating better.**
Talk to your dietitian, nurse or doctor about hints for eating better.

- **Try to consume a third of your daily protein and calorie requirements at breakfast.**
If this is too much for one sitting, eat two smaller breakfasts, two or three hours apart. Appetite is usually best in the morning; it decreases as the day progresses. (See pages 101–111 in the Recipes section for breakfast food ideas.)

- **Eat frequent small meals.**
Consuming frequent small meals is the best way to ensure that you get enough food. Eating only small amounts is especially helpful if you have difficulty tolerating food.

- **Snack between meals.**
Keep nutritious, high-protein, high-calorie snacks on hand for nibbling, e.g., milkshakes, malts, and commercial high-protein supplements. (See pages 167–173 in the Recipe section for energy-rich shakes and fruit cups, and General Dietary Guideline 2, *A High-Protein/High-Calorie Diet*, on pages 38–44.

- **Appeal to your sense of smell.**
Cook dishes with tantalizing aromas and special sauces. Gravies and sauces are aromatic and enhance the taste of food. They also add calories and make swallowing easier. But avoid foods whose odors trigger queasiness. Trust past experience in planning your meals.

- **Be creative with desserts.**
Take advantage of the appeal of desserts and load them with calories. (See the section on desserts, pages 149–159, under Recipes.)

- **Follow your own preferences in eating.**
Within any dietary restriction, there is still room to improvise and to choose foods that you like and mealtimes that suit your appetite.

- **Vary your diet.**
At a time when you have little interest in food, your menus may tend to be repetitive. Variety will help spark your interest.

- **Exercise before meals.**
Light exercise for 5 to 10 minutes about a half-hour before mealtime will help stimulate your appetite. The exercise need not be strenuous; any movement, such as walking or stretching, will help.

- **Have an aperitif before meals.**
If to your liking, a glass of wine just before meals will help you relax and will stimulate your taste buds. Check with your physician first, however, because some chemotherapy drugs interact with alcohol, causing a sick feeling.

- **Relax for a few minutes immediately before meals.**
Ask your doctor or nurse for specific relaxation exercises, or just set aside some quiet time before dining. Meditation helps some people.

- **Hints to improve taste.**
Mouth-rinsing before meals may improve taste.

- **Have family or friends visit for company at mealtime.**
Try to make mealtime a social time. Dine with family or friends, but avoid stressful topics of conversation.

- **Make your mealtimes pleasant.**
Your mealtime atmosphere affects your appetite. If you are alone, turn on the radio, television, or music for company. Set an attractive table. Anything that adds eye appeal, such as fresh flowers, attractive colors, and garnishes, can help your appetite.

- **Certain drugs may help to stimulate appetite, *but only under the direction of your doctor.***
Progesterone—Megace® (40 mg to 80 mg in divided doses) or Marijuana—Marinol® (tetrahydrocanabinol) smoked or in cookies or brownies or suppositories 30 minutes before meals may increase your appetite. Metochlopromide (Reglan®) stimulates movement in the gastrointestinal tract and may cause a sensation of hunger before meals. (See Specific Problem 2, *Nausea and Vomiting*, page 8.)

- **If mouth or swallowing pain makes eating difficult, mouth analgesics (pain relievers) or washes before eating can help.**
See Specific Problem 4, *Sore or Ulcerated Mouth or Throat*, page 14, and Specific Problem 5, *Difficulties in Chewing and Swallowing*, page 18.

Important Tips

- Eat small portions 4 to 6 times per day.
- Choose energy-rich foods and fluids for meals and snacks, so what you eat *counts*.
- Allow family and friends to help in food preparation.
- Indulge in favorite foods, desserts and/or wine with meals to perk up your appetite.
- Relax, take the time to enjoy your meal.
- Ask your physician and dietitian for further ideas.

Problem 2

Nausea and Vomiting

NOTE: Not everyone has nausea, and it may not occur every time you receive chemotherapy!

Nausea is a feeling of stomach distress accompanied by the urge to vomit. Both nausea and vomiting, though common side effects of chemotherapy, can sometimes be prevented by the use of anti-nausea and anti-emetic (anti-vomiting) drugs (for example, Compazine®, Thorazine®, Torecan®, Tigan®, and Reglan®).

Continued vomiting, of course, makes eating impossible, but it is often possible to prevent vomiting by quelling the nausea. There are also ways to reduce exhaustion and residual nausea after prolonged vomiting.

Attempts to reduce nausea/vomiting are vital, as psychologic anticipatory nausea/vomiting can occur even before taking chemotherapy. Relaxation exercises or meditation may help.

To Prevent Vomiting and Nausea

- **Take an anti-nausea drug and a sedative, such as Valium® or Ativan®, one-half to one hour before you receive an intravenous chemotherapy drug.**
  Take additional anti-nausea medication one-half to one hour before meals if you feel nauseated or have a queasy stomach. When you are unable to keep pills down because of vomiting, you may be able to take the medication (e.g., Compazine®, Dramamine® or Torecan®) in suppository form. If nausea is severe, several doses of anti-nausea medication may be needed up to 24 hours before a treatment. REMEMBER: DO NOT DRIVE IF THE DRUG SEDATES YOU.

- **If you know your chemotherapy drug causes intense vomiting, take a sedative immediately before or during chemotherapy and arrange for someone to drive you home from your treatment.**
  Rest in a cool, dark room away from noise (avoid hot rooms), light, and aromas until the acute effect of the chemotherapy drug wears off. Calm music can be soothing and may distract your attention from the feeling of nausea. Eating smaller

portions of soft, bland foods (see "Swallowing Training Program," pages 173–181, in the Recipe section) for 1 to 3 days after a chemotherapy treatment may help reduce symptoms.

- **Change the room in which you receive chemotherapy—avoid distasteful smells such as an alcohol skin-wipe odor.**

- **For many people, marijuana reduces nausea effectively, but not everyone can tolerate the side effects of this drug.**
  The effects include euphoria, silliness, a sense of time-distortion, sensations of coldness, and paranoia. People who have used marijuana recreationally appear to have fewer problems with the side effects than those inexperienced with the drug. Marijuana can be smoked (a poor option), taken in suppositories, ingested in capsules, or included in food. The use of the drug has been legalized for medical use in most jurisdictions.

  A synthetic version of marijuana's active ingredient, THC (tetrahydrocanabinol) or Marinol® is available by prescription. This is a much safer option than using marijuana bought from questionable sources, which may be contaminated with fungi that can cause lung infections, or with paraquat, a poisonous spray that actually causes nausea. And smoking marijuana may cause lung cancer. If you grow your own marijuana (which is not advised), bake it at 350 degrees for at least one hour before using it to kill any biological contaminates. Heat also may help make it more active.

  In recent years, marijuana use has been almost completely replaced by combinations of anti-emetics such as Ativan® or Reglan®, with Compazine® or other drugs.

- **Avoid eating for several hours before chemotherapy.**
  If the "dry heaves" are a problem, eat something light and starchy, such as crackers, Melba toast or dry toast, before the drug is administered. Avoid fatty or spicy foods.

- **Nausea patterns are variable.**
  Some people do better eating lightly before and after chemotherapy; others can't eat for many hours. Try to learn your own pattern.

- **Do not ingest favorite or particularly healthful foods before chemotherapy.**
  If chemotherapy makes you vomit, you could develop a conditioned aversion to these foods. They then will not only

lose their appeal, but even the sight or smell of them will stimulate the memory and experience of nausea. Try eating hard sugar-free candies, mints, or sugar-free lemon drops between a meal and chemotherapy, so if a food aversion occurs, it will relate to the candy rather than the more nutritious foods. Where vomiting does result in food aversion, behavioral treatment by a psychologist can be very helpful.

- **Sitting up or walking after meals may help reduce nausea caused by activating bowel activity.**
- **Avoid overpowering aromas.**
  If food odors trigger nausea, you may find foods served chilled or at room temperature more appealing. Their odors are usually less intense than those of hot foods. To reduce the odor of beverages, drink them through a straw.
- **Eat and drink slowly.**
- **Eat frequent small meals.**
  You are less likely to be nauseated when the amount of food in your stomach is small. But be sure to eat often to meet your calorie and protein needs.
- **Suck on ice chips or popsicles.**
- **Eat breakfast every day.**
  Appetite is usually best and nausea less of a problem in the morning. (See Specific Problem 1, *Loss of Appetite,* page 4.)
- **Avoid liquids at mealtimes.**
  Liquids, especially sweet ones, in combination with food may aggravate nausea. Drink before or after meals instead of during meals.
- **Rest after eating, but keep your head higher than your feet.**
  Do not lie down flat for at least two hours after eating.

If Vomiting has Occurred

Try a new approach with your next therapy. *If actively vomiting*—lie on your side to avoid choking on the vomitus.

- **Carbonated beverages may help.**
  Carbonated beverages help neutralize an alkaline stomach and reduce residual nausea. Citrus-flavored soft drinks or ginger ale are usually easiest to tolerate. Avoid carbonated beverages,

however, if gas is a problem. Or try stirring soda to release most of its carbonation before you drink it.

If carbonated beverages are not helpful, it might help to buy cola syrup, available from your pharmacist; pour it directly over ice, and sip it slowly. Another option is to eat clear, cool foods and beverages such as flavored gelatin, Kool-Aid®, Gatorade®, popsicles, frozen fruit drinks (slushes), tea, chicken or beef broth. Mint has also proved helpful in reducing nausea.

- **Replace fluid and electrolytes lost.**
  (See Specific Problem 9, *Dehydration*, page 26). Be sure to drink extra fluids before a chemotherapy treatment.

- **Keep your mouth clean and blow your nose to rid yourself of the sensation and taste of vomiting.**
  Sometimes brushing your teeth or sucking on sugar-free hard candy helps to quell the feeling of nausea.

To Control Residual Nausea

High-carbohydrate, low-fat foods may help.

- **Avoid fatty and fried foods, and also spicy foods, or foods with a strong odor.**
  Fatty foods stay in the stomach for a long time, and may contribute to nausea. Substitute baked, broiled, or steamed foods.

Important Tips

- Drink plenty of fluids before chemotherapy and for 1 to 3 days following treatment, especially bland drinks such as tea, broth, juices, Jell-O® and popsicles.
- The day of chemotherapy—eat a bland, low-fat, light diet—for example, tea, toast with jelly, crackers, Jell-O® and broth.
- **Avoid your favorite foods on the day you have chemotherapy.**
- Avoid heavy, greasy or spicy foods.
- Choose dry, bland foods such as toast, crackers and unsalted pretzels.
- Eat small, frequent snacks rather than 2 to 3 large meals.
- Ask your physician about anti-nausea, anti-emetic medications.

Problem 3

Taste Changes

"Taste blindness," or an altered sense of taste and smell, can be a side effect of some chemotherapy drugs. Changes vary with individuals, but the most common complaints are of foods tasting too sweet or too bitter, or of a continuous metallic taste or smell. The following hints may help.

If Foods Taste Too Sweet

- **Use coffee or sour fruit juices to mask sweetness.**
- **Dilute fruit juice or other sweet beverages with half water or ice.**
- **Eliminate concentrated sweets.**
- **Avoid sweet fruits.**
  Vegetables may be more appealing.
- **Try Gymnema Sylvestra, an herbal tea from India used by professional tasters before eating.**
  It will deaden the taste buds to sweet tastes for about 20 minutes if it is held in the mouth for about 5 minutes before eating.

If Foods Taste Too Bitter

- **Add sweet fruits to meals.**
  Add honey or NutraSweet® to foods and beverages.
- **If hot meat tastes bitter.**
  Try eating meats cold or at room temperature.
- **If meat tastes too bitter, substitute blandly-prepared chicken and fish, mild cheeses, eggs, dairy products, or tofu.**
  All these foods may taste better when prepared in casseroles or stews. (See pages 111–114 in the Recipe section for ideas on preparing meatless dishes.)
- **Marinating foods may make them taste better.**
  Marinate meats, chicken, or fish in pineapple juice, wine, Italian dressing, lemon juice, soy sauce, or sweet-and-sour sauces to make them taste better.

- **Mouth care can help, such as brushing teeth several times a day, using mouth rinses (saline solution of water mixed with salt, hydrogen peroxide or bicarbonate of soda or diluted Cepacol® or Chloroseptic®).**
  See section on *Mouth and Dental Care,* p. 375.

If Foods Taste "Off"

- **Simply drinking liquids, such as water, tea, ginger ale, or fruit juices mixed with club soda may remove some of the strange tastes in your mouth.**
  It might also help to suck on hard candies, such as sugar-free mints. Sugar-free gum or hard candies are often very helpful in reducing after tastes due to Cytoxan or other drugs used in IV therapy.
- **Add wine, beer, mayonnaise, sour cream, or yogurt to soups and sauces to cover the off-tastes of other foods.**
  (Check with your physician before using alcohol to make sure it is permissible.)
- **Eat starchy foods, such as bread, potatoes, rice, and plain pasta noodles.**
  Do not add butter, margarine, or other fatty substances to these foods.
- **Choose bland foods.**
  Eggs, cheeses (including cottage cheese), hot cereals, puddings, custards, tapioca, cream soups, toast, potatoes, rice and peanut butter are less likely to taste strange than foods with more distinctive tastes.
- **You may have cravings for spicy or salty foods.**
  Spicy, highly-seasoned foods are irritating to many. However, if your doctor does not advise against such foods, and if you can tolerate them, by all means satisfy such urges. Often flavorings such as herbs, spices or food seasonings may help. Also, *acid foods* such as grapefruit may stimulate taste buds (if they do not irritate).
- **High-protein foods and supplements become particularly important *when taste blindness discourages eating.***
  (See General Dietary Guideline 2, *A High-Protein/High-Calorie Diet,* page 38.)
- **A relaxed and pleasant atmosphere.**
  Can help reduce problems of taste blindness.

Problem 4

Sore or Ulcerated Mouth or Throat (Stomatitis/Mucositis)

The lining, or mucosa, of the gastrointestinal tract, which includes the inside of the mouth and throat, is one of the most sensitive areas of the body. Mucositis, or sores or ulcerations of this lining, is a side effect of many chemotherapy drugs, and of radiation therapy to the head and neck. Mouth or throat infections, for example, monila thrush, can also cause sore mouth. Pain control is particularly important in order to maintain good nutritional intake.

Mouth care is very important in treating mucositis, along with a high-protein, high-calorie diet which will speed healing. (See General Dietary Guideline 2, *A High-Protein/High-Calorie Diet,* page 38.) NOTE: Alcohol and tobacco irritate the mouth—avoid them. Adequate fluid intake helps mouth sores.

This is particularly important with "dry mouth," a reduction in saliva or change in salivary composition that encourages plaque and gum disease—and can lead to loss of teeth. (See the next succeeding discussions on cleansing and swallowing, and also the separate discussion of *Mouth and Dental Care,* Appendix A, p.375.)

- **Use a soft-bristled toothbrush.**
  The brush can be softened by soaking it in warm water. A solution paste of baking soda and water may be less irritating than commercial toothpaste.

- **If brushing your teeth is too painful, try using a cotton swab or gauze instead of a toothbrush.**
  You can also buy sponge-tipped Toothettes® impregnated with dentrifice. Or you can wrap a piece of gauze around your finger, soak it in salt water, and wipe your mouth and teeth clean. Sensodyne-F® toothpaste may help sensitive teeth. Also, Biotene™, a dry-mouth toothpaste, produces hydrogen peroxide, a protective antiseptic.

- **Avoid commercial mouthwashes.**
  They are stringent and will burn or sting. Lemon glycerine (Lemon-Glycerine Pakette-Tomac®) has been used, but glycerin is a drying agent and can promote dry mouth.

- **Prepare your own mouthwash.**
  Liquid Xylocaine (or 1 to 2 tablespoons of baking soda) and 1 teaspoon salt dissolved in 1 quart of warm water and swished in the mouth and spit out, used before meals, will lessen irritation. Cool yogurt may also be soothing. Mix equal parts of water and hydrogen peroxide for a frequent gargle (dilute 1:3 or 1:4 if irritating).

- **Useful commercial preparations.**
  Include Oral Balance™, a moisturizing gel that coats and protects tissue, Zilactine® and Orabase® for pain relief from ulcers and lesions, and Ulcerease™, a non-prescription soothing oral anesthetic.

- **Try mild anesthetics to reduce pain.**
  Anesthetic gels such as Viscous Xylocaine®, mouth sprays such as Hurricaine®, lozenges, or systemic analgesics such as Tylenol® or codeine tablets may be needed to help relieve pain. Benadryl® elixir used as a rinse is effective in reducing mouth pain. A mixture of Benadryl® and Hydrocortisone can reduce mouth irritation and promote healing.

- **Remove dentures and rinse mouth several times a day.**
  Dentures should be cleaned. Avoid denture "glues" if mouth is irritated.

- **Try medications such as Milk of Magnesia®, Carafate®, Aludrox®, Maalox®, or Mylanta® (1 tablespoon swished around the mouth), Orabase® (with or without Kenolog®), or a methylcellulose solution (e.g., Cologel®).**
  These will stick to ulcerations and give them a protective coating.

- **Drink through a straw.**

- **Ways to freshen your mouth.**
  Suck sugar-free sour lemon hard candies or mints to freshen your mouth.

- **Care for your mouth carefully after each meal and at bedtime.**

- **A Water-Pik® to cleanse the mouth is helpful.**

- **Examine your mouth with a flashlight each day in the mirror.**
  Report sores and white patches to your physician. This could be an early thrush (fungus) infection, which is *easily* treated.

- **You may have to adjust the way you smile to keep from irritating your mouth.**
  Chapstick® or moisturizing lipstick helps dry, or cracked lips.

Things to Avoid

- **Very hot or very cold foods.**
  Foods served at room temperature are often the least irritating.
- **Citrus fruits.**
  Grapefruit, lemons, oranges, and tomatoes may burn the mouth.
- **Salty foods.**
  Can cause a burning sensation in the mouth.
- **Hot, spicy foods.**
  Avoid foods containing such hot or strong spices as pepper, chili powder, curry powder, nutmeg, and cloves.
- **Coarse, rough foods.**
  Raw vegetables, nuts, seeds, or coarse breads or grains can irritate a sensitive mouth and throat.
- **Very dry foods, such as toast, dry crackers, or chips.**
- **Alcoholic beverages and coffee.**

Foods to Emphasize

- **Try a softer diet.**
  Choose bland foods such as mashed potatoes, yogurt, scrambled eggs, custards, milkshakes, puddings, gelatins, creamy hot cereals, cream pasta dishes, and macaroni and cheese. See General Dietary Guideline 14, *A Soft-Food/Pureed-Food Diet,* page 86, and related recipes in Chapter 3.
- **Blenderize or puree foods in a blender if a soft diet is still too harsh.**
  Use soups and gravies liberally.
- **Try a full-liquid diet if solid or pureed foods are still too irritating.**
  See your physician or dietitian for a full-liquid diet.

- **Consume fruits that are low in acid.**
  Fruits such as bananas, canned pears and canned peaches, and drink fruit nectar juices.
- **If you have difficulty swallowing.**
  Swallow small amounts of well-chewed or soft food, or use a straw to drink a liquid formula. *(See Specific Problem 5,* Difficulties in Chewing and Swallowing and Dry Mouth, *page 18.)*
- **Cold food from the ice box may help reduce mouth pain. Ice chips or sorbet before meals often help.**
- **If you are not getting enough protein and calories, use fortified milk—made by adding 1 cup non-fat dry milk to 1 quart whole milk—for drinking and in all recipes calling for milk.**
  If lactose intolerance is a problem, see General Dietary Guideline 6, *A Lactose-Free/Lactose-Restricted Diet,* page 61. Also, consider adding a high-protein diet supplement to your menu. (See General Dietary Guideline 2, *A High-Protein/High-Calorie Diet,* page 38.)
- **Drugs are often difficult to swallow with a sore mouth or throat.**
  Use liquid drugs, crushed tablets or pills mixed in 1/2 to 1 ounce of applesauce or pudding; fruit juices may be helpful as well.
- **Oxygen causes nasal and mouth dryness.**
  Oil or neosporin in your nose 3 to 4 times a day can help.

Important Tips

- Practice good mouth care, including careful, gentle toothbrushing, oral rinses, and/or the use of special protective moistening gels.
- Drink plenty of bland fluids—usually tolerated best if taken at room temperature and sipped through a straw.
- Choose soft or blenderized foods.
- Do not eat spicy or coarse, crunchy foods.

Problem 5

Difficulties in Chewing and Swallowing (Dysphagia) and Dry Mouth (Xerostomia)

Some chemotherapy drugs may cause jaw pain or a weakening of the throat muscles, resulting in difficulties in chewing and/or swallowing. Chemotherapy may also reduce saliva production, resulting in mouth dryness. The following dietary hints will help with these problems.

- Try to improve oral hygiene (see the preceding discussion beginning on page 14, on Sore or Ulcerated Mouth and Throat).
- Drink 8 to 10 glasses of fluids daily.

If You Have Difficulty Chewing and/or Swallowing

- **Eat soft, moist foods.**
  You will find such foods as custards, high-protein milkshakes, puddings, stews, and casseroles easiest to eat. (See General Dietary Guideline 14, *A Soft-Food/Pureed-Food Diet*, page 86.)

- **Add plenty of liquids to foods to soften them.**

- **Cut foods into small pieces.**
  Make pieces small enough to be swallowed with a minimum of chewing. Add gravies and sauces to meats and add minced meat, vegetables, rice, and potatoes to cream soup for ease of swallowing.

- **Do not use a full-liquid diet if you are having difficulty swallowing.**
  Thin liquids could go down your windpipe and cause choking or gagging. Make sure all beverages are of milkshake consistency to avoid this problem.

- **To make sure you get enough protein and calories, use high-protein liquid dietary supplements prescribed by your physician or dietitian.**
  Thicken liquid supplements with ice cream for added calories.

If You Have a Dry Mouth

- AVOID: Dry, sticky foods such as peanut butter; hard, dry foods, such as crackers, nuts, and popcorn; and raw vegetables.
- AVOID: Commercial Mouthwashes.
- **Use creams, sauces, gravies, dressings, and liquids to moisten your food.**
  Add nutrients to your gravies and sauces by making them with the water in which vegetables have been cooked.
- **Try sucking on sugar-free hard candy or popsicles or chewing sugar-free gum.**
  This may help to stimulate saliva production.
- **Drink generous amounts of liquids with meals.**
  However, be sure your beverages contain nutrients, because liquids are filling. (See Chapter 3, Recipes, beginning on page 167, for high-protein/high-calorie beverages.)
- **For severe, prolonged dry mouth, ask your physician or dentist to prescribe an artificial saliva product, such as MouthKote®, Saliva-Aid®, or Xero-Lube®.**
- **Pay meticulous attention to oral hygiene.**
  When your mouth has dried, you have lost the natural protection of your saliva. Your oncology nurse can give you some tips on mouth care. Consult your dentist about fluoride mouthwashes or gels to protect your teeth against decay. (See the discussion of Sore or Ulcerated Mouth Care in preceding Specific Problem 4 for information on mouth care, swabs, and artificial saliva.)

Recommended Commercial Preparations

- Moi-Stir® (Kingswood Laboratories, Inc.), an oral swabstick as an aid to mouth care and oral hygiene, contains a moistening solution of chemicals and water similar to natural saliva (supplied in an 8-ounce plastic bottle).
- MouthKote™ is an oral natural saliva substitute for dry mouth (Xerostomia) caused by medication, smoking, surgery and irradiation. Swish 1 or 2 teaspoons in mouth 8 to 10 seconds, then swallow. WARNING: Discontinue use and consult a physician if rash appears. Keep out of reach of children. Store at room temperature.

Problem 6

Diarrhea

Certain chemotherapy drugs (and abdominal radiotherapy) are toxic to the cells lining your stomach and intestines and can cause diarrhea. When you have diarrhea, food passes through the gut more quickly, so many nutrients are not absorbed. You also lose fluids and electrolytes, which are vital to the fluid balance of your body. Your physician may prescribe drugs to stop the diarrhea if it is severe. Imodium®, Lomotil®, codeine, Kaopectate®, and Pepto Bismol® are available in drugstores, but such anti-diarrheal drugs can cause constipation.

The following tips will help reduce diarrhea while allowing you to maintain a good nutritional status. (If diarrhea persists, call your physician. It could be due to a variety of causes, including an intestinal blockage, antibiotics or the cancer.)

- **Replace lost fluids and electrolytes.**
  See the Specific Problem 9 discussion of Dehydration (page 26) for potassium-rich foods and fluids.

- **Since water-soluble vitamins are lost with diarrhea, it is important to replace them, especially B vitamins, by taking a one-a-day type of vitamin supplement.**
  NOTE: High doses of vitamin C (more than 100 milligrams a day) may aggravate diarrhea. Do not use megadoses of any vitamin—that is, doses greater than two times the U.S. Recommended Dietary Allowance (U.S. RDA.) (See General Dietary Guideline 4, *Food Sources of Vitamins*, page 52.) Do not take vitamins on an empty stomach. This can cause nausea.

- **Avoid milk or milk products unless milk has been treated with Lactaid® or is lactose-free.**
  (See General Dietary Guideline 6, *A Lactose-Free/Lactose-Restricted Diet*, page 61.)

- **Non-spiced applesauce and bananas are helpful in treating diarrhea.**

- **Reduce your intake of foods that are high in roughage and residue.**
  See General Dietary Guideline 5, *The Fiber and Residue Contents of Foods*, page 58.

- **Consume foods that are high in protein and calories, such as creamed dishes and puddings, as tolerated.**
  See General Dietary Guideline 2, *A High-Protein/High-Calorie Diet,* page 38, and recipes for recommended foods in Chapter 3.

- **If nutritional supplements are needed to maintain your protein and calorie levels, use such products as Isocal®, Osmolite®, and Vivonex T.E.N.® *(most of which are* lactose-free).**
  Ask your nutrition advisor or pharmacist which products have low osmolality, since these products may be better tolerated.

- **Avoid spicy, rich, gas-producing foods such as beans.**

- **Avoid laxatives!**

- **Ileostomy and colostomy diarrhea.**
  This may be severe enough to require physician guidance and anti-diarrhea medicine, as well as dietary intervention.

- **Protect your rectum.**
  Use with creams such as A&D Ointment® or Diaperene®. Tucks® can help clean the anal area. Sitz baths (a warm-hot water bath 6" deep) to bathe an inflamed anus are also helpful.

- **Black or bloody stools.**
  Call your physician immediately if your stools look black or bloody, or if you notice any significant change in their appearance.

Problem 7

Protecting the Gastrointestinal Tract (Enteritis)

Certain chemotherapy drugs (and abdominal radiotherapy) are toxic to the cells lining your stomach and intestines and may result in bleeding and ulceration. This gastrointestinal bleeding may cause you to lose iron and other nutrients. Also, your intestines may not be able to utilize bile salts, which are necessary for the absorption of fats and the fat-soluble vitamins A, D, E, and K. The following hints will help you replace such nutrient losses.

- **Eat foods rich in iron.**
  (See General Dietary Guideline 3, *Food Sources of Minerals*, page 45.) Unless diarrhea is a problem, consume foods or drinks rich in vitamin C, such as orange juice, when you eat iron-rich foods, to aid absorption of the iron. Avoid drinking black tea, since it contains a substance called tannin, which inhibits the absorption of iron.

- **Maintain your intake of water-soluble vitamins and minerals by eating foods rich in these nutrients and taking a one-a-day type of multiple-vitamin/mineral supplement.**
  If you have diarrhea, avoid high doses (more than 100 milligrams a day) of vitamin C. Do not use megadoses—that is, doses greater than twice the U.S. Recommended Daily Allowances (U.S. RDA) of any vitamin or mineral. (See General Dietary Guidelines 3 and 4, *Food Sources of Minerals* and *Food Sources of Vitamins*, pages 45 and 52, respectively.)

- **Ask your pharmacist for the fat-soluble vitamins A, D, E and K in their water-soluble carrier forms.**
  In this form, they can be absorbed without the aid of bile salts. NOTE: Do not take megadoses of these vitamins. Even in their water-soluble carrier forms, vitamins A, D, E, and K are still stored in the fatty tissues of the body and can accumulate to toxic levels.

- **If you have diarrhea, follow the instructions in the Specific Problem discussion of Diarrhea.**

- **Your physician or dietitian may advise that you need to substitute medium-chain triglyceride fats for long-chain triglycerides.**
  If so, see General Dietary Guideline 8, *A Long-Chain Triglyceride-Restricted/Medium-Chain-Triglyceride Fat Diet,* page 68.

- **If kidney stones begin to develop, you may need a special diet.**
  (See general Dietary Guideline 10, *How To Prevent Kidney Stone Formation*, page 74.)

Important Tips

- Drink plenty of fluids to replace losses from diarrhea.
- If you have diarrhea, avoid milk products, fresh fruits and vegetables and very coarse, rough foods, which can be difficult to digest.
- Eat slowly.
- Try eating more frequent, small snacks rather than 2 to 3 large meals per day.
- Avoid alcohol.

Problem 8

Constipation

Some chemotherapy drugs depress intestinal reflexes, reducing the normal-movement of stools, and causing constipation. You may also experience such related symptoms as headache, foul breath, abdominal distention, loss of appetite, flatulence (gas), and a general malaise. Stools are infrequent and often hard.

Use laxatives only on the advice of your physician; some can do more harm than good—for instance, if you are taking narcotics, bulk-forming laxatives (such as bran, Metamucil®, or Konsyl®) will increase constipation. Certain other laxatives, when used on a continual basis, cause irritation of the digestive tract and often make it difficult to regain normal bowel habits once the laxative is discontinued. Mineral oil will reduce absorption of the fat-soluble vitamins.

The following dietary hints will help prevent or relieve constipation.

- **Eat foods that are high in fiber and bulk (unless they cause other problems).**
  These include fresh fruit and vegetables (raw or cooked with skins and peels on), dried fruit, whole-grain breads and cereals, and bran. (But raw fruits and vegetables are to be avoided when white blood cell count (WBC) is lower than 1800.) See General Dietary Guideline 5, *The Fiber and Residue Contents of Foods*, page 58. NOTE: Any high-fiber diet should be started *before* a chemotherapy drug that causes constipation is administered.

- **Drink plenty of fluids (8 to 10 glasses a day).**
  AVOID DEHYDRATION! (See Specific Problem 9, *Dehydration*, page 26.) Try to drink highly nutritional fluids (milkshakes, eggnogs, and juices, as opposed to water), since liquids can be filling and may reduce your appetite. Apple juice or prune juice may be particularly helpful, especially if heated.

- **Add bran to your diet gradually.**
  Start with 2 teaspoons per day and gradually work up to 4 to 6 teaspoons per day. Sprinkle bran on cereal or add it to meatloaf, stew, pancakes, baked goods and other foods. Both wheat germ and oat bran are helpful.

- **Avoid refined foods.**
  Examples are white bread, sugar, starchy desserts, and candy. Chocolates, cheeses, and eggs may be constipating.

- **Take prunes or a glass of prune juice in the morning or at night to increase regularity.**
  Prunes contain a natural laxative substance as well as fiber. Warmed prune juice and stewed prunes are most effective.

- **Eat a large breakfast.**
  Eat a large breakfast with some type of hot beverage, such as herbal tea, hot lemon water, or decaffeinated coffee.

- **Rest and relaxation.**
  Get adequate rest and eat at regular times in a relaxed atmosphere.

- **Regular exercise.**
  Regular exercise will stimulate your intestinal reflexes and help restore normal elimination.

- **Your doctor may find it necessary to prescribe medications (stool softeners and/or laxatives/enemas) to prevent or treat constipation, especially if you are on narcotics for pain control.**

Important Tips

- Include high-fiber breads and cereals, and fresh fruits and vegetables in each meal.
- Drink plenty of fluids, including water, prune juice, fruit drinks, and other non-caffeine beverages.
- Plan some form of daily exercise.
- Consult your physician before taking any laxatives.

Problem 9

Dehydration

Dehydration is a lack of fluid in the body. Common symptoms include feelings of dryness in your mouth, eyes and tongue, tiredness, difficulty swallowing, fever and reduced urine output.

Chemotherapy or its side effects such as diarrhea, sweating, or vomiting—or an inability to drink fluids—can lead to dehydration, muscle cramps, and exhaustion. Certain minerals called electrolytes—such as sodium, potassium, and magnesium—may also be lost. Replacing lost fluid and electrolytes is *very important*, because fluid losses of as little as 2% can cause problems with blood circulation and body temperature. It is essential that you consume adequate fluids to prevent the harmful effects of dehydration.

The following hints will help you replace fluids and electrolytes.

- **Drink lots of water.**
  Sometimes just plain water is best for immediate fluid replacement, because it enters the circulation faster than fluids containing other substances. Cold water leaves the stomach fastest, though iced or cold water sometimes causes abdominal pain. Ice chips or popsicles may help you swallow better. (If made from Citrotene® or Vivonex T.E.N.®, the ice chips or popsicles will add important nutrients.)

- **Keep fluids (water, juices, and other liquids) handy at the bedside.**

- **Avoid sugar and sugar-containing drinks.**
  Sugar causes fluid to stay in the stomach longer. Orange juice, soft drinks, and most fruit drinks are high in sugar and should be diluted with three parts water. Even electrolyte-replacement drinks such as Gatorade® and ERG® contain sugar and salts. Dilute such drinks to half their strength.

- **Do not rely on salt tablets.**
  Salt tablets are rarely beneficial, and should only be taken on the advice of your physician.

- **Frequently throughout the day, drink liquids or eat foods that become liquid in the stomach.**
  Examples are juice, fruit-ades, punch, soft drinks, tea, milk, milkshakes, eggnogs, soup, broth, Jell-O®, ice cream, sherbet,

fruit ices, popsicles, and fruits with a high fluid content, such as grapes or watermelon.

- **Eat lots of fruits and vegetables.**
  They can contain up to 95% water and also tend to be good sources of potassium and magnesium, minerals that prevent muscle weakness.

- **Eat foods that are high in potassium.**
  Potassium losses can cause fatigue, muscular cramping, and muscular weakness, so potassium must be replaced if large amounts of body fluids are lost. Speak to your physician before taking a potassium supplement, however.

  Muscle cramps that are not cured by potassiumm replacement may clear up if you increase your calcium and/or magnesium intake. See General Dietary Guideline 3, *Food Sources of Minerals,* page 45.

- The following chart gives you good sources of potassium. NOTE: Food sources high in potassium also tend to be high in sodium.

Very High Potassium Content (500 mg per serving)	***High Potassium Content (250 mg per serving)***
1 teaspoon cream of tartar (added to juice just before taking)	1 nectarine
1 medium banana	1/2 cup rhubarb
1/2 cup raisins	2 cups Postum® cereal beverage
6 apricots	3 cups coffee, tea, or decaffeinated coffee
1/2 cantaloupe	1/4 cup beans or peas
1 large potato	1/4 cup summer squash
2/3 cups spinach	1 medium raw tomato
1/4 cup powdered non-fat milk	4 ounces vegetable juice cocktail
1-1/2 teaspoon salt substitute (potassium chloride)	1 medium artichoke
5 medium dates	1/4 avocado
1 slice honeydew melon (2" × 6")	1/3 papaya
6 ounces prune juice	6 spears asparagus
1 large artichoke	2/3 cup broccoli
1/2 cup cooked beans (chili, kidney, lima)	4 large leaves lettuce
5 ounces tomato juice	1 medium orange
10 ounces orange juice	

- **Skin lotions may help dry skin. Mouth care is important for dry mouth.**
  (See Specific Problem 4, *Sore and Ulcerated Mouth or Throat,* page 14.)
- **Treat diarrhea, vomiting, and dehydration actively.**
  (See Specific Problem 2, *Nausea and Vomiting,* and Problem 6, *Diarrhea,* pages 8 and 20, respectively.)
- **Try to normalize fever to reduce excessive fluid loss.**
- **If dehydration persists, consult your physician. More aggressive treatment may be needed.**

Chapter 2

General Dietary Guidelines

1. ***Basic Nutrition for the Cancer Patient***
2. ***A High-Protein/High-Calorie Diet***
3. ***Food Sources of Minerals***
4. ***Food Sources of Vitamins***
5. ***The Fiber and Residue Contents of Foods***
6. ***A Lactose-Free/Lactose-Restricted Diet***
7. ***A Gluten-Restricted/Gliadin-Free Diet***
8. ***A Long-Chain-Triglyceride-Restricted Medium-Chain-Triglyceride Fat Diet***
9. ***A Cholesterol and Fat-Restricted Diet***
10. ***How To Prevent Kidney Stone Formation (Acid Ash/Alkaline Ash Diet)***
11. ***A Transient Glucose Intolerance/Diabetic Diet***
12. ***A Sodium-Restricted Diet***
13. ***A Tyramine and Dopamine-Restricted Diet***
14. ***A Soft-Food/Pureed-Food Diet***

Guideline 1

Basic Nutrition for the Cancer Patient

As a cancer patient undergoing chemotherapy, you will encounter certain drug side-effects that may interfere with your intake of food. The "General Dietary Guidelines" section of this book provides you with particular dietary programs designed to help reduce specific side-effects. These, along with Chapter 1, *How to Deal With Specific Problems*, will help you make your food choices from The Basic Four groups.

One of the most important ways that you, as a cancer patient, can help yourself get well is to eat the right amounts of certain important types of foods. Your body needs the nutrients in these foods to repair its tissue and maintain its weight. As with any type of serious illness, when you have cancer, your body's first need is for calories—those units of energy a food gives your body when it is "burned" for fuel. If you do not consume enough calories, your body will begin to break down its own tissues to obtain more.

With the exception of water, all foods have calories. Some foods, like most sweets and alcohol, give you mostly calories and little else, while others, such as milk and eggs, give you calories plus many necessary nutrients.

The components of foods that supply calories are carbohydrates, proteins, and fats, but they have other functions as well. Protein, for instance, is essential for rebuilding vital tissues and maintaining proper body function.

To keep from using precious protein for energy, it is critical that we supply our bodies with enough carbohydrates and fats. Fats are a particularly concentrated source of energy, yielding more than twice as much energy per gram as carbohydrates and proteins. Fats also insulate our bodies, line our nerves, and form a part of our cell membranes.

Some 40 other nutrients do not provide energy but have other vital functions. Vitamins and minerals, for example, are called energy facilitators. Some of them help release energy from foods, though they do not provide energy themselves. Although vitamin and mineral supplements are often popularly regarded as compensation for poor nutrition, they cannot provide adequate energy and will not prevent your body from breaking down its tissues for fuel if you do not eat enough energy foods.

Everyone must consume minimum amounts of the different nutrients in foods to maintain normal body functions. Recommended Dietary Allowances, or RDAs, are estimates of the amounts necessary to prevent nutrient deficiency diseases among a range of people.

Many people erroneously use RDAs as personal prescriptions on which to base their nutrient intake, but RDAs tell us little about a particular individual's needs, especially when clinical conditions such as cancer are involved. Besides, when most of us make our diet choices, we choose foods, not nutrients.

Translating RDAs into daily meal plans takes a great deal of time and training. Those not trained in nutrition can use the "Daily Food Guide" prepared by the U.S. Department of Agriculture (USDA) to help them choose the kinds and amounts of foods to eat for good nutrition, but those with cancer need more specialized information and diet plans.

Still, good nutrition for cancer patients is rooted in basic nutritional principles. For example, no one single food can give us all the nutrients we need in the necessary amounts, which means that we need variety in our diets. With a variety of food we can balance our food choices to meet our needs. Moderation prevents overconsumption of food components that are necessary in limited amounts but detrimental in excessive amounts. These principles apply as much to cancer patients as to the general population.

The same is true for the USDA "Daily Food Guides"—all the dietary information and food choices assembled here for cancer patients are drawn from this comprehensive guide. The guide classifies foods into four broad nutritious groups, called The Basic Four, and a fifth group containing foods that supply lots of calories but few nutrients. These groups are as follows:

1. Milk and dairy products
2. Meat or meat equivalents
3. Fruits and vegetables
4. Breads and cereals
5. Fats, alcohol, and sweets

The Basic Four Food Groups

The Basic Four groups contribute large amounts of the major nutrients that are needed for health, with each particular group being selected because it contains certain kinds of nutrients. Many of The Basic Four foods are nutrient-dense, meaning that they contain a large proportion of nutrients in relation to their caloric value.

It is very important for you as a cancer patient to know which foods are nutrient-dense, because your need for nutrients is unusually great. By consuming food from the first four groups each day in recommended amounts, you will be meeting your daily nutrient needs while ensuring that your diet is varied, balanced, and moderate.

The foods in the fifth group are considered calorie-dense—they have lots of calories but few nutrients. In your effort to supply your body with nutrients as well as calories, you are encouraged to learn which foods fall into this category, and, on the whole, to limit them.

A diet consisting of the recommended amounts of foods from The Basic Four food groups is known as a foundation diet. The foundation diet supplies about 90% of the essential nutrients and about 75% (approximately 1,200 to 1,300 daily) of the necessary calories. You can add calories to the diet simply by including more servings from The Basic Four food groups. Cancer patients undergoing drug treatment should take most of these additional calories from the dairy foods group (if tolerated), and/or the meat and meat-substitutes group for added protein and fat.

What follows is a simple overview of The Basic Four food groups, their major nutrients, and recommended uses. Take this opportunity to become acquainted with these four categories of nutritious foods, their nutritional characteristics, and their dietary uses, and use this section as a general reference guide when you plan your daily menus.

The Milk and Dairy Products Group

One serving equals:

1 8-ounce cup of fluid or reconstituted dry milk, whole, low-fat, or skim milk, buttermilk, or evaporated milk.

Daily servings recommended:

Child, under age 9: 2 to 3

Child, aged 9 to 12: 3 or more

Teenager: 4 or more

Adult: 2 or more

In general, the major nutritional contributions of dairy foods are calcium, high-quality protein, and riboflavin (vitamin B_2). They also contribute other nutrients, such as vitamins B_1, B_6, B_{12}, A, and D (if fortified), plus niacin and the mineral magnesium. Milk protein is inexpensive, easily digested if you are not subject to lactose intolerance (covered below), and of high quality. It's important to keep milk out of the light, because light can destroy some of its riboflavin content. Milk is low in iron, manganese, copper, and vitamin C.

Skim or low-fat milk should be substituted for whole milk if you want to reduce fat and/or calorie intake, but use whole milk if you want to increase calories. Children under the age of two should always drink whole milk. Children two to six should be given 2%, low-fat milk. Over the age of six, either 1% or 2% low-fat or skim milk is encouraged.

These milk equivalences match the calcium content (but not necessarily the calorie content) of milk in the portions shown:

Milk Equivalents

1 cup plain yogurt	= 1 cup milk
1 ounce shredded cheddar/Swiss cheese (1-1/3 ounce = 1 cup)	= 3/4 cup milk
1-inch cube cheddar/Swiss cheese	= 1/2 cup milk
1/2 cup ice cream or ice milk (1-2/3 cup ice cream = 1 cup milk)	= 1/3 cup milk
1 tablespoon or 1/2-ounce processed cheese spread or 1 tablespoon Parmesan cheese	= 1/4 cup milk
1/2 cup cottage cheese	= 1/4 cup milk

Milk used in cooked foods—such as creamed soups, sauces, and puddings—can count toward your daily intake of this group, too. See the recipes for soups, beverages, desserts and meatless meals in Chapter 3, *Useful Recipes and Tables.*

If you have lactose intolerance (diarrhea from milk), substitute milk treated with lactase enzyme (e.g., Lactaid®) or cheese, yogurt, or ice cream. You may have to avoid other dairy products and you may need to take a calcium and riboflavin supplement to meet your needs. See General Dietary Guideline 6, *A Lactose-Free/Lactose-Restricted Diets,* page 61.

NOTE: An imitation dairy product, such as Mocha-Mix®, Poly Rich®, Ponan® or non-dairy creamer, is one that resembles a real milk product, especially in flavor and cooking characteristics, but does not contain milk solids which provide the nutritional value in real milk. Imitation dairy products will generally not contribute high-quality protein or calcium, and many contain *more* saturated fat than cream.

The Meat and Meat-Equivalent Group

One serving equals:

2 to 3 ounces of lean cooked meat, poultry, or fish; or

2 eggs; or

1 to 1-1/2 cups cooked dried beans or peas; or

2-1/2" × 2-1/2" square tofu (soybean curd)

2 tablespoons of peanut butter may replace 1/2 serving of meat.

Daily servings recommended: 2 or more

According to the USDA Daily Food Guide, we should eat two or more servings from the meat and meat-equivalent group each day. In general, two servings of meat provide approximately 50% of the protein, 20% to 50% of the iron, 25% to 30% of vitamins B_1 and B_2, and 30% of the niacin we need.

Meat is not a good source of vitamins A or C or the mineral calcium. The iron and other minerals in meat vary according to meat type. Muscle meats are high in iron, organ meats are even higher, while chicken (white meat), and fish have relatively low iron levels. Muscle meats contribute zinc and phosphorus in addition to iron.

Non-meat alternatives such as beans, peas, and peanut butter contain less protein than meat but are inexpensive, and provide good protein values when eaten with other protein foods. Eggs, cheese, and peanut butter contain a lot of fat, but the protein in eggs and cheese is of good to excellent quality. Beans and peas are also good sources of fiber.

The fat content in the meat group may vary from 1% to 40%, depending upon the animal feed, slaughter weight, cut of meat, extent of fat trimmed off, and method of preparation. Usually, the higher the grade of meat, the higher the fat content. The following list classifies meat and meat substitutes by fat content, listing low, medium, and high-fat categories:

Low-Fat

Beef: Baby beef (very lean), chipped beef, chuck, flank steak, tenderloin, plate ribs, plate skirt steak, round, all cuts rump, spareribs, tripe

Lamb: Leg, rib, sirloin, loin (roast and chops), shank shoulder

Low-Fat (CONTINUED)

Pork: Leg (whole rump, center shank)

Veal: Leg, loin, shank, shoulder, cutlets

Poultry: Meat without skin of chicken, turkey, Cornish hen, guinea hen, pheasant

Fish: Any fresh or frozen (except salmon); canned tuna, mackerel, crab, or lobster (packed in water), clams, oysters, sardines (drained)

Cheeses: Those containing less than 5% butterfat

Cottage cheese: Dry and 2% fat

Dried beans and peas

Tofu

Medium-Fat

Beef: Lean ground (15% fat), corned beef (canned), rib eye, round (ground commercial)

Pork: Loin (all cuts tenderloin), shoulder arm (picnic), shoulder blade, Boston butt, Canadian bacon, boiled ham

Liver, heart, kidney, and sweetbreads (NOTE: These meats are high in cholesterol)

Creamed cottage cheese

Cheese: Mozzarella, ricotta, farmer's cheese, Neufchatel, Parmesan

Eggs (NOTE: Yolks are high in cholesterol)

Fish: Shrimp, salmon (fresh or water-packed)

High-Fat

Beef: Brisket, corned beef, regular ground beef (greater than 15% fat), hamburger, chuck (ground commercial), roasts (rib), steaks (club and rib)

Lamb: Breast

Pork: Spareribs, loin (back ribs), ground pork

Veal: Breast

Poultry: Capon, duck (domestic), goose

Cheese: Cheddar, Swiss types

Cold-cuts

The Fruit and Vegetables Group

One serving equals:

1/2 cup of vegetable or fruit; or

1 medium apple, banana, or potato; or half a medium grapefruit or cantaloupe.

Daily servings recommended: 4 or more, including:

(a) 1 good or 2 fair sources of vitamin C daily

Good sources: Grapefruit or grapefruit juice, orange or orange juice, cantaloupe, guava, mango, papaya, raw strawberries, broccoli, Brussels Sprouts, green pepper, sweet red pepper

Fair sources: Honeydew melon, lemon, tangerines, watermelon, asparagus, cabbage, cauliflower, collards, garden cress, kale, kohlrabi, mustard greens, potatoes, sweet potatoes cooked in the jacket, rutabagas, spinach, tomatoes, tomato juice, turnip greens

(b) 1 good source of vitamin A at least every other day

Good sources: Dark green and deep orange or yellow vegetables or fruits (e.g., apricots, broccoli, cantaloupe, carrots, collards, cress, kale, mango, persimmon, pumpkin, spinach, sweet potatoes, turnip greens and other dark green leaves, winter squash)

Fruits and vegetables provide some of your iron and most of your vitamins A and C, and are good sources of folic acid and magnesium as well. Fruits may help stimulate the appetite, and their organic acid content helps in the absorption of iron and calcium.

Most fruits and vegetables are nutrient-dense, low in calories, low in fat, and high in fiber. Fruit juices are higher in calories and lower in fiber than the comparable fruit.

Fruits and vegetables high in vitamins A and/or C, and the cruciferous vegetables (cabbage, kale, kohlrabi, broccoli, Brussels Sprouts, and cauliflower) are recommended to help prevent cancer (but have not as yet been shown to have any role in its treatment).

The Whole-Grain Breads and Cereals Group

One serving equals:

1 slice of whole-grain bread, or an equivalent serving of whole-grain baked goods; or

1 cup ready-to-eat high-fiber cereal; or

1/2 to 3/4 cup cooked cereal, pasta, or macaroni (all whole-grain only)

Daily servings recommended: 4 or more per day

Four or more servings of whole-grain products are recommended each day to contribute carbohydrate calories, fiber, and the vitamins niacin, B_1, and B_2. This group contains all grains served in the whole-grain form, including wheat, corn, oats, buckwheat, rice, and rye made into such products as breads, biscuits, muffins, waffles, pancakes, cooked or ready-to-eat cereals, noodles, pasta, rice, rolled oats, etc.

The proteins in grains are incomplete—that is, they do not contain all the essential amino acids that are the building blocks of proteins. Different grains can be combined to meet protein needs, but doing so requires a thorough knowledge of grain complements and special menu planning. Do not attempt to meet protein needs through grains alone without the guidance of a dietitian or other qualified nutritionist.

This group provides calories in an inexpensive way. If you need additional calories, but not protein, you can add servings of whole-grain foods to your daily diet.

If you are interested in adding fiber to your diet, see General Dietary Guideline 5, *The Fiber and Residue Contents of Foods,* on page 58.

Guideline 2

A High-Protein/High-Calorie Diet

Purpose

This diet is designed to reverse the effects of weight loss and tissue-wasting, but to do so it must be continued until body weight has been restored. The diet is essentially normal, except that it is supplemented with high-protein, high-calorie foods. Extra servings of milk, meat, and eggs are included. You can use special high-protein/high-calorie commercial liquid supplements where indicated. If you need to increase calories, add more carbohydrates and fat.

Instructions

Use the following foods or their nutritional equivalents in the recommended amounts daily:

- 1quart whole milk or equivalent. Use milk with Lactaid® if lactose intolerance is a problem (see General Dietary Guideline 6, *Lactose-Free/Lactose-Restricted Diets,* page 61). Use skim milk if you do not need extra calories, but need protein.
- 8 ounces of medium-fat meat, fish, poultry, or cheese. Choose from the following:

  Beef: Ground (15% fat), canned corned beef, rib eye, round

  Pork: All cuts tenderloin, shoulder arm, shoulder blade, Boston butt, Canadian bacon, boiled ham

  Liver, heart, kidney, sweetbreads (NOTE: All are high in cholesterol)

  Cheese: Creamed cottage, mozzarella, ricotta, Neufchatel, Parmesan, farmer's

  Fish: Any fresh or frozen

  Poultry: Any meat of chicken, turkey, Cornish hen, guinea hen, pheasant
- 2 whole eggs. If high cholesterol is a problem, use only egg whites or egg substitutes. (NOTE: Do not use raw eggs; they may contain *Salmonella* bacteria, which cause food-poisoning that can be especially dangerous to cancer patients).

- 4 servings of vegetables to include the following:

  1 serving (1/2 cup) dark green, deep yellow/orange vegetable (e.g., broccoli, carrots, tomatoes, etc.)

  1 to 2 servings (approximately 1/2 to 2/3 cup each) starchy vegetables (e.g., corn, lima beans, potatoes, winter squash)

  1 to 2 servings (1/2 cup each) other non-starchy vegetables (e.g., bean sprouts, cabbage, cauliflower, eggplant, summer squash)

- 3 servings fruit, including one citrus, if tolerated. (Serving size varies with type of fruit.)
- 7 servings whole-grain bread, whole-grain cereal, or dried beans, peas, or lentils. Serving sizes are 1 slice for bread and 1/2 cup for cereal or dried/cooked beans, peas, and lentils.
- 5 servings fat, including butter, margarine, oil, or mayonnaise (1 serving = 1 teaspoon); nuts (1/4 cup); light or sour cream (2 tablespoons); heavy cream or salad dressing (1 tablespoon)
- The following high-protein nutritional supplements can help you consume a sufficient quantity of high-protein food:

  Ensure® (Ross Laboratories)
  Ensure Plus® (Ross Laboratories)
  Sustacal® (Mead Johnson)
  Citrotein® (Sandoz Nutrition)
  Meritene® (Sandoz Nutrition)
  Resource® (Sandoz Nutrition)
  Magnacal® (Sherwood Medical)

  Other products are also available (see Table 2, p 187). You can add extra powered milk to creamed potatoes, creamed soups, gravies, and cottage cheese to increase protein content. You can also drink and use double-strength milk in cooking; make it by adding 1 cup powdered milk to 1 quart whole or low-fat milk.

- See the Recipe Index (page 387), and the section on Cooking with Commercial Supplements (page 167) for high-protein recipes. Also contact the National Cancer Institute (1-800-4-CANCER), your local American Cancer Society unit, or other organizations for cancer patients and their families for publications containing high-protein recipes and diets.

High-Protein Supplements

If you are unable to eat enough food to supply the protein and calories you need, if you are losing weight, or if you are having difficulty in eating normal foods, you might be advised to add one of the high-protein supplements listed in Table 2 (page 187) to your diet as a between-meal snack. In addition to protein, these supplements contain fat, carbohydrates, vitamins, and minerals, and are high in calories.

High-protein supplements come in a variety of flavors and forms: in a canned milkshake form, ready to drink; or in powdered form, to be mixed with milk or water. Instant Breakfast is available in the supermarket; the rest are available without prescription in drugstores and some supermarkets. In some areas, the American Cancer Society also carries high-protein supplements.

In choosing one of these supplements, you should consider:

- Their comparative cost.
- Their taste. Some will be more palatable to you than others.
- The amount of protein you will be getting. Several of the high-protein supplements do not contain much more protein per quart than milk (1 quart of whole milk contains 32 grams of protein). However, some of these products (Citrotein®, Ensure®, Resource® liquid, and Magnacal®) are lactose-free (milk-free) and may be needed if your physician tells you that you have milk (lactose) intolerance (see the General Dietary Guideline 6, *Lactose-Free/Lactose-Restricted Diets,* page 61). If you do not need a lactose-free product, you will get the most protein from Instant Breakfast, Meritene®, Sustacal®, or Sustagen®.

In addition to the supplements listed in Table 2, *High-Protein Supplements,* page 187, many other brands of protein drinks and protein powder are available in supermarkets and drugstores. If you prefer to use one of these products, you should compare it to those listed in Table 2 to make sure you are getting comparable amounts of protein and calories.

Liquid predigested protein has also been used as a high-protein supplement in hospital settings, where a patient's condition can be closely monitored. It supplies 15 grams of protein per 2 tablespoons. Although available without prescription in health food stores, **liquid predigested protein should only be used under medical supervision because of possible serious side effects.**

If your physician advises the use of liquid predigested protein, you may improve its rather poor taste by using one of the flavored varieties (cherry is recommended) and by using it chilled. Mixing it with apple juice, ice cream, or yogurt may also improve its taste. You may find it easiest to get it over with quickly, treating it as a bad-tasting medicine, by tossing down the 2-tablespoon dose from a small cup.

High-Calorie Supplements

High-Calorie Supplements (see Table 3, page 189) contain no protein. They supplement the diet with extra calories derived from fat and carbohydrates. High-calorie supplements come as liquid, powder, or oil and are easily mixed with your regular foods. All are available without prescription in drugstores.

Elemental Diets

Elemental (nutritionally complete) diets (see Table 4, page 190) are recommended only when a clear liquid diet must be the sole source of nutrition. All are low-residue and lactose-free. They are available only by prescription and are more expensive than the high-protein supplements recommended to add protein and calories to your regular diet.

Cooking With Convenience Foods

If you must prepare your own meals, you may sometimes feel too ill from your disease or your therapy to do much cooking. However, with the help of the many convenience foods available, you can still prepare appetizing, nutritionally adequate meals with little time and effort.

A major drawback is their expense, and it's worthwhile checking to see how much you are really getting for your money—and looking for alternatives if they are out of your price range. Many canned, frozen, and packaged foods have a high salt content and may not be suitable for people with water-retention problems or people who must otherwise be on a salt-restricted diet. Check the label!

Frozen dinners and canned or frozen main dishes and vegetables take minimum preparation. Serve them with fruit or juice, milk, and bread for a satisfying and nutritious meal. For economy, and to build up a resource to fall back on, cook larger quantities and freeze the leftovers in individual serving sizes. If practical financially, a microwave oven can shorten heating and cooking times dramatically.

Shortcuts

Many canned and frozen convenience foods can be combined with other food to make quick, easy, and appetizing meals. For example:

- Melt cheese over broccoli or asparagus; or mix cheese into a white sauce, add broccoli or asparagus, and serve on toast or crackers.
- Make a patty out of canned corned beef hash, top with a pineapple slice and grill.
- To canned spaghetti, add cooked ground meat, tuna, diced chicken or ham, dried beef, or sliced frankfurters, heat or bake to blend the flavors, and, starting from a basic canned item, you have an appetizing meal.
- Mix canned gravy or canned white sauce with tuna, canned shrimp, or diced cooked chicken or turkey.
- Add tuna or chicken and chopped onion and green pepper to undiluted condensed chicken soup. Top with an unbaked baking powder biscuit and bake until biscuit is brown and dish is heated through.

Frozen Foods

If you have a freezer, keep commercially frozen food on hand. You can also freeze individual servings of uncooked foods, such as hamburger patties, chops, chicken pieces, or fish fillets. Homemade stews, casseroles, and other mixed dishes can also be put into individual serving containers and kept in the freezer. You can have a week's basic meals prepared and frozen for daily use. Then you need only heat the major entree and prepare side dishes.

Canned and Packaged Foods

Stock up on non-perishable foods. A supply of canned and packaged foods not needing refrigeration will save you trips to the supermarket and also offer you a ready variety of foods to meet whatever your taste preference may be at the moment. Many of these products now come in a one-serving size and are especially good for between-meal snacks to increase your calorie and protein intake. Some foods you might want to stock are listed below.

Beverages
Canned and dry milk
Instant hot cocoa mix
Instant breakfast mix
Instant coffee
Tea, regular and herbal
Instant beef or chicken broth
Fruit and vegetable juices
Fruit-ades (Kool-Aid®, Gatorade®, etc.)
Carbonated drinks

Breads, Cereals, and Cereal Products
Dry cereal
Instant hot cereal
Instant pancake mix
Muffin mixes
Crackers (saltines, grahams, etc.)

Desserts
Instant pudding
Canned pudding
Jell-O®
Unflavored gelatin
Cake and cookie mixes

Fruits and Vegetables
Canned fruit
Dried fruit
Canned vegetables
Canned vegetable soups
Pureed baby foods

Meat and Other Protein Foods
Canned meat, poultry, or fish
Canned mixtures of meat, poultry or fish with vegetables, noodles, spaghetti, rice, macaroni, or beans
Canned soups made with meat, poultry or fish, peas, lentils, or other beans
Peanut butter

Sauces and Seasonings

Canned gravy

Packaged gravy mixes

Packaged seasoning mixes

Canned sauces

Snacks and Sweets

Instant Breakfast bars*

Granola bars*

Nuts*

Candy

Jam and jelly

Honey

***These foods may be difficult for some to tolerate and are clearly inappropriate for those with chewing and swallowing difficulties.**

Guideline 3

Food Sources of Minerals

Use these listings to familiarize yourself with the necessary dietary minerals.

Phosphorus

Recommended Dietary Allowance: *Adult*: Before age 25, pregnant and lactating women—1200 mg; after age 25 (except as above)—800 mg
Major functions in the body: Helps release energy from fuel nutrients, activates enzymes and vitamins, aids in absorption and transport of nutrients, maintains acid-base balance, part of structure of cell membranes and compounds such as DNA and RNA
Deficiency symptoms: Rickets, osteomalacia, muscle weakness, bone pains, anorexia
Overconsumption symptoms: High blood phosphate, low blood calcium and magnesium, tetany, loose bowels, convulsions
Significant sources: *High*—200 to 1200 mg per 100 g—tuna, mackerel, pike, red snapper, sardines, whitefish, liver, rabbit, turkey, beef brains, chicken, eggs, pistachio nuts, pumpkin, lentils, popcorn, grains (except corn), chocolate, yeast, low-fat yogurt, American cheese
Medium—100 to 200 mg per 100 g—perch, shrimp, squid, clams, swordfish, tongue, veal, beef, chicken, gizzards, heart, lamb, pork, Macadamia nuts, barley, white rice, prunes, raisins, corn, peas, cheese, mushrooms, almonds, oysters, eggs
Fair—50 to 100 mg per 100 g—chestnuts, coconuts, dates, figs, collards, watercress, endive, horseradish, kale, kohlrabi, leeks, artichokes, asparagus, broccoli, buttermilk, cream cheese, cream, milk, molasses, lima beans

Calcium

Recommended Dietary Allowance: Adult: Before age 25, pregnant and lactating women—1200 mg; after age 25 (except as above)—800 mg
Major functions in the body—Necessary for bone and tooth formation, part of intercellular substance, helps transmit nerve impulses,

helps substances to enter and leave cells, part of blood-clotting mechanism

Deficiency symptoms—Tetany, muscle cramps, convulsions, osteoporosis, stunted growth, prickly skin sensation, laryngeal spasm, irritability

Overconsumption symptons—Nontoxic except as a oa-arsenate, oa-molybdynate, oa-chloride, hypothyroidism, vitamin D overdose

Significant sources—*High*—200 to 400 mg per 100 g—sardines, pilchards, caviar, egg yolks, almonds, sesame seeds, filberts, kale, collards, mustard greens, turnip greens, soybeans, cheeses, blackstrap molasses, kelp, Brewer's yeast, milk chocolate, ice cream, low-fat yogurt, Dolomite

Medium—100 to 200 mg per 100 g—shrimp, salmon, mackerel, anchovies, scallops, Brazil nuts, pistachio nuts, sunflower seeds, oats, buckwheat, wheat bran, figs, cabbage, chard, broccoli, milk, and dairy products, tofu, oysters

Fair—50 to 100 mg per 100 g—whole eggs, wheat germ, brown sugar, Romaine lettuce, lima beans, almonds

M *Magnesium*

Recommended Dietary Allowance: Adult—350 mg (M); 280 mg (F) except, 320 mg pregnant, and 355 mg (1st 6 mos.), and 340 mg (2nd 6 mos.) lactating

Major functions in the body: Part of bone structure, helps get energy to cells, has a part in muscle relaxation, helps some hormones to function, necessary for function of heart and skeletal muscles and nerves

Deficiency symptoms: Poor growth, irritability, convulsions, tetany

Overconsumption symptoms: Nausea, malaise, muscle weakness and paralysis, paralysis of respiration, heart, and CNS

Significant sources: *High*—100 to 400 mg per 100 g—almonds, Brazil nuts, cashews, soybeans, parsnips, buckwheat, wheat bran and germ, chocolate, cocoa, blackstrap molasses, Brewer's yeast, kelp

Medium—100 to 200 mg per 100 g—filberts, hickory nuts, peanuts, pecans, pistachio nuts, walnuts, sesame seeds, barley, millet, oats, rye, wheat, wild rice, beet greens, corn, peas, carrots, brown sugar, tofu

Fair—50 to 100 mg per g—shrimp, tuna, clams, brown rice, apricots, dates, figs, lima beans, chard, parsley, collards, spinach, molasses, baker's yeast, coconuts, raw sugar

Potassium

Recommended Dietary Allowance: Not set. Estimated minimum requirement 1600–2000 mg/day*
Major functions in the body: Necessary to maintain water balance, functions in nerve impulses, helps keep heartbeat regular, role in protein and carbohydrate metabolism
Deficiency symptoms: Muscle weakness, irregular heartbeats, paralysis, fragile bones, sterility, decreased growth rate, loss of weight, death
Overconsumption symptoms: Depression of heart and central nervous system, mental confusion, weakness, vomiting, tingling, paralysis of extremities, disruption of normal heart function
Signficant sources: *High*—400 to 1000 mg per 100 g—halibut, herring, ling cod, sardines, goose, pecans, sesame seeds, sunflower seeds, walnuts, almonds, cashews, avocados, dates, figs, prunes, raisins, watercress, garlic, lentils, parsley, potatoes, spinach, artichokes, greens, sweet potato
Medium—200 to 400 mg per 100 g—haddock, perch, salmon, shrimp, tuna, liver, chicken, duck, beef kidneys, lamb, coconut, brown rice, wheat, kumquats, cantaloupes, plums, apricots, bananas, rhubarb, carrots, cauliflower, celery, chives, kale, asparagus, green beans, peas, green peppers, squash, tomato juice
Fair—50 to 200 mg per 100 g—caviar, lobster, oysters, eggs, beef heart, liver, tongue, barley, pears, tangerines, berries, apples, oranges, milk, cheeses, pickles, maple syrup, vinegar, cooked oatmeal

Iron

Recommended Dietary Allowance: *Adult:* Males—10 mg; Females, under 50—15 mg; over 50—10 mg; pregnant—30 mg
Major functions in the body: Carries oxygen to cells in blood and provides oxygen to muscles, necessary for collagen synthesis, production of antibodies, removal of fat from blood, conversion of provitamin A to vitamin A, role in detoxification of drugs in liver, helps turn fuel nutrients into energy

*Estimated minimum requirement derived from the report of the subcommittee of the Food and Nutrition Board accompanying the 10th edition of the RDA's. National Academy Press (1989).

Deficiency symptoms: Listlessness, fatigue, sore tongue, depressed growth, thin, concave nails, decreased resistance to infection, retarded mental development, anemia
Overconsumption symptoms: *Acute*—rapid increase in pulse and respiration, pallor, drowsiness, prostration, coma, death from cardiac failure, black stools
Chronic—hemorrhaging GI tract, liver injury, prolonged blood clotting time
Significant sources: *High*—5 to 18 mg per 100 g—clams, oysters, caviar, liver and kidney, nuts, chives, parsley, dry soybeans, wheat germ and bran, enriched white rice, blackstrap molasses, Brewer's yeast, sorghum syrup
Medium—1 to 5 mg per 100 g—deep sea fish, scallops, shrimp, chicken, duck, turkey, eggs, pork, veal, beef, tongue, heart, nuts, barley, brown rice, rye, wheat, oats, buckwheat, dates, figs, raisins, prunes, olives, spinach, artichokes, lima beans, lentils, cauliflower, broccoli, Cheddar cheese, mushrooms, green beans
Fair—0.1 to 1.1 mg per 100 g—carp, salmon, flounder, crab, lobster, enriched white rice, lemons, limes, bananas, melons, apples, corn, cucumbers, butter, cheeses, cream, milk, oils

Sodium

Recommended Dietary Allowance: Not established. Estimated minimum requirement for adults—500 mg/day*
Major functions in the body: Necessary for proper distribution of body fluids and function of nerve impulses
Deficiency symptoms: Anorexia, nausea, muscle atrophy, retarded bone development, poor growth, weight loss
Overconsumption symptoms: Diarrhea, salivation, exhaustion, respiratory failure, inhibition of growth, edema, hypertension, anemia
Significant sources: *High*—100 to 700 mg per 100 g—tuna, clams, caviar, lobster, sardines, scallops, shrimp, brains, eggs, beef liver, beet greens, celery, Swiss chard, olives, peas, butter, buttermilk, cream cheese, Parmesan cheese, swiss cheese, Cheddar and cottage cheese, pickles, table salt, kelp, Brewer's yeast, canned soup, frozen dinners, high processed foods, baking soda

*Estimated minimum requirement derived from the report of the subcomittee of the Food and Nutrition Board accompanying the 10th edition of the RDA's. National Academy Press (1989).

Medium—30 to 100 mg per 100 g—flounder, haddock, halibut, oysters, red snapper, goose, beef heart, lamb, beef, chicken, duck, pork, turkey, liver, veal, sesame seeds, beets, kale, spinach, turnips, watercress, milk
Fair—1 to 50 mg per 100 g—clams, coconuts, filberts, peanuts, berries, beans, broccoli, Brussel sprouts, cabbage, onions, parsley, peas, barley, brown rice, rye wheat, mushrooms, yeast, chocolate, molasses, limes

 Zinc

Recommended Dietary Allowance: *Adult*: Males—15 mg; Females—12 mg except, 15 mg pregnant; lactating: 19 mg (1st 6 mos.), and 16 mg (2nd 6 mos.)
Major functions in the body: Helps enzymes that release dioxide from lungs, part of insulin, necessary for synthesis of protein and collagen, growth, wound healing
Deficiency symptoms: Growth failure, anorexia, dwarf gonads, dermatitis, impaired wound healing, spoon nails, taste changes
Overconsumption symptoms: Lassitude, slow tendon reflexes, diarrhea, CNS, depression, tremors, paralysis of extremities, bloody inflammation of the intestines, vomiting
Significant sources: *High*—4 to 10 mg per 100 g—oysters, herring, beef, lamb, beef and pork liver, sunflower seeds, pumpkin, cheese, wheat, yeast, maple syrup, bone meal, gluten, tea
Medium—0.4 to 4 mg per 100 g—lobster, crab, shrimp, tuna, perch, chicken, turkey, pork, veal, livers, eggs, peanuts, cashews, oats, barley, wheat, brown rice, rye, avocados
Fair—0.1 to 0.4 mg per 100 g—apples, grapes, oranges, bananas, bean butter, cream, milk, oil, white sugar, honey, dates, mushrooms, cucumber

 Copper

Recommended Dietary Allowance: Not established. Estimated safe and adequate daily dietary intake for adults—1.5–3 mg
Major functions in the body: Stimulates iron absorption, storage, and releases, hemoglobin synthesis, necessary for synthesis of collagen, helps maintain nerve sheath
Deficiency symptoms: Anemia, bone disease
Overconsumption symptoms: *Acute*—hypernuria, coma, CV collapse, hypotension, sporadic fever, death
Chronic—nausea, vomiting, stomach, pain, yellow watery diarrhea, dizziness, jaundice, green stools, saliva, and vomitus

Significant sources: *High*—1 to 10 mg per 100 g—oysters, crabs, bluefish, calf, duck, lamb, pork, beef liver and kidney, nuts, soybeans, wheat germ and bran, yeast, gelatin, cornmeal, margarine, mushrooms
Medium—0.1 to 1 mg per 100 g—halibut, flounder, tuna, snapper, trout, peanuts, turkey, barley, wheat, oats, rye, rice, apples, bananas, lemons, dates, apricots, asparagus, corn, kale, onions, potatoes, spinach, lentils, sweet potatoes
Fair—less than 0.1 mg per 100 g—sardines, salmon, beef, grapes, oranges, pears, peaches, carrots, cabbage, milk, cheeses, white sugar, lettuce, cauliflower, cottage cheese

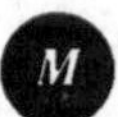

Selenium

Recommended Dietary Allowance: Adult—70 μg* (M); 55 μg (F) except, 65 μg pregnant, 75 μg lactating.
Major functions in the body: Part of enzymes, antioxidant, "spares" vitamin E, protects against cirrhosis in liver, counteracts effects of heavy metals
Deficiency symptoms: Possible, but not known: alcoholic liver failure, neonatal jaundice, cancer
Overconsumption symptoms: Not-studied in humans; severe neurological symptoms in animals
Significant sources: *High*—30 to 100 μg per 100 g—oysters, tuna, lobsters, shrimp, trout, cod, flounder, liver, kidney, cashew nuts, peanuts, wheat germ and bran, brown rice, barley, Brewer's yeast
Medium—10 to 30 μg per 100 g—beef, lamb, liver, heart, egg, chicken, pork, walnuts, white rice, oats, alfalfa, garlic, dry lentils, Cheddar cheese, molasses, mushrooms
Fair—1 to 10 μg per 100 g—egg white, chestnuts, almonds, raisins, apples, bananas, oranges, pears, lettuce, okra, turnips, tomatoes, cabbages, milk, cottage and Swiss cheese, beer, margarine, sugar

Iodine

Recommended Dietary Allowance: Adult—150 μg; except, 175 μg in pregnancy and 200 μg in lactation
Major functions in the body: Part of thyroid hormone that regulates growth and development and controls the basal metabolic rate (rate at which the body uses energy for fuel)

*μg = microgram; 1/10 of mg

Deficiency symptoms: Pituitary tumors, decreased basal metabolic rate, increased blood lipids, goiter

Overconsumption symptoms: *Acute*—GI irritation, skin hemorrhages, hypersensitivity

Chronic—brassy taste, burning in mouth and throat, symptoms of head cold, skin lesions, diarrhea

Significant sources: *High*—30 to 50 μg per 100 g—ocean fish and shellfish, sunflower seeds, kelp, moss, cod liver oil, mushrooms, iodized salt

Medium—10 to 50 μg per 100 g—eel, catfish, sardines, tuna, mackerel, crab, salmon, eggs, beef, liver, peanuts, pineapple, spinach, turnip greens, asparagus, Cheddar cheese, chocolate, iodized salt, mayonnaise

Fair—1 to 10 μg per 100 g—carp, river bass, lake trout, river perch, walnuts, almonds, cashews, raisins, pears, apples, bananas, broccoli, mustard greens, rice, wheat, barley, oats, rye, wheat germ, milk, cheese, butter, molasses, margarine

Guideline 4

Food Sources of Vitamins

Use these listings to familiarize yourself with the necessary vitamins.

Fat-Soluble Vitamins

Vitamin A (retinol, retinic acid, provitamin A-Carotides, Beta Carotene)

Recommended Dietary Allowance: *Adults*—1000 µg. RE* (M); 800 µg RE(F); except lactating: 1,300 µg 1st 6 mos.; 1,200 µg 2nd 6 mos.
Major functions in the body: Integrity of immune system, skin and mucous membranes; promotes bone and tooth development; forms visual purple in sight processes; may protect against cancer through roles in immune system and epithelial tissue
Deficiency symptoms: Slowed growth in children; night blindness; diarrhea; intestinal infections; xeropthalmia-blindness
Overconsumption symptoms: Nausea, irritability, blurred vision, growth retardation; enlargement of liver and spleen; loss of hair; joint pain; increased pressure in skull; skin changes
Significant sources: *High*—10,000 to 76,000 IU per 100 mg—liver, liver oil, carrots, mint, kohlrabi, parsley, spinach, turnip greens
Good—1000 to 10,000 IU per 100 mg—butter, cheese, egg yolk, margarine, powdered milk, cream, white fish, eel, kidney, mangoes, apricots, yellow melons, peaches, nectarines, beet greens, pumpkin, sweet potato, watercress, tomatoes, lettuce, squash, Swiss chard, whole milk, winter squash

Vitamin D (Calciferol, "sunshine vitamin")

Recommended Dietary Allowance: *Adult*—Under 25 (and in pregnancy and lactation at any age): 400 IU; Over 25: 200 IU
Major functions in the body: Promotes bone and teeth formation, increases intestinal absorption of calcium; activated vitamin D is considered a hormone

*RE = retinol equivalents

Deficiency symptoms: Delayed growth, loss of minerals from bones (rickets in children, osteomalacia in adults)
Overconsumption symptoms: Nausea, weight loss, irritability, mental and physical growth retardation, kidney damage, deposition of calcium from bones in soft tissue
Significant sources: *Best*—1000 to 25,000 IU per 100 g—liver oils
Good—100 to 1000 IU per 100 g—egg yolk, fortified margarine, lard, herring, salmon, mackerel, pilchards, sardines, tuna, shrimp, kippers
Fair—10 to 100 IU per 100 g—grain and vegetable oils, cod, fish roe, halibut, butter, cream, eggs, cheeses, liver, beef, veal, vitamin D fortified milk and dairy products
NOTE: 1/2 hour total sun exposure on skin each day will provide adequate provitamin D

Vitamin K

Recommended Dietary Allowance: *Adult*—Over 25: 80 μg (M); 65 μg (F)
Major functions in the body: Role in blood clotting
Deficiency symptoms: Increased bleeding, increased clotting time, hemorrhage
Overconsumption symptoms: Blood clot, vomiting
Significant sources: *Best*—100 to 300 μg per 100 g—cabbage, cauliflower, soybeans, spinach, pork, beef liver, beef kidney, Brussels Sprouts
Good—10 to 100 μg per 100 g—potatoes, strawberries, tomatoes, alfalfa, wheat, egg yolk, green tea
Fair—0 to 10 μg per 100 g—corn, carrots, green peas, parsley, mushrooms, milk, brewed coffee or tea

Vitamin E (Tocopheral)

Recommended Dietary Allowance: *Adult*—10 mg α TE(M); 8 mg α TE(F); except, 10 mg in pregnancy, and 12 mg (1st 6 mos.), and 11 mg (2nd 6 mos.) in lactating
Major functions in the body: Functions as an antioxidant, protecting vitamins A and C and unsaturated fatty acids from destruction; protects cell memranes
Deficiency symptoms: Hemolytic anemia in newborns, poorly developed muscles, yellowing and hardening of gall bladder
NOTE: deficiency is rare

Overconsumption symptoms: High blood pressure, allergies, gastrointestinal distress, nausea, abnormal iron metabolism
Significant sources: *Best*—50 to 300 mg per 100 g—vegetable oils, margarines, mayonnaise, sunflower seeds
Good—5 to 50 mg per 100 g—coconuts, peanuts, olives, cod liver, palm oil, walnut oil, wheat germ, alfalfa, barley, dry soybeans, lima beans, poppy and sesame seeds, chocolate, rosehips, cocoa butter, peanut butter, mint, corn, sweet potatoes, nuts, beef liver
Fair—0.5 to 5 mg per 100 g—Brussels Sprouts, carrots, parsnips, mustard greens, brown rice, lettuce, cauliflower, peas, turnip greens, kale, asparagus, kohlrabi, green peppers, spinach, cabbage, bacon, beef, lamb, pork, veal, eggs, butter, cheeses, whole wheat flour, dried navy beans, cornmeal, oatmeal, coconut, blackberries, pears, apples, olives, yeast

Water-Soluble Vitamins

Vitamin C (Ascorbic Acid)

Recommended Dietary Allowance: *Adult*—60 mg; except in pregnancy, 70 mg; in lactation, 95 mg (1st 6 mos.), and 90 mg (2nd 6 mos.)
Major functions in the body: Functions in collagen to hold cells together, strengthens blood vessels, promotes healing of wounds and bones, functions in immune system to increase resistance to infection, aids in absorption of iron and calcium
Deficiency symptoms: Edema, failure of wounds to heal, bleeding gums, weakness, listlessness, rough skin, aching joints, easy bruising (scurvy)
Overconsumption symptoms: Deficiency symptoms when megadoses stopped; diarrhea, gut discomfort, kidney stones, reproductive failure, dependency on high dose of vitamin, inactivation of Vitamin B_{12}
Significant sources: *Best*—100 to 300 mg per 100 g—broccoli, Brussels Sprouts, collards, horseradish, kale, parsley, green peppers, turnip greens, black currants, guava, rosehips
Good—50 to 100 mg per 100 g—beet greens, cabbage, cauliflower, chives, kohlrabi, mustard greens, watercress, spinach, lemons, oranges, papayas, strawberries
Fair—25 to 50 mg per 100 g—asparagus, lima beans, beet greens, okra, peas, potatoes, radishes, summer squash, gooseberries, grapefruit,

limes, mangoes, cantaloupe, honeydew melons, tangerines, raspberries, tomatoes, kumquats

Vitamin B_6 (Pyridoxine, Pyridoxal, Pyridoxamine)

Recommended Dietary Allowance: *Adult*—2 mg (M); 1.6 mg (F), except in pregnancy, 2.2 mg, and in lactation, 2.1 mg
Major functions in the body: Necessary for protein metabolism, helps convert tryptophan to niacin, fatty acid metabolism, and red blood cell formation
Deficiency symptoms: Dermatitis near eyes, anemia, convulsions, irritability, muscle twitchings, kidney stones
Overconsumption symptoms: Some evidence of neurological symptoms
Significant sources: *High*—1000 to 10,000 μg per 100 g—liver, herring, salmon, walnuts, peanuts, wheat germ, brown rice, yeast, blackstrap molasses
Medium—100 to 1000 μg per 100 g—bananas, avocados, grapes, pears, barley, cabbage, corn, oats, peas, beef, lamb, pork, veal, cod, flounder, halibut, mackerel, whale, sardines, tuna, butter, eggs, shellfish
Fair—10 to 100 μg per 100 g—apples, cantaloupes, grapefruit, lemons, oranges, peaches, raisins, strawberries, watermelons, cherries, currants, asparagus, beans, beet greens, lettuce, onions, cheese, milk

Vitamin B_{12} (Cobalamin)

Recommended Dietary Allowance: *Adult*—2 μg, except in pregnancy, 2.2 μg, and in lactation, 2.6 μg
Major functions in the body: Necessary for nucleic acid synthesis, development of normal red blood cells, and maintenance of nerve tissues
Deficiency symptoms: Poor growth, pernicious anemia, inflamed tongue, neurological disorders
Overconsumption symptoms: None reported
Significant sources: *High*—50 to 500 μg per 100 g—kidney, liver, brain
Medium—5 to 50 μg per 100 g—chicken liver, beef, chicken heart, egg yolk
Fair—0.5 to 5 μg per 100 g—cod, flounder, haddock, halibut, shrimp, lobster, scallops, tuna, swordfish, whale, beef, pork, lamb, chicken, cheeses, milk, eggs

Vitamin B_1 (Thiamin)

Recommended Dietary Allowance: *Adult*—Males under 50: 1.5 mg; Males over 50: 1.2 mg; Females under 50: 1.1 mg; Females over 50: 1.0 mg. pregnant: 1.5 mg; lactating: 1.6 mg
Major functions in the body: Helps to break down carbohydrates for fuel, promotes synthesis of ribose, a normal functioning of nervous system
Deficiency symptoms: Impaired growth, wasting of tissues, loss of reflexes, tingling in fingers and toes, mental confusion, depression, swelling, weight loss, severe deficiency called beriberi
Overconsumption symptoms: Edema, nervousness, sweating, increased heart rate
Significant sources: *High*—1000 to 10,000 µg per 100 g—wheat germ, rice bran, soybean flour, yeast, ham, fortified grain products, nuts
Medium—100 to 1000 µg per 100 g—gooseberries, plums, raisins, asparagus, beans, beet greens, broccoli, Brussels Sprouts, cauliflower, beef, calf, chicken, pork, lamb, turkey, mushrooms, eggs, milk, carp, clams, cod liver
Fair—10 to 100 µg per 100 g—fruits, vegetables, cheeses, fish

Vitamin B_2 (Riboflavin)

Recommended Dietary Allowance: *Adult*—Males under 50: 1.7 mg; Males over 50: 1.4 mg; Females under 50: 1.3 mg; Females over 50: 1.2 mg; Pregnant: 1.6 mg; Lactating (1st 6 mos.): 1.8 mg; Lactating (2nd 6 mos.): 1.7 mg
Major functions in the body: Helps cells use oxygen for the release of energy from food, promotes good vision and healthy skin
Deficiency symptoms: Inflammation of lips, mouth, tongue, skin of face, cracks in corners of the mouth, lesions of cornea
Overconsumption symptoms: None reported in humans
Signficiant sources: *High*—1000 to 10,000 µg per 100 g—beef, veal, chicken, pork, sheep liver and kidneys, yeast, milk, yogurt, cottage cheese
Medium—100 to 1000 µg per 100 g—avocados, currants, asparagus, beans, beet greens, broccoli, cauliflower, corn, kale, parsley, peas, spinach, bacon, beef, chicken duck, goose, fortified grain products
Fair—10 to 100 µg per 100 g—apples, apricots, bananas, blackberries, cranberries, raspberries, strawberries, cherries, grapes

Niacin (Nicotinamide, Nicotinic Acid)

Recommended Dietary Allowance: *Adult*—Under 50: 19 mg (M); 15 mg (F); Over 50: 15 mg (M); 13 mg (F); pregnant, 17 mg; lactating, 20 mg
Major functions in the body: Important for fat synthesis, tissue function and utilization of carbohydrates for energy, promotes healthy skin, nerves, digestive tract; aids digestion and promotes normal appetite
Deficiency symptoms: Sun-sensitive skin lesions, diarrhea, anorexia, weakness, vertigo, irritability, disorientation, severe case called pellagra
Overconsumption symptoms: Nicotine acid: nausea, headache, flushing, cramps
Significant sources: *High*—10 to 100 mg per 100 g—beef, pork, sheep liver, chicken liver, lamb, kidney, eggs, herring, cod ovary, wheat germ, bran, dried peas, peanuts, yeast, royal jelly
Medium—1 to 10 mg per 100 g—avocados, dates, figs, prunes, asparagus, beans, broccoli, corn, kale, almonds, cashew nuts, chestnuts, walnuts, barley, oats, wheat, rye, brown rice, beef, veal, chicken, duck, lamb, mushrooms
Fair—0.1 to 1 mg per 100 g—apples, apricots, bananas, berries, cherries, figs, grapes, grapefruit, lemons, melons, oranges, peaches, pears, pineapple, plums, raisins, tangerines

Panthothenic Acid

Recommended Dietary Allowance: Not set; Adult safe and adequate daily intake—4–7 mg
Major functions in the body: Involved in energy metabolism
Deficiency symptoms: Fatigue, sleep disturbance, nausea
Overconsumption symptoms: None reported
Significant sources: *High*—2 to 10 mg per 100 g—beef, pork, sheep livers, chicken liver, lamb, kidney, eggs, herring, wheat germ, whole grain, dried peas, peanuts, yeast, royal jelly
Medium—0.5 to 2 mg per 100 g—salmon, clams, mackerel, walnuts, broccoli, soybeans, oats, lima beans, cauliflower, peas, beef, pork, chicken, lamb, mushrooms, wheat, cheeses
Fair—0.1 to 0.5 mg per 100 g—bananas, oranges, peaches, pears, onions, kidney beans, cabbage, lettuce, almonds, oysters, lobsters, shrimp, veal, milk, honey, molasses

Guideline 5

The Fiber and Residue Contents of Food

Purpose

The foods listed here are recommended to help you prevent or treat constipation. These foods are (1) high in dietary fiber (the portion of plant materials that is not digested), (2) high in connective tissue (the rough, fibrous parts of meat and gristle), and/or (3) high in residue (meaning they are low-fiber foods that increase stool weight and bulk by other than fiber). If diarrhea is a problem, lowering fiber and residue intake will help decrease the frequency of evacuation.

Instructions

For controlling *constipation,* emphasize the foods on the high-fiber/high-residue list. For controlling *diarrhea,* emphasize foods on the low-fiber/low-residue list.

High-Fiber/High-Residue Foods

Beverages
Milk, drinks made from high-fiber vegetables, and fruits

Bread and Cereal Products
Have 5 or more servings daily to control constipation. Coarse whole-grain breads and cereals, especially wheat bran, oatmeal, cracked wheat, baked products incorporating seeds and nuts, brown rice, and coconut; avoid highly-refined products

Meat and Meat Substitutes
Tough, fibrous meats with gristle (e.g., stew meat, seasoned meat, and fried meat, smooth or chunky peanut butter, dried peas and beans, nuts and seeds)

Vegetables
Eat 2 or more servings of raw vegetables and 2 servings of cooked vegetables daily to control constipation. Any,

especially peas, parsnips, rutabagas, broccoli, Brussels sprouts, cabbage, onions, raw carrots, turnips, cauliflower, fresh tomatoes, zucchini, corn, and sweet potatoes or potatoes with jackets

Fruits

Have 2 or more servings of raw fruits and, if desired, 1 serving of cooked or canned fruit (peel on) to control constipation. Any, especially dates, figs, prunes, boysenberries, blackberries, kumquats, pineapple, rhubarb, avocados, grapes, apples, peaches, pears, and guava, fresh grapefruit and orange sections

Fats and Oils

Nuts, olives

Desserts

Those containing raisins, dried or fresh fruit, coconut or nuts; avoid highly-refined products

Miscellaneous

Chocolate nut bars, peanut brittle, pickles, sesame seeds, any soups (except consommé)

Low-Fiber/Low-Residue Foods

Beverages

Carbonated beverages, cereal drinks, cider, coffee, tea (preferably decaffeinated), 2 or fewer cups of milk

Bread and Cereal Products

Enriched white bread and toast, Melba toast, crackers and bagels, cereals (not bran, granola, or whole-grain), waffles, French toast, refined cereals (e.g., Cream of Wheat®, Cream of Rice®, baby cereals), French bread, noodles, white rice, and potatoes without skin.

Meat and Meat Substitutes

Ground or well-cooked tender beef, ham, veal, lamb, pork, poultry, tender steaks, fish, oysters, shrimp, lobster, clams, liver, crab, organ meats, eggs, cheese, and cottage cheese (include in total milk servings)

Vegetables

Strained vegetable juice, lettuce, cooked vegetables (e.g., asparagus tips, string beans, beets, carrots, eggplant, tomato, lima beans, spinach, potatoes, pumpkin, squash, artichokes; **do not use raw vegetables, corn or lima beans**

Fruits

Strained fruit juices (except prune), canned fruits, applesauce, stewed or cooked fruits; **do not use raw fruits**

Fats and Oils

Butter, margarine, salad oils, mayonnaise, cream, crisp bacon, plain gravies, plain salad dressings with allowed foods, smooth peanut butter

Desserts

Plain cakes and cookies, gelatin, plain puddings, custard (made from allowed milk), any plain dessert made from allowed foods without nuts or coconut (e.g., ice cream, ices, popsicles, etc.)

Miscellaneous

Soups made from allowed foods or strained soups and consommés; candy made from allowed foods, honey, molasses, sugar, catsup, vinegar, prepared mustard. The following spices are recommended:

Allspice	Oregano
Basil	Paprika
Bay leaves	Parsley flakes
Celery salt, powder, or leaves	Pepper, black, ground
Cinnamon	Rosemary
Cumin powder	Sage
Ginger	Savory
Mace	Tarragon
Marjoram	Thyme
Onion powder	Turmeric

On a low-residue diet, it is advisable to reduce your intake of fats. Prepare your food by baking, broiling, stewing, poaching or boiling; **do not fry foods**.

If diarrhea persists after making these dietary changes, consult your physician.

Guideline 6

A Lactose-Free/Lactose-Restricted Diet

Purpose

This diet guides you in controlling lactose (milk sugar) intolerance caused by certain chemotherapy drugs. The symptoms of such an intolerance are diarrhea and excessive gas. Drug-induced lactose intolerance is temporary and usually disappears after chemotherapy has ceased and the intestinal tract has healed.

Instructions

Lactose is found in many foods, and is added to some drugs as a filler or a sweetening agent. Often, when there is lactose in a drug it is not identified on the label. Ask your pharmacist about this if you think medication may be causing you gas or diarrhea. Also, make a practice of reading food labels and be on the lookout for the word *lactose*. Lactic acid or lactate will probably not be a problem, but lactose could be causing you real difficulty.

Lactose intolerance results from lack of the enzyme lactase, which breaks down the sugar lactose. You can buy lactase enzyme at your drugstore without a prescription in the form of a product called Lactaid®, made by the Sugar-Lo Company. This enzyme will break down a large portion of the lactose in milk if mixed according to directions.

NOTE: There are different degrees of lactose intolerance. To determine the degree of your sensitivity, first eliminate *all* sources of lactose. Three days later, add back milk treated with Lactaid®. Every two or three days, add Lactaid® to a single previously excluded food, and try it again in your diet. If you tolerate that food, keep using it; if you don't, exclude it for the present, and try it again later. Follow this regimen as long as diarrhea is a problem. If you were not previously lactose-intolerant, once treatment has ceased and your intestinal tract has healed, you should be able to return to your normal diet.

Base your food choices on the following lists of allowed and prohibited foods.

Foods Allowed

Beverages

Isomil®, Prosobee®, Mocha-Mix®, Polyrich®, meat-based formulas used as milk substitutes, carbonated drinks, coffee, freeze-dried coffee, fruit drinks, some instant coffees (read the labels), Lidalac®, and other lactose-free milks or milks treated with lactase enzyme (Lactaid®), and lactose-free products such as Ensure®, Ensure Plus®, Citrotein®, Resource®, and soy milk

Breads and Cereals

Breads and rolls made without milk, bagels, Italian bread, some cooked cereals, prepared cereals (read the labels), macaroni, spaghetti, rice, and soda crackers

Meat, Fish, Poultry, etc.

Plain beef, chicken, turkey, lamb, veal, pork, and ham, strained or junior meats or vegetables, and meat combinations that do not contain milk or milk products; kosher frankfurters; all eggs prepared without milk or prepared with Lactaid®-treated milk, and tofu

Vegetables

Fresh, canned, or frozen artichokes, asparagus, broccoli, cabbage, carrots, cauliflower, celery, corn, cucumbers, eggplant, green beans, kale, lettuce, mustard greens, okra, onions, parsley, parsnips, pumpkin, rutabagas, spinach, squash, tomatoes, white and sweet potatoes, yams, lima beans, and beets (**beware of cream-based sauces**)

Fruits

All fresh, canned, or frozen that are not processed with lactose (read the labels)

Fats

Margarine and dressings that do not contain milk or milk products, oils, bacon, some whipped toppings, some non-dairy creamers (read the labels), nut butters, and nuts

Soups

Clear soups, vegetable soups, consommés, cream soups made with Mocha-Mix®, or Lactaid® or non-dairy creamers

Desserts

Water and fruit ices, frozen fruit bars (read label), gelatin, angel food cake, homemade cakes, pies and cookies made from allowed ingredients, puddings made with water or milk treated with lactase enzymes

Miscellaneous

Soy sauce, carob powder, popcorn, olives, pure sugar candy, jelly or marmalade, sugar, corn syrup, carbonated beverages, gravy made with water, baker's cocoa, pickles, pure seasonings and spices, wine, molasses (made from beet sugar), pure monosodium glutamate, instant coffees that do not contain lactose (read the labels)

Foods Prohibited

Beverages

All untreated milks of animal origin and all milk-containing products (except lactose-free milk), such as skim, dry, evaporated, or condensed milk, yogurt, ice cream, sherbet, malted milk, Ovaltine®, hot chocolate, some cocoas and instant coffees (read the label), powdered soft drinks with lactose, curds and whey; milk that has been treated with *Lactobacillus acidophilus* culture rather than lactase

Breads and Cereals

Some prepared mixes such as muffins, biscuits, waffles, pancakes, cornbread, some dry cereals, such as Total®, Special K®, Cocoa Krispies® (read the labels), Instant Cream of Wheat®, commercial breads and rolls to which milk solids have been added, zwieback, French toast made with milk, Bisquick® mix

Meat, Fish, Poultry, etc.

Creamed or breaded meats, fish, or fowl, sausage products such as frankfurters, liver sausage, cold cuts containing non-fat milk solids or cheese, eggs, omelettes, and souffles containing milk, cheese, cottage cheese

Vegetables

Any to which lactose is added during the processing: peas, creamed, breaded, or buttered vegetables, instant potatoes, corn curls, frozen French fries processed with lactose

Fruits

Any canned or frozen fruits processed with lactose (read the labels)

Fats

Margarine and dressings containing milk or milk products, butter, cream, cream cheese, peanut butter with milk-solid fillers, salad dressings containing lactose (read the labels), sour cream

Desserts
Commercial cakes, cookies, mixes, custards, puddings, sherbet, ice cream made with milk, ice milk, frozen yogurt, anything containing chocolate, pie crust made with butter, gelatin made with carrageen, whipped cream

Miscellaneous
Chewing gum, chocolate, some cocoas, coffee, peppermint, butterscotch, caramels, some instant coffees, dietetic preparations (read the labels), certain antibiotics and vitamin and mineral preparations, spice blends if they contain milk products, MSG extender, artificial sweeteners containing lactose such as Equal®, Sweet 'n Low®, and some non-dairy creamers (read the labels), dips made with milk products

Guideline 7

A Gluten-Restricted/Gliadin-Free Diet

Purpose

Certain proteins in certain cereal grains (glutens and gliadins) may interfere with the absorption of food by susceptible patients on chemotherapy. An intolerance to gluten may result from severe toxic effects of the chemotherapy drug on the intestinal mucosa. If this is the case, temporary gluten/gliadin restriction in the diet may help, but it is important first to rule out lactose intolerance and fat malabsorption before you commit yourself to this very restricted diet. If you had gluten intolerance before your chemotherapy, see a dietitian or other nutritionist for more explicit instructions.

Instructions

Because a chemotherapy-induced gluten intolerance is not an allergy to gluten per se, you may be able to tolerate some gluten-containing foods and not others. Try foods from the limited foods list below, one at a time, to determine your tolerance for them.

Foods Allowed

Beverages
Carbonated drinks, cocoa (no wheat flour added), coffee, decaffeinated coffee (no wheat flour added), fruit juices and drinks, nectars, milk, tea

Bread and Flour Products
Bread products made only from arrow wheat, buckwheat, soybean flour, or gluten-free wheat starch, cornmeal, cornbread, corn muffins and corn pone with no wheat flour, cornstarch, gluten-free macaroni products, gluten-free porridge, rice wafers, soybean wafers, pure rice, sago, and tapioca

Cereals
Corn or rice cereals (read the labels)

Meats
All

Desserts
Cakes, cookies, pastries, etc., prepared with permitted low-gluten flours or instant potato granules, custard, gelatin desserts, homemade cornstarch and rice puddings, ice cream and sherbet if they do not contain gluten stabilizers (read the labels), tapioca pudding, wheat starch cookies

Fats
Butter, corn oil, French dressing (pure), fortified margarine, mayonnaise (pure), olive oil, other animal and vegetable fats and oils, olives, nuts, bacon

Soups
Broth, bouillon, clear meat and vegetable soups, creamed soups, soups thickened with cream, allowed starches or flours

Miscellaneous
Pepper, pickles, popcorn, potato chips, sugar, syrups, vinegar, molasses

Foods Limited

Beverages
Ale, beer, cereal beverages such as Postum® and Ovaltine®, commercial chocolate milk with cereal additives, instant coffee containing wheat, root beer

Bread and Flour Products
Breaded foods, breads, rolls, doughnuts, pastries, egg noodles, crackers, etc., made from wheat, rye, oats, or barley, commercial gluten bread, commercially prepared mixes for biscuits, cornbread, muffins, pancakes, buckwheat pancakes, waffles, etc.

Foods to Check (read the labels)

All-purpose flour, baking powder, biscuits, barley flour, bran, bread crumbs, bread flour, cake mixes, cookie mixes, cracker meal, graham flour, macaroni, malt, matzos, noodles, pancakes, pastry flour, pretzels, rye flour, Rye-Krisp®, spaghetti, flour, self-rising flour, vermicelli, waffles, wheat, cracked wheat and whole-wheat, wheat germ, zwieback

Cereals
All cereals containing malt, bran, or wheat germ or made of rye, wheat, oats, or barley (read the labels)

Meats
None

Desserts
Cakes, cookies, commercial ice cream containing gluten stabilizers, doughnuts, ice cream cones, pie, prepared mixes, prepared pudding thickened with flour

Fats
Commercial salad dressings containing gluten stabilizers, homemade cooked salad dressings if thickened with flour

Soups
All soups thickened with wheat products or containing barley, noodles, or other wheat, rye, and oat products in any form

Guideline 8

A Long-Chain-Triglyceride-Restricted/Medium-Chain-Triglyceride Fat Diet

Purpose

This diet is designed to reduce the malabsorption of fat and relieve the symptoms of fat in the stool (steatorrhea). The excess fat in the stool results from chemotherapy toxicity to the gut, which prevents the absorption of the fat into the body. This diet will help increase the absorption of calcium, fat-soluble vitamins, and fat calories.

The diet RESTRICTS the fats known as long-chain triglycerides (LCTs); medium-chain triglycerides (MCTs) are allowed.

Instructions

To control fat in the stools, follow these steps:

- Consume no more than 5 ounces of very lean meat, fish, or poultry daily (see foods lists for allowed meats).
- Limit your intake of whole eggs or egg yolks (no limit on egg whites) to 3 a week. For each egg yolk eaten, subtract 1 ounce of meat.
- If vitamin supplements are necessary or desired, use fat-soluble vitamin supplements prepared in their water-soluble form. NOTE: These vitamins will be fat-soluble once they are in the body and *can* still be toxic if taken in excess.
- Foods ordinarily prepared with the addition of oils can be prepared using MCT® oil (Mead Johnson). Recipe books are available from Mead Johnson (Evansville, Indiana 47721). You can purchase the oil from your pharmacist.
- In place of milk recipes use skim milk, or MCT-based supplements such as Pregestimil® and Portagen® (both from Mead Johnson).
- Avoid deep-frying or sauteeing foods. Use non-stick sprays such as Pam® and teflon-coated pans for cooking.

- Design your diet by choosing Basic Four foods (see Guideline 1, page 30) from the "allowed" list below.

Foods Allowed

Beverages
Skim milk, cereal beverages, coffee, tea, soft drinks

Bread and Bread Substitutes
Hamburger rolls, hard rolls, enriched white bread, whole-wheat bread, pumpernickel or rye bread (bread products contain some LCTs but are permitted in order to add palatability and variety to the diet), cooked or dry cereals, macaroni, noodles, rice, spaghetti

Meat and Meat Substitutes
Skim milk, cottage cheese, egg whites as desired, egg yolks, and whole eggs only in prescribed amounts, lean and well-trimmed skinless meat, canned fish packed in water only, poultry only in prescribed amounts

Fruits
All except avocados

Vegetables
All to which no fat except MCT® is added

Soups
Fat-free broths, bouillon, consomme, fat-free vegetable soups, soups made with skim milk

Fats
Only MCT® oil

Desserts
Water ices, frozen fruit juice bars, angel food cake, gelatin, meringue, any made from special MCT® recipes, frostings with no fat, fruit whips, mixes only if they contain no LCTs, butter or margarine in prescribed amounts, gravies made with clear soups and MCT® oil

Miscellaneous
Pickles, salt, spices, jellies, syrup, sugars, any special recipe for which MCTs are substituted for LCT, cocoa (limited to 1 tablespoon dry cocoa per day)

Foods Limited

Beverages
Whole milk, buttermilk, partially skimmed milk, light, heavy, or sour cream

Bread and Bread Substitutes
Commercial biscuits, coffee cake, cornbread, crackers, doughnuts, muffins, sweet rolls

Meat and Meat Substitutes
Frankfurters, cold cuts and sausages, any cheese other than skim milk cheese, cottage cheese, fatty meats, fish canned in oil, whole eggs and egg yolks except as prescribed, goose, duck soups, cream soups made from whole milk, soups containing stock from fatty meats

Fruits
Avocados

Vegetables
Creamed vegetables or those prepared with fats other than MCT®

Soups
All except those allowed

Fats
Palm and coconut oil, oils and shortenings of all types, sauces, and gravies except for those made with MCT® oil, commercial salad dressings, mayonnaise, whipped toppings

Desserts
Commercial cakes, pies, cookies, pastries, puddings, custards

Miscellaneous
Butter, chocolate, coconut or cream candies, creamed dishes, commercial popcorn, frozen dinners, homemade products containing whole milk and fats, mixes for muffins, biscuits and cakes, olives, nuts, commercially fried foods such as potato chips, French fried potatoes, and fried fish

Guideline 9

A Cholesterol and Fat-Restricted Diet

Purpose

This diet is designed to reduce the serum levels of cholesterol and triglycerides by controlling both food sources of cholesterol and triglycerides and the fats manufactured by the body. This low-cholesterol, modified-fat diet limits cholesterol intake to 300 mg daily. The ratio of polyunsaturated fat to saturated fat in this diet varies from 2.8:1 to 1.8:1.

Instructions

Limit daily food choices to the groups and servings outlined in the plan below. Choose your foods from the "Foods Allowed" list.

Food Group	*Number of Servings*
Milk and dairy group (skim only)	2
Meat Group (cooked poultry, fish or lean, trimmed meat)	2 to 3
Whole-grain bread and cereal	7 or more
Vegetable and fruit (include 1 serving citrus fruit, 1 serving dark green or yellow vegetable, and 1 or more others)	5
Fats (vegetable oils, olive oil, Puritan oil, or margarine only)	6 to 9 teaspoons
Desserts and sweets (made with vegetable oils and margarine only)	6 to 9 teaspoons

Foods Allowed

Milk

Non-fat dry or skim milk, non-fat evaporated milk, buttermilk, plain or low-fat or non-fat yogurt

Eggs
2 eggs, maximum per week (count as a meat serving), egg white as desired, low-cholesterol commercial egg substitutes as desired

Meat and Meat Alternatives
Broiled, roasted, braised, or stewed lean beef, lamb, veal, liver, chicken/turkey (without skin), lean pork/ham, non-oily fish, low-fat luncheon meats, tofu, dried beans and peas

Cheese
Uncreamed low-fat cottage cheese, cheese made with non-fat milk

Breads and Cereals
Whole-grain breads, whole-grain cereals, water bagels, yeast breads, saltines, graham crackers, Melba toast, noodles, pasta, rice, potatoes

Vegetables
Fresh, frozen, canned vegetables and juices (avoid frozen vegetables made with cream sauces)

Fruits
All except avocados and coconuts

Soups
Low-fat meat or vegetable-based soups, creamed soups made with non-fat milk or from fat allowance

Desserts
Sugar sweets, sherbet, fruit ice, angel food cake, gelatin, meringues, pudding made with non-fat milk, fruit whips, frozen yogurt, frozen fruit juice bars

Foods Limited

Milk
Whole milk, "evaporated milk," eggnog, milkshakes, malts (made from whole milk), ice cream, high-fat yogurt, condensed milk, cream, half-and-half, non-dairy creamers, imitation and regular sour cream

Eggs
More than 2 whole eggs per week; fried eggs not fried in low-oil pan spray

Meats
Most luncheon meats: pastrami, corned beef, sausage, goose, duck, fried meats or fish, fish packed in oil, bacon, Canadian bacon

Cheese
All except those listed on the allowed list

Breads and Cereals
Quick breads (muffins, biscuits, waffles, pancakes), most crackers, doughnuts, sweet rolls, egg noodles, croissants

Vegetables
Olives, those cooked in oil, butter, or salt pork

Fruits
Avocados, coconut

Soups
Most commercial creamed soups, fat-containing soups

Desserts
Ice cream, ice milk, frozen desserts, cakes, pies, pastries, whipped cream, chocolate, nuts, coconut, cooked custards

Guideline 10

How to Prevent Kidney Stone Formation (Acid Ash/ Alkaline Ash Diet)

Some drugs can cause particular patients to form kidney stones. There may be no symptoms, or patients may have an ashen pallor combined with very severe back pain (flank to groin). The degree of pain depends on the amount of urine backed up behind the obstruction caused by the kidney stone.

Some stones are small enough to pass through the urinary tract and if excreted, should be collected by the patient. It is very important that the physician determine the type of kidney stone formed before a special diet is begun, since one type might call for a diet that acidifies the urine, while another might call for an alkaline urine.

If the kidney stones are found to be of the *calcium oxalate* type, follow these steps to *acidify* the urine (with an acid ash diet):

- Limit foods high in calcium, such as milk, cheese and other milk products.
- Limit foods high in phosphate, such as milk products, eggs, organ meats, and whole-grains.
- Limit foods high in oxalic acid, such as asparagus, spinach, cranberries, plums, tea, cocoa, and coffee.
- Drink at least 10 to 12 glasses of water a day, unless the local water is hard. "Hard water" contains more calcium and magnesium. If the local water is "hard," substitute distilled water.
- Take vitamin B_6 supplements.
- Take magnesium supplements.

If you have a *uric acid* stone (the most common type caused by chemotherapy), the urine will need to be *alkalinized.*

- Emphasize alkaline-forming foods such as dairy products, fruits (especially dried fruits), vegetables (especially green beans and peas), and breads prepared with baking soda or baking powder.

- Limit your consumption of meat, eggs, fish, poultry, cereals, breads, pasta, rice, cranberry juice, prune juice, and plums.

Your physician may find it necessary to prescribe the drug allopurinol to prevent uric acid precipitates.

Foods that are neutral—that is, that are neither acid or alkaline-forming—can be used freely for any type of kidney stones. Neutral foods include butter, margarine, shortening, oils, sugar, hard candies, gum drops, honey, and pure starches.

For all types of stones, drink plenty of fluids with meals and snacks and choose foods with a high water content. Drink large amounts of water and fluids throughout the day and night—approximately 10 to 12 glasses every 24 hours (see the advice on previous page regarding hard water).

Guideline 11

A Transient Glucose Intolerance/ Diabetic Diet

Purpose

Some chemotherapy drugs (e.g., Prednisone) may induce temporary glucose intolerance. This diet guide will help control blood glucose levels and keep them as near to normal as possible.

Education regarding basic nutrition, food selection and preparation, daily food plans, and the nutrient composition of foods are the keys to treatment where transient glucose intolerance develops. You will probably be able to meet your nutrient needs by adhering to the principles of sound nutrition, without having to rely on special "dietetic" or "diabetic" foods. **However, if you were prediabetic before treatment and clinical diabetes is suspected, it is IMPERATIVE that you see a diabetes specialist and clinical dietitian for a full work-up and consultation.**

Instructions

If you develop drug-induced glucose intolerance, you will probably need to control your calorie intake as well as your nutrient composition. Also note that meal regularity is important, as is balancing meals and engaging in regular physical activity.

The primary objective of this diet is to limit the intake of simple sugars. Simple sugars are found in fruits, desserts, sweets, and even such processed foods as white bread. Learn to read food labels on packaged products and look for words that end in *ose*, such as *fructose*, *glucose*, and *lactose*. The *ose* ending indicates simple sugars.

The point of the diet is to substitute starches and fiber, also known as complex carbohydrates, for the simple sugars. Therefore, emphasize whole-wheat and whole-grain breads and cereals as opposed to more highly-refined products, and favor vegetables over fruits.

For a true diabetic diet, a system of food exchanges is used, but this plan for controlling transient glucose intolerance is much simpler. It recommends an 1,800-calorie diet composed of foods in The Basic Four groups as follows:

Food Group	***Daily Servings***
Milk (skim or low-fat)	2
Vegetables	2 or more vegetables
Fruits	2 fruits
Whole-grain breads and cereals	4 or more
Meat	2 or more

See Dietary Guideline 1, *Basic Nutrition for the Cancer Patient*, page 30, for The Basic Four food groups.

NOTE: Once more, it is important to emphasize that if a true state of clinical diabetes is suspected, it is vital that your physician refer you for further testing and detailed dietary counseling.

- Eat 3 meals daily; space meals evenly throughout the day, and do not skip meals.
- Combine carbohydrate and protein foods at every meal.
- Avoid concentrated sweet foods such as honey, brown or white sugar, syrups, jelly and jam, desserts.
- Ask your physician to discuss with you signs of transient glucose intolerance such as dizziness, trembling, and excessive thirst.

Diabetic Diet

It is especially important to control diabetes when you are receiving chemotherapy so your body can better tolerate and respond to the chemotherapy treatments. With this in mind, each person's diabetic regimen should be individualized, taking into consideration the medications chosen, meal patterns, and eating habits. Your physician and dietitian can help you individualize a diabetic plan appropriate for you.

My Plan

Breakfast: ________AM

_____ Servings bread or _____ biscuit

_____ Servings cereal (1/2 cup dry or 3/4 cup cooked)

_____ Cup milk (non-fat/low-fat)

_____ Cup juice or _____ small piece of fruit

_____ Teaspoon margarine

_____ Egg or _____ oz. cheese

Snack: ________AM

Lunch: ________PM

______ Servings bread or ______ cup starchy vegetable (potato, corn, peas), or ______ cup rice, pasta, noodles
______ Oz. lean meat/poultry/fish/cheese
______ Cup vegetables
______ Cup juice or ______ small piece of fruit
______ Teaspoon margarine or ______ tablespoon salad dressing
______ Cup of milk (non-fat/low-fat)

Snack: ________PM

Dinner: ________PM

______ Servings bread or ______ cup starchy vegetable or ______ cup rice/pasta/noodles
______ Oz. lean meat/poultry/fish/cheese
______ Cup vegetables
______ Cup juice or ______ small piece of fruit
______ Teaspoon margarine or ______ tablespoon salad dressing
______ Cup milk (non-fat/low-fat)

Snack: ________PM

The following foods may be included with meals or snacks.

Free Foods
Coffee
Tea
Diet gelatin
Consommé/bouillon
Diet "sugar-free" soft drinks
Pickles
Plain lettuce
Lemons
Sugar substitutes—Nutrasweet®, Equal®, Sweet 'n Low®
Water

Guideline 12

A Sodium-Restricted Diet

Purpose

Follow this diet if you are retaining water and salt as a result of chemotherapy. It is similar to, but not as restrictive as a diet to control high blood pressure.

This diet is NOT meant to take the place of a restricted-sodium diet that you must follow if you have hypertension, and it should not be used if your doctor puts you on a restricted-sodium diet for reasons other than limiting water retention from drug-treatment side effects. Rather, consult your physician or dietitian for a more complete diet.

This diet restricts your consumption of foods containing large amounts of natural sodium, as well as commercially processed foods to which a sodium-containing component has been added. Its objective is to limit sodium to about 3,000 to 4,000 mg daily. The aim is to restore a normal sodium balance in the body by getting rid of excess sodium and water.

NOTE: *Severe* sodium restriction is *not* necessary when the retention is related to chemotherapy, and diuretics are not usually appropriate. Diuretics should be used only under a doctor's care.

NOTE: Too-little sodium in the diet can produce muscle cramps, dizziness, reduced blood pressure, convulsions, and other problems. If you have any of these symptoms, stop this diet and consult your physician.

Instructions

In addition to the sodium that is present in foods naturally, there are many sodium-containing compounds in processed foods, such as monosodium glutamate (MSG), baking powder, sodium chloride, baking soda, disodium phosphate, sodium proprionate, and sodium benzoates. Read food labels for references to sodium and make your food choices accordingly.

NOTE that in this diet foods are not "allowed" or "prohibited," but rather "emphasized" and "deemphasized." Since the sodium restriction in this plan is not radical, you are encouraged to use your judgment based on the two complementary lists.

Foods Emphasized

Milk
Skim, low-fat, whole, evaporated (low-sodium)

Vegetables
Fresh, frozen, or canned with no salt or other sodium compounds added

Fruits
Fresh, frozen, canned, or dried

Bread
Low-sodium breads, cereals, and cereal products, breads and yeast rolls made without salt, quick breads made with sodium-free baking powder or potassium bicarbonate without salt or made from low-sodium mix, low-sodium or unsalted crackers, plain matzos, unsalted yeast waffles

Cereals
Long-cooking, unsalted, dry cereal such as puffed rice, puffed wheat, shredded wheat, barley, cornmeal, cornstarch

Meats and Meat Alternatives
Meat not on "deemphasized" list, poultry, eggs (1 per day), low-sodium cheese and peanut butter, liver (only once every 2 weeks), fresh tongue, fresh bass, bluefish, catfish, cod, eels, flounder, halibut, rockfish, salmon, sole, trout, salmon, canned low-sodium water-packed tuna, unsalted cottage cheese

Fat
Unsalted spreads, oils, cooking fats

Miscellaneous
Beverages: Cocoa made with allowed milk, instant freeze-dried, or regular coffee, coffee substitutes, lemonade, Postum®, tea, fruit juices or nectars, non-cola sodas (diet or regular), sodium-free or low-sodium mineral waters

Candy: Homemade, salt-free, special low-sodium, plain unflavored gelatin

Leavening agents: Cream of tartar, sodium-free baking powder (potassium bicarbonate), yeast, rennet dessert powder (not tablets)

Flavoring aids: Allspice, almond extract, anise, basil, bay leaf, bouillon cubes (low-sodium), caraway seed, cardamom, chives, cinnamon, cloves, cocoa (1 to 2 teaspoons), cumin, curry, dill, fennel, garlic, ginger, horseradish (prepared without salt), juniper, lemon juice or extract, mace, maple extract, marjoram, mint, mustard (dry), nutmeg, onion, fresh slices of orange or orange extract, oregano, paprika, parsley, pepper, peppermint extract, poppy seeds, poultry seasoning (without salt), rosemary, saffron, sage, salt substitute (only with doctor's approval), savory, sesame seeds, sorrel, sugar, tarragon, thyme, turmeric, vanilla extract, vinegar, walnut extract, wine (if doctor approves)

Foods Deemphasized

Milk
Commercial foods made with milk, milk solids or whey

Vegetables
Canned vegetables or juices (except low-sodium ones), artichokes, beet greens, celery, Swiss chard, dandelion greens, kale, mustard greens, sauerkraut, spinach, beets, carrots, frozen peas (if processed with salt), white turnips, frozen lima beans (if processed with salt), hominy, potato chips, vegetables prepared with salt pork

Fruits
Crystallized or glazed fruits, Maraschino cherries, dried fruits with sodium sulfite added

Bread and Cereals
Yeast bread, rolls, or Melba toast made with salt or from commercial mixes, quick breads made with baking powder, baking soda, salt, or monosodium glutamate, or made from commercial mixes, quick-cooking, instant, and enriched cereals containing sodium compounds (read the labels), dry cereals except as listed, graham crackers or any other except low-sodium crackers, salted popcorn, self-rising cornmeal or flour, pretzels, potato chips, corn chips, waffles containing salt, baking power, baking soda, or egg white solids, instant mashed potatoes

Meat and Meat Alternatives
Brains or kidneys, canned, salted, or smoked meats, bacon, bologna, chipped or corned beef, frankfurters, ham, kosher meats, luncheon meat, salt pork, sausage, smoked tongue, frozen fish fillets, canned, salted, or smoked fish, anchovies, caviar, salted or dried cod, herring, canned, salted salmon

(except dietetic low-sodium), shellfish (clams, crabs, lobster, oysters, scallops, shrimp, etc.), cheese except low-sodium dietetic, egg substitutes, frozen or powdered, peanut butter unless low-sodium dietetic, frozen dinners, frozen potatoes

Fats

Salted butter or margarine, bacon fat, olives, commercial French or other dressings (except low-sodium), commercial mayonnaise (except low-sodium), salted nuts, dips, commercial gravies, and sauces

Miscellaneous

Beverages: Cola beverages, instant cocoa mixes, prepared beverages and mixes (including fuit-flavored powdered), vegetable juices

Desserts: Commercial candies, cakes, and cookies, commercial sweetened gelatin desserts and mixes of all types, pastries, chocolates

Leavening agents: Regular baking powder, baking soda (sodium bicarbonate), rennet tablets, pudding mixes, molasses

Flavoring aids: Barbecue sauce, bouillon cubes, regular catsup, celery salt, seeds, or leaves, chili sauce, sodium cyclamate, sodium, saccharin, garlic salt, horseradish prepared with salt, meat extracts, sauces in general, tenderizers, monosodium glutamate, prepared mustard, onion salt, pickles, relish, sauerkraut, table salt, soy sauce, sugar substitutes containing sodium, Worcestershire sauce, dried soup mixes, canned soups, instant soup (Cup-A-Soup®, Top Ramen®)

Sodium Content of Some Foods

500 mg or more of sodium per serving

Scant 1/4 teaspoon of salt

3/4 teaspoon monosodium glutamate

1/2 bouillon cube

1 cup tomato juice

1/2 cup cooked rice, spaghetti, noodles, hominy, etc., seasoned with salt

1/2 cup drained sauerkraut

1 cup canned soup

1 average frankfurter (1-1/2 oz.)

1 day's supply of drinking water if the water contains 220 mg sodium per quart

Approximately 250 mg of sodium per serving

1 ounce canned tuna

2 ounces canned sardines or salmon

2/3 cup buttermilk

1/2 cup canned or regularly seasoned carrots, spinach, beets, celery, kale, or white turnips

5 salted crackers

3/4 cup tomato juice

1 day's supply of drinking water if the water contains 120 mg sodium per quart

Approximately 200 mg of sodium per serving

1 slice regular bakery bread or roll

2 thin slices of bacon, crisp and drained

3 ounces canned shrimp, cooked in salted water

1/2 cup canned or regularly seasoned vegetables

1 day's supply of drinking water if the water contains 100 mg sodium per quart

1/2 cup frozen peas or lima beans

1 ounce natural cottage cheese

1 tablespoon catsup

Approximately 100 mg of sodium per serving

1/2 cup of the following: unsalted vegetables, beets, frozen mixed peas and carrots, Swiss chard

1 ounce fresh kosher meat

1 ounce frozen fish fillets

Approximately 50 mg of sodium per serving

1/2 cup of the following: vegetables—fresh, frozen, or canned without salt, one artichoke (edible base and leaves), beets, carrots, celery, dandelion greens, kale, mustard greens, black-eyed peas, spinach, succotash, turnip greens, white turnip

1 day's supply of drinking water if the water contains 40 mg sodium per quart

Guideline 13

A Tyramine and Dopamine-Restricted Diet

Purpose

The purpose of this diet is to restrict foods that contain chemicals called monamines, if you are taking drugs that are monamine oxidase inhibitors (MAOI). Monamines, which are found in certain foods, are potentially hazardous substances that can cause constriction of blood vessels and an abnormal elevation of blood pressure.

Normally they are not a threat, since our bodies are equipped with monamine-detoxification enzymes. But a person taking a MAOI drug such as procarbazine (Matulane®), temporarily loses this natural protection. For this reason, foods high in such monamines as tyramine and dopamine **must be eliminated or restricted during the period of drug administration**.

Foods that have been fermented, or aged, or in which there has been protein breakdown to increase the flavor are not permitted on this diet. Most cheeses are particularly high in tyramine. Broad beans, pods, avocados, and bananas contain dopamine, so they are restricted, too. Although yogurt is a fermented product, it is not excluded from this diet because no adverse side effects of yogurt have been reported by people taking MAOI drugs.

Foods Prohibited

Beverages
Alcoholic beverages

Bread and Bread Substitutes
Homemade yeast breads with substantial quantities of yeast, breads or crackers containing cheese

Fats
Sour cream

Fruits
Bananas, red plums, avocados, figs, raisins

Meats
Aged game, liver, canned meats, yeast extracts, commercial meat extracts, stored beef liver, chicken livers, salami, sausage, salt-dried fish such as herring, cod, pickled herring

Cheese
Aged blue cheese, blue Boursault, brick, Brie, Camembert, Cheddar, Colby, Ementaler, Gouda, mozzarella, Parmesan, provolone, Romano, Roquefort, Stilton

Vegetables
Italian broad beans (pods contain tyramine), green bean pods, eggplant

Miscellaneous
Yeast concentrates, soup cubes, products made with concentrated yeasts, commercial gravies or meat extracts, soups containing items that must be avoided, soy sauce, any protein-containing food that has been stored improperly or that may have become spoiled

Foods Allowed

Beverages
All except alcoholic beverages; limit caffeinated coffee or tea to 1 to 2 cups per day

Bread and Bread Substitutes
All those not on "prohibited" list

Fats
All except sour cream

Fruits
Limit of 1 small orange (2-1/2" diameter), which provides 1 mg tyramine, any other fruits not on "prohibited" list

Meats
Cottage cheese and meats not on "prohibited" list, eggs

Vegetables
Tomato (limit 1/2 cup daily), all vegetables not on "prohibited" list

Miscellaneous
Anything not on "prohibited" list

Guideline 14

A Soft-Food/Pureed-Food Diet

Purpose

This diet is composed entirely of semi-liquid or soft foods. No spicy foods that might irritate the mouth are included. This diet is recommended when you are having difficulty chewing and swallowing or if you have soreness in the mouth, throat, or jaws.

Instructions

You can buy pureed food in the form of baby food or puree foods yourself using a food mill, food processor or electric blender. Experiment to find the consistency that works best for you.

If you are experiencing a loss of appetite or fill up easily, try eating frequent small meals instead of three large meals a day. Adding eggnogs (but not containing raw eggs), milkshakes, and liquid high-protein diet supplements as between-meal snacks will increase your protein and calorie intake. (See *Special Shakes,* page 95, and *Cooking with Commercial Supplements,* page 167 of the Recipe chapter.)

If you have a problem with **lactose intolerance, refer to General Dietary Guideline 6, page 61, which deals with that problem**, because this diet relies heavily on milk-based foods to provide large amounts of high-quality protein.

NOTE that the following lists are headed "Foods to Emphasize" and "Deemphasized Foods." There are no restrictions here. You are encouraged to eat whatever is comfortable and non-irritating for you. However, some foods on the "Deemphasized Foods" list are difficult to digest.

Foods to Emphasize

Ripe avocados, bananas, and papayas

Cooked cereals and dry cereals with cream, milk, or fortified milk

Cottage cheese, cream cheese, mild processed cheeses

Custard, pudding, gelatin

Eggnogs and boiled, poached, or scrambled eggs
Tender baked, broiled, roasted, poached or stewed fish
Meat and poultry served in broth or cream sauce
Canned, pureed, or stewed fruit
Fruit and vegetable juices and nectars
Mashed, cooked vegetables (yam, potato, carrots)
High-protein diet supplement
Ice cream, sherbet, frozen yogurt
Milk drinks (especially fortified milk), flavored yogurt, strained cream soups, and broths

Deemphasized Foods

Bread containing hard crusts, nuts, seeds, or whole-grains
Coconut, nuts, raisins, dates
Fried foods
Dried fruit
Excessive amounts of herbs and spices
Horseradish, olives, pickles, relish
Rich pastries
Popcorn, potato chips, and pretzels
Whole fish, meat, poultry
Smoked, spiced, or processed meats, such as bacon, luncheon meats, or sausage
Pepper, chili powder
Raw fruit that is not pureed, except ripe avocados, bananas, and papayas
Raw vegetables
Jams and preserves containing tough skins and seeds
Tart juices

Chapter 3

Useful Recipes and Tables

Janine Bernat, R.D.
Carol Stitt, R.D.
Ernest H. Rosenbaum, M.D.
Janet L. Ramstack, Dr.P.H.
Isadora Rosenbaum

The following collection of recipes has been chosen with the needs and problems of the cancer patient in mind, and incorporates recommendations we have made in this book. These recipes are suggestions and examples, and not an exclusive listing of the foods you should eat. Rather, we hope they will give you suggestions for appetizing dishes that are high in protein and calories and are also easy to eat and digest when you are having dietary problems.

We have included both traditional American recipes and recipes of ethnic origin. Other recipes reflect the popularity of "natural" and "health" foods. We have also included a special section on cooking with convenience foods to give you ideas for shortcuts to nutritious meals when you are not feeling well enough to do much cooking.

A section on cooking with high-protein and high-calorie commercial supplements provides information for those for whom they are prescribed. Recipes helpful to those having difficulty in swallowing are also included.

Some of these recipes may not be advisable for some; each of you has a different problem and different tolerances. So, before using any recipe, check with your physician or other nutrition advisor and consult Chapter 1, *How to Deal with Specific Problems,* and Chapter 2, *General Dietary Guidelines.* They refer you to foods best for your situation. However, you will want to experiment, within the guidelines you are given, because that is how you will best get to know your individual preferences and tolerances.

Remember that variety stimulates the appetite. We hope you will try some of these recipes and experiment with changes to make them fit your preferences. Even if you do not use the recipes themselves, reading through them may give you many ideas on preparing your own recipes with added nutritional value.

Breakfasts

Breakfast can be your best meal of the day. Most breakfast foods are easy to eat because they are soft, moist, bland, and light. They make good meals at any time of the day. Remember them when you are not feeling up to heavier food. The recipes beginning on page 101 offer some appetizing variations on common breakfast foods and show you ways to cook a nutritious high-protein, high-calorie breakfast.

Beverages

The beverage recipes are high in protein and calories and make nutritious additions to your diet as between-meal snacks. You will also find them soothing when you have a sore or dry mouth.

To increase the protein and calorie content of recipes calling for milk, 2 tablespoons of non-fat dry milk solids (50 calories, 5 grams protein) or 2 tablespoons of a protein powder (70 calories, 15 grams protein) may be added. If you must restrict the fat content of your diet, you can use skim milk or fortified skim milk instead of whole milk. If you have milk (lactose) intolerance, you can use a milk substitute such as Mocha Mix®, Poly Rich®, or Dairy Rich®, or IMO® in place of sour cream, or you can make reduced-lactose milk by adding Lactaid®.

Condiments

If you are advised to avoid salt in your diet, you can find salt substitutes (made with potassium instead of sodium) such as Nu Salt®, Co-Salt® or Adolf's Salt Substitute® in the supermarket. It is a good idea to consult your doctor before using a salt substitute.

In place of pepper and other irritating seasonings you can use the mild herbs and spices listed below:

Cheese dishes: bay leaves, oregano, parsley, paprika

Egg dishes: oregano, parsley, paprika, rosemary, sweet basil, thyme

Fish: bay leaves, lemon juice, oregano, parsley, paprika, rosemary, sweet basil, thyme

Meat: allspice, bay leaves, cinnamon, lemon juice, oregano, parsley, paprika, rosemary, sweet basil, thyme

Poultry: bay leaves, cinnamon, lemon juice, oregano, parsley, paprika, rosemary, sweet basil, thyme

Salads: lemon juice, oregano, parsley, rosemary, sweet basil, thyme

Sauces: bay leaves, lemon juice, oregano, parsley, paprika, rosemary, sweet basil, thyme

Soups: bay leaves, lemon juice, oregano, parsley, paprika, rosemary, sweet basil, thyme

Vegetables: bay leaves, lemon juice, oregano, parsley, paprika, rosemary, sweet basil, thyme

Desserts

Desserts are an especially appealing part of a meal and are therefore a good way to get needed calories and protein. Have a dessert with lunch and dinner and also for a between-meal or bedtime snack. Custards and puddings are especially high in protein since they use eggs and milk. They are also soft and moist and easy to eat. The dessert recipes include many old favorites, along with ideas for adding variety and increasing their nutritional value.

Dairy and Egg Dishes

Milk, cheese, and eggs are high in protein and calories. The dairy and egg dishes make satisfying light meals and are soft and moist and easy to eat. Try them as a change from meat, poultry, and fish.

Main Dishes

Meat, poultry, and fish are some of your chief sources of protein, and the recipes featuring these foods show you how to prepare them so they are soft, moist, and high in calories. Some of the recipes are bland; others are spicier for a variation in taste. If you do not feel like eating meat, poultry, or fish, see *Dairy and Egg Dishes* (page 111), for meatless main dish suggestions.

Salads

You will find the high-protein salad recipes cool and refreshing, especially if you need soft, moist foods or if you are finding the aroma of cooked foods difficult to tolerate.

Snacks

The snack suggestions are high in protein and calories. Most are of a soft consistency that you will find easy to swallow and digest.

Soups

Often when you don't feel like eating solid food, but want to eat something substantial, you will find that soup is a good answer.

Sauces

Sauces add calories and are a good way to moisten meat, vegetables, noodles, and rice to make swallowing easier.

Cooking With Commercial Supplements

These recipes use commercial high-protein and high-calorie supplements for added nutritional value. Ensure®* adds both protein and calories. It is lactose-free and therefore can be used even if you have milk (lactose) intolerance. Polycose®* is a tasteless and odorless source of calories; it can be added to foods and beverages without significantly changing their natural flavors or volume. Vivonex T.E.N.®* is used to fortify clear liquid diets. See Table 2 High-Protein Supplements, page 187 for a more complete description of these products. Ask the dietitian member of your healthcare team if you have questions about supplements or have difficulty locating them in stores.

Special Shakes

Suggestions for adding more protein to your shakes: Make "double-strength" milk. Add 1 cup of non-fat dry milk to 1 quart of milk. Use this "double-strength" milk in your soups, custards, puddings, and milkshakes.

Mr. Trewin's Old-Fashioned Chocolate Milkshake

1/2 cup whole milk
1/2 cup chocolate ice cream
1 tablespoon chocolate syrup
1 tablespoon malted milk powder
*515 calories**, 11 grams protein*

*Ensure® and Polycose® recipes from "Nutrition: A Helpful Ally in Cancer Therapy," courtesy of Ross Laboratories. Vivonex T.E.N.® recipes courtesy of Eaton Laboratories.

**Adopting popular usage, "calories" will be used for kilocalories of energy.

Tofu Shake

1/4 lb. tofu
1/2 banana
1/2 cup orange juice
2 teaspoons honey to taste
235 calories, 11 grams protein

Cafe-Chocomalt

1 teaspoon instant coffee dissolved in 1 oz. hot water
1/2 cup chocolate ice cream
1 tablespoon malted milk powder
1/2 cup whole milk
540 calories, 15 grams protein

Peanuts and Bananas

1 tablespoon peanut butter
1/2 banana
1/2 cup vanilla ice cream
1/2 cup milk
354 calories, 12 grams protein

Melon Shake

1/2 cup chopped cantaloupe, honeydew, or watermelon
1/2 cup half-and-half
1/2 cup vanilla ice cream
1 tablespoon honey (if desired)
402 calories, 8 grams protein

Beverages

These beverage recipes are high in protein and calories and make nutritious additions to your diet as between-meal snacks. You will also find them soothing when you have a sore or dry mouth.

Fortified Milk

Use this extra-high-protein milk for drinking and in all recipes calling for milk.

1 cup non-fat dry milk powder

1 quart whole milk

Combine ingredients and mix until smooth.

880 calories, 56 grams protein per quart; 220 calories, 14 grams protein per cup

Fortified Skim Milk

If you must restrict the fat content of your diet, you can make fortified milk with skim milk.

1 cup non-fat dry milk powder

1 quart skim milk

Combine ingredients and mix until smooth.

596 calories, 56 grams protein per quart; 149 calories, 14 grams protein per cup

Easy Hot Chocolate Mix

1 1-lb. box Nestle's Quik®

1 9-oz. box instant milk (or Dairy Rich® or Mocha Mix®)

1 3-oz. jar non-dairy creamer

1/2 cup powdered sugar

Mix ingredients well and store in a dry place in air-tight container. For single serving, fill serving cup 1/2 full of dry mixture and add boiling water to fill.

220 calories, 17 grams protein

Berry Milk

1/2 cup strawberries, fresh or thawed frozen
1/4 cup blackberry nectar
1 tablespoon sugar
1 cup milk

Combine all ingredients in a blender and blend until smooth. Serves 1.

200 calories, 9 grams protein

Strawberry-Banana Milk

1/2 cup strawberries, fresh or thawed frozen
1/2 ripe banana, sliced
1 teaspoon sugar
1 cup milk

Combine ingredients in a blender and blend until smooth. Serves 1.

220 calories, 9 grams protein

Pineapple Buttermilk

1/4 ripe banana, sliced
1/2 cup canned crushed pineapple
1 cup buttermilk

Combine all ingredients in a blender and blend until smooth. Serves 1.

235 calories, 10 grams protein

Milkshake

3/4 cup milk
1 cup vanilla ice cream
1 to 2 tablespoons chocolate or strawberry syrup or 1/2 ripe banana, sliced

Combine all ingredients in a blender and blend to desired thickness. Serves 1.

Variation: Omit flavoring and substitute your favorite ice cream for the vanilla ice cream.

405 calories, 13 grams protein

Almond-Peach Milkshake

1 cup milk
1 cup sliced peaches
1/4 teaspoon salt
1 to 3 drops almond extract
1 cup vanilla ice cream

Combine all ingredients in a blender and blend to desired thickness. Serves 1.

Variation: Marinate peaches in 1 tablespoon brandy before adding to other ingredients.

650 calories, 15 grams protein

Sherbet Shake

This is a lighter shake than the milkshake and is a good snack for a fat-restricted diet.

3/4 cup non-fat milk
1 cup sherbet, any flavor

Combine ingredients in a blender and blend to desired thickness. Serves 1.

325 calories, 8 grams protein

Orange Juice Shake

1 cup orange juice
1/2 cup vanilla ice cream

Combine ingredients in a blender and blend to desired thickness. Serves 1.

260 calories, 5 grams protein

Orange Freeze

3/4 cup orange juice
1 tablespoon lemon juice
1 cup orange sherbet

Combine ingredients in a blender and blend to desired thickness. Serves 1.

340 calories, 3 grams protein

Orange Buttermilk Shake

1 cup buttermilk

1/2 cup orange juice

2 tablespoons brown sugar

1 cup vanilla ice cream

Combine ingredients in a blender and blend to desired thickness. Serves 1.

530 calories, 15 grams protein

Ice Cream Soda Float

3/4 cup root beer, cola, or fruit-flavored soda

1/2 cup vanilla ice cream

Place a large scoop of vanilla ice cream in a tall glass and add soda until glass is almost full. Serve with a straw. Serves 1.

230 calories, 3 grams protein

Orange Juice Float

3/4 cup orange juice

1/2 cup orange sherbet

Pour orange juice into a tall glass and top with a scoop of orange sherbet. Serve with a straw. Serves 1.

215 calories, 2 grams protein

Peach Yogurt Shake

1 cup sliced peaches

1 cup plain yogurt

1 cup skim milk

2 tablespoons honey

Combine ingredients in a blender and blend until smooth. Serves 1.

Variations: Instead of peaches, use 1 cup of sliced bananas, fruit cocktail, strawberries, raspberries, or blackberries. If you use raspberries or blackberries, strain after blending to remove seeds.

535 calories, 21 grams protein

Apricot Yogurt Smoothie

1 cup chilled apricot nectar

1 cup plain yogurt

Combine ingredients in a blender and blend until smooth. Serves 1.

Variations: Instead of apricot nectar, use peach or pear nectar or your favorite fruit juice. Add honey to taste.

265 calories, 12 grams protein

Hi-Protein Smoothies

These smoothies are like milkshakes, thin or thick, depending on the temperature.

Blend until smooth:

1 cup cottage cheese

1 cup yogurt

Add one of the following:

1 banana + some strawberries + 1 teaspoon vanilla + honey to taste

1 peach + some strawberries + 1 teaspoon vanilla + honey to taste

1 banana + 2 tablespoons peanut butter + 1 teaspoon vanilla + honey to taste

Serves 1.

Variations: Substitute your favorite fruit or jam. Substitute chocolate or other flavoring for vanilla. If you want it thinner, add milk or more yogurt. If you want it colder, blend with a cracked ice cube. Serves 1.

475 calories, 43 grams protein

Alcoholic Beverages

A decision to drink alcoholic beverages is obviously a personal matter; in addition, the alcoholic ingredients and some of the listed spices can be irritating to some. They are included here for those who can tolerate them, wish to try them, and for whom they have been professionally recommended.

Cold Milk Punch

2 tablespoons brandy
1 cup cold milk
1-1/2 tablespoons powdered sugar
1/8 teaspoon vanilla
Ground nutmeg*

Combine brandy, milk, sugar, and vanilla in blender and blend until smooth. Pour into a tall glass and sprinkle with ground nutmeg. Serves 1.

290 calories, 8 grams protein

Hot Eggnog

1 cup hot milk
1 egg
3 teaspoons sugar
2 tablespoons brandy or rum
Ground nutmeg*

Combine milk, egg, sugar, and brandy in a blender and blend until smooth. Pour into a large mug and sprinkle with ground nutmeg. Serves 1.

350 calories, 15 grams protein

*May be irritating.

Hot Milk Toddy

1 cup hot milk

2 tablespoons rum

1-1/2 teaspoons sugar

1-inch piece of cinnamon stick

Ground nutmeg*

Place sugar, cinnamon stick, and rum in a large mug and stir to dissolve sugar. Pour into the hot milk and sprinkle with nutmeg. Serves 1.

250 calories, 8 grams protein

Tom-and-Jerry

1 egg

1 tablespoon sugar

1 tablespoon Jamaican rum

2 tablespoons bourbon

3/4 cup hot milk

Dash of ground cinnamon*

Dash of ground cloves*

Put all ingredients except milk into a blender and whip at high speed until frothy and light-yellow. Remove cover and add hot milk gradually while blender is going. Serves 1.

340 calories, 13 grams protein

Breakfasts

Cooked Cereal

When making cooked cereal, add extra protein and calories by using *fortified milk*** or half-and-half instead of water. Top cereal with a pat of butter and serve with fortified milk or half-and-half.

1 cup fortified milk adds 220 calories, 14 grams protein

1 cup half-and-half adds 324 calories, 8 grams protein

1 tablespoon butter adds 100 calories

*May be irritating.

**Recipe on page 95.

Nutty Fruity Cereal

1/2 cup 100% bran cereal

1/4 cup nut pieces

1/8 cup dried fruits (raisins, apricots, etc.)

Mix ingredients together and add milk. (It even tastes good adding hot water—similar to Wheatena or Postum®.) Eat a 1/2-portion at a time—or the whole thing. 1 or 2 bowls of cereal.

233 calories, 6.94 grams protein

Mammaliga

This traditional Rumanian cornmeal dish is very high in protein and calories and is good for breakfast, lunch, or dinner.

2 cups water

1/2 teaspoon salt

1/2 cup cornmeal

3 tablespoons butter

1-1/2 cups cottage cheese

Add salt to water and bring to a boil. Slowly sprinkle in cornmeal so water never stops boiling and stir until cornmeal is completely moistened. Reduce heat and simmer, stirring only enough to keep cereal from sticking; too much stirring makes it gummy. When liquid is absorbed and cornmeal is tender, stir in butter and cottage cheese. Eat hot, right away. Serves 2.

470 calories, 28 grams protein per serving

Variations: Add extra protein and calories by using fortified milk or half-and-half instead of water.

690 calories, 42 grams protein per serving with fortified milk

794 calories, 36 grams protein per serving with half-and-half

Cottage Cheese Pancakes

You will find that French toast, waffles, and pancakes are easy to chew and swallow, especially with butter and syrup on them. Cottage cheese gives these pancakes added protein.

3 eggs

1/2 cup cottage cheese

1/4 cup flour

2 to 3 tablespoons milk

Separate eggs. Beat yolks and combine with other ingredients. Beat egg whites and fold into mixture. Spoon onto hot griddle. Cook on both sides until golden brown. Serves 4.

80 calories, 7 grams protein per serving

Finnish Oven Pancake

2 eggs

1 tablespoon sugar

1/2 teaspoon salt

1/3 cup flour

2 tablespoons butter

1-1/3 cups milk

Heat butter and milk until butter is melted. Beat eggs and sugar until fluffy. Stir in salt and flour. Add milk and butter gradually. Pour into 8-inch square baking dish that has been heated in oven with at least 1 tablespoon butter. Bake 30 minutes at 400 degrees. Serves 2.

394 calories, 15 grams protein per serving

Tofu Pancakes

1/2 cup tofu (soybean curd)

1 egg

Pinch of salt

Drain tofu and mash smooth with a fork. Add egg and salt and beat well. Drop by tablespoonfuls on buttered griddle, hot enough so a drop of cold water bounces around on it. When pancake is bubbly, turn and cook until golden. Serve with butter and apricot jam or yogurt and applesauce. Serves 1.

156 calories, 14 grams protein

Apple Pancakes

2 eggs
1 apple, cored and cut into small pieces
2 tablespoons flour
1/2 cup 100% bran cereal
1/4 teaspoon cinnamon* or nutmeg,* or both
1/4 teaspoon vanilla

Mix ingredients in blender. Grease a Teflon skillet with butter. Pour batter in preheated skillet. Cook, and don't rush to turn. 4 large or 6 small pancakes.

421 calories, 17.6 grams protein per serving

Vita Pancakes

1 cup unbleached flour
2 teaspoons baking powder
1 teaspoon sugar
1 cup 100% bran cereal
2 tablespoons wheat germ
1/4 cup Egg Beaters® or Second Nature®
1 cup apple juice or orange juice
2 tablespoons safflower oil
Optional: 1 stiffly-beaten egg white

Thoroughly stir together flour, baking powder and sugar. Stir in cereal and wheat germ. Mix Egg Beaters®, oil and juice. Stir into flour mixture until moistened. (Fold in stiffly-beaten egg white.) Bake on Pam®-greased hot griddle. When bubbly, turn once. Makes 12 medium to large pancakes.

125 calories, 3 grams protein per pancake

*May be irritating.

Buttermilk French Toast

2 eggs
1 cup buttermilk
1/8 teaspoon salt
1 teaspoon sugar
1/2 cup 100% bran cereal
4 slices bread

In a shallow pan, beat 2 eggs slightly. Add buttermilk, salt, and sugar. Combine so that there are no streaks of egg showing. Add four slices white bread, cut in halves. Allow to soak 10 minutes, turning once or twice so that the bread becomes soaked with the mixture. Lift carefully with spatula and coat both sides with cereal. Butter generously a shallow pan. Place toast in pan and pour melted butter over the top of the toast. Set in a hot oven (450 degrees). Bake about 15 minutes or until crisp and brown. Serve hot with maple syrup. Serves 2.

350 calories, 23.8 grams protein per serving

French Toast

1 egg
1/4 teaspoon salt
2 tablespoons half-and-half
1-1/2 teaspoons sugar
2 slices thick white bread
2 tablespoons butter

Beat together with egg, salt, cream, and sugar. Dip bread in mixture and fry in melted butter until browned on both sides. Serve with butter and syrup. Serves 1.

441 calories, 11 grams protein

Popovers

Popovers are easy to make and delicious served hot from the oven, filled with butter and jam.

3 eggs
1 cup milk
1 cup flour
Pinch of salt

Mix ingredients and pour into greased, deep muffin or popover tins. Fill cups half-full and bake 25 to 30 minutes at 450 degrees.

100 calories, 3 grams protein per popover

Bran Muffins

These hearty bran muffins will add bulk and fiber to your diet.

2 cups whole wheat flour
1-1/2 cup bran*
2 tablespoons sugar
1/4 teaspoon salt
1-1/4 teaspoons baking soda
2 cups buttermilk
1 egg, beaten
1/2 cup molasses
1/4 cup melted margarine
Optional: 1 cup raisins

Mix together until blended, the flour, bran, sugar, salt, and baking soda. Beat together the buttermilk, egg, molasses, and melted margarine and add to dry ingredients, stirring only until just mixed. Add raisins. Fill well-greased muffin cups 2/3 full and bake 25 minutes at 350 degrees. Makes 20 2-inch muffins.

100 calories, 3 grams protein per muffin

*May be irritating.

Sugar-Free/Diabetic Fiber Nut Muffins

3/4 cup whole wheat flour
1/2 cup white flour
1/4 teaspoon salt
1/2 teaspoon low-cal sweetener (Sweet 'n Lo®)
1 cup milk
1 egg
3 tablespoons vegetable oil
1 cup 100% bran cereal
1 cup chopped raw apples
1/2 cup raisins
1/2 cup chopped walnuts
1/4 teaspoon cinnamon*
1 tablespoon baking soda

Preheat oven to 400 degrees. Stir flour, baking powder, cinnamon, and salt together. Set aside. In a large mixing bowl, combine bran cereal, milk, and sweetener. Add egg and oil. Beat well. Add flour mixture using minimal stirring. Add apple, raisins and walnuts. Pour batter into greased muffin pans, or use paper liners. Bake at 400 degrees for 25 minutes or until lightly browned. Makes 15 muffins.

100 calories, 4 grams protein per muffin

Lazy Man Muffins

1 (generous) cup 100% bran cereal
1 cup milk (use Acidophilus milk for those with lactose intolerance)
2 eggs
1-1/4 cup biscuit mix (such as Jiffy® or Bisquick®)

Preheat oven to 400 degrees. Mix bran cereal, milk, and eggs. Let set 1 to 2 minutes while you grease the muffin pan. Add biscuit mix. Stir only until combined. Spoon evenly into 12 muffin cups. Bake 20 to 25 minutes at 400 degrees or until lightly browned. Makes 12 muffins.

100 calories, 4 grams protein per muffin

*May be irritating.

Refrigerator Bran Muffins

2-1/2 cups 100% bran cereal

1 cup boiling water

2 eggs, slightly beaten

2 cups buttermilk

1/2 cup salad oil

2 cups raisins, currants, chopped pitted dates or chopped pitted prunes; or use 1 cup of favorite fruit and 1 cup nuts

2-1/2 teaspoons baking soda

1/2 teaspoon salt

1 cup sugar

2-1/2 cups regular all-purpose flour, unsifted

In a large bowl mix bran cereal with boiling water, stirring to moisten evenly. Set aside until cool. Add eggs, buttermilk, oil, and fruit (and nuts if desired), and blend well. Stir together the baking soda, salt, sugar, and flour, then stir into bran mixture. Spoon batter into buttered 2-1/2-inch diameter muffin cups, filling 2/3 to 3/4 full. Bake in a 425 degree oven for about 20 minutes or until top springs back when lightly touched. Serve hot. Makes about 3 dozen muffins.

NOTE: You can bake muffins now or refrigerate the batter in a tightly-covered container for as long as two weeks, baking muffins at your convenience. Stir batter to evenly distribute fruit before using.

135 calories, 3 grams protein per muffin

Apricot Nut Bread

1 package Pillsbury Nut Bread Mix

1/2 cup chopped dried apricots

1/2 cup crushed 100% bran cereal

Increase water by 2 tablespoons and prepare according to directions on box. Bake as directed. (May take a little longer to bake than directed.) 12 slices

Tastes better the next day!

100 calories, 2 grams protein per slice

High-Protein/High-Vitamin Crunchy Granola

5 cups old-fashioned oatmeal (not instant)
1 cup cut almonds*
1 cup unrefined sesame seeds*
1 cup hulled sunflower seeds*
1 cup unsweetened shredded coconut*
1 cup soy flour
1 cup powdered non-fat milk
1 cup wheat germ
1 cup honey
1 cup safflower, cottonseed, or soy oil

Combine dry ingredients in a large bowl. Mix oil and honey in a separate bowl and combine with dry ingredients. Spread on cookie sheets and bake at 250 degrees, stirring occasionally, until lightly browned. Mixture burns very easily, so watch it. Makes 15 cups.

270 calories, 8 grams protein per 1/2 cup

Matzo Brie

2 eggs
2 matzos
1 tablespoon butter or margarine
1/2 teaspoon salt
2 teaspoons grated onion or instant minced onions

Beat eggs, salt, and onion together. Hold matzos under running water to soften, then drain and crumble into eggs. Mix well. Melt butter in skillet and pour into matzo mixture. Scramble with fork while frying until lightly browned but not dry. Serves 1.

490 calories, 18 grams protein

*May be irritating.

Melon Bowl

1/2 cantaloupe

1 cup plain or fruit yogurt

Scoop out cantaloupe seeds from center and fill with your favorite flavor of yogurt. Serves 1.

350 calories, 11 grams protein

Heavenly Ham 'n Eggs 'n Cheese

2 eggs

1/4 cup sour cream

2 oz. ham, chopped

1/2 cup cheese, grated

1 tablespoon butter or margarine

Beat eggs with sour cream. Heat butter in frying pan, add ham, and saute. Pour in eggs beaten with sour cream. When eggs are half set, top with grated cheese. Cover and cook a few more minutes until eggs are set and cheese is melted. Slide out of pan, folding over in half onto warm plate. Serves 1.

615 calories, 38 grams protein

Eggs Benedict

1 English muffin half

1 slice cooked ham

1 poached egg

1/2 cup Hollandaise sauce

Toast English muffin, cover with ham, and top with poached egg. Serve hot, covered with Hollandaise sauce (see *Sauces* section, page 144, or use canned sauce). Serves 1.

462 calories, 28 grams protein

Breakfast Suggestions

Foods you do not usually think of for breakfast can give variety and awaken your appetite:

Eggnogs and milk drinks (see *Beverages* section, page 95)
English muffin with melted cheese or cream cheese
Sandwiches
Soups
Steak

Dairy and Egg Dishes

Avocado and Cheese Omelette

2 eggs
1/4 cup sour cream
1 tablespoon melted butter or margarine
1/2 cup grated cheese
1/2 avocado, sliced

Beat eggs with sour cream. Pour into hot frying pan in which butter has been melted. When eggs are half set, sprinkle with cheese and layer avocado slices on top. Cover and cook for a few more minutes until eggs are set and cheese is melted. Slide out of pan, folding over in half onto warm plate. Serves 1.

790 calories, 31 grams protein

Scrambled Egg Casserole

6 eggs
1 tablespoon butter
1/2 can cream of mushroom soup
1/3 cup half-and-half
4 slices bacon, fried and crumbled
13-oz. jar of mushrooms
2 oz. sharp cheddar cheese, grated

Beat eggs and half-and-half, then scramble in melted butter. Place in 1-quart casserole dish. Pour on soup, mushrooms and cheese; top with bacon. Bake at 250 degrees for 45 minutes. Serves 2 to 3.

395 calories, 18 grams protein per serving

Spinach Pudding

1 10-oz. package frozen spinach, defrosted and drained

2 cups drained cottage cheese

2 eggs

1 teaspoon salt

1 tablespoon Parmesan cheese

Mix all ingredients together until well blended. Pour into buttered 1-1/2-quart casserole and bake 30 minutes at 350 degrees. Serve sprinkled with Parmesan cheese. Serves 6.

171 calories, 19 grams protein per serving

Quiche Lorraine

1 frozen 9-inch pie shell

3/4 cup grated Swiss cheese

3 eggs

1 cup heavy cream

Salt and pepper to taste

Sprinkle bottom of pastry shell with cheese. Beat eggs until well blended. Beat in cream and add salt and pepper. Pour mixture over the cheese. Bake at 375 degrees 30 to 40 minutes or until set. Serves 6.

Variations: Add chopped ham, chopped, cooked bacon, sliced fried mushrooms (cooled), or chopped olives. Omit cheese and add 3/4 cup of any cooked vegetable or meat.

195 calories, 7 grams protein per serving

Fried Cheese, Italian Style

8 oz. mozzarella cheese

1/3 cup whole wheat flour

1 egg, lightly beaten

Oil

Cut cheese into eight cubes. Dredge with flour, dip in beaten egg, and coat with flour again. Make sure cheese is well-coated with egg and flour. Heat oil to cover surface of skillet generously. When hot, quickly brown cheese on all sides, about 3 minutes per side, remove from heat, and serve.

157 calories, 7 grams protein per cube

Cheese Strata

12 slices bread
6 slices American cheese
4 eggs
2-1/2 cups milk
1/2 teaspoon salt
Pepper to taste

After trimming crusts from bread, arrange 6 slices of bread in the bottom of a baking dish. Cover with cheese, then cover with remaining slices of bread. Beat eggs and add milk and seasonings, mixing well. Pour over bread and cheese and let stand 1 hour. Bake at 325 degrees until lightly browned and puffed. Approximately 45 minutes. Serves 4.

556 calories, 27 grams protein per serving

Cheese Fondue

1 cup dry white wine
1 clove garlic*, minced
2 tablespoons flour
1 can condensed cheddar cheese soup
4 slices natural Swiss cheese, cut into pieces
Bite-size bread cubes (French bread is good)

Simmer wine and garlic in a fondue pot or a saucepan. Combine flour and cheese and gradually blend into wine. Heat until cheese melts, stirring occasionally. Blend in soup and heat until smooth. Spear bread with a fork and dip into fondue. Serves 4.

150 calories, 8 grams protein per serving

*May be irritating.

Welsh Rarebit

1 tablespoon butter
1-1/2 cups diced aged cheddar cheese
1/3 teaspoon salt
1/4 teaspoon dry mustard*
1 teaspoon Worcestershire sauce
1/2 to 3/4 cup cream
1 egg yolk

In the top of a double-boiler, melt butter, then stir in cheese. When cheese is melted, add salt, mustard, and Worcestershire sauce. Stir in cream gradually. When mixture is hot, remove from heat and stir in egg yolk. Serve hot over hot toasted crackers or bread. Serves 4.

340 calories, 13 grams protein per serving of sauce

Noodle Ring

8 oz. broad noodles
1/2 teaspoon salt
1 tablespoon margarine or oil
1 medium onion cut into small pieces
3 celery stalks cut into small pieces
2 eggs, well beaten
1 cup grated or diced cheddar cheese

Cook noodles in boiling water to which salt and oil have been added. Drain and rinse in cold water. Saute onion and celery for 8 to 10 minutes. Add to noodles. Add eggs and cheese to noodle mixture and put into well-greased casserole. Bake 15 to 20 minutes at 375 degrees. Serves 8.

Variations: Add mushrooms, diced chicken, turkey, beef, chopped ham, or tomato sauce. The addition of meat or poultry will increase the protein content of the recipe.

110 calories, 8 grams protein per serving

*May be irritating.

Main Dishes

Swiss Steak

1 lb. round steak, 1-1/2" thick

1 cup stewed tomatoes

Flour, salt, pepper and chopped garlic*

Season meat with salt, pepper and garlic and sprinkle with flour. Pound flour into meat with a meat mallet or the edge of a heavy plate to tenderize. Heat cooking oil in heavy skillet and brown meat well on both sides. Add stewed tomatoes to cover meat, cover pan, and cook very slowly on top of stove or in 325 degree oven until meat is very tender (at least 2 hours). Add a little water from time-to-time if necessary to keep meat covered. Serves 3.

Variations: Add chopped sliced onions, green peppers or sliced mushrooms to meat with stewed tomatoes.

322 calories, 31 grams protein per serving

Ground Beef Stroganoff

Serve this softer version of beef stroganoff over noodles, rice, mashed potatoes, or toast.

1/4 cup butter

1/2 cup onions, minced

1 lb. ground beef

1 clove garlic*, chopped

2 tablespoons flour

2 teaspoons salt

1/4 teaspoon pepper

1/2 lb. mushrooms, sliced

1 can condensed cream of mushroom soup

1 cup sour cream

Melt butter in a skillet and cook minced onions until soft. Add ground beef and chopped garlic and stir until slightly browned. Stir in flour, salt, pepper, and mushrooms and cook 5 minutes. Add soup and simmer 10 minutes. Stir in 1 cup sour cream and heat. Serves 4.

622 calories, 25 grams protein per serving

*May be irritating.

Chinese Beef Tomato

If you are experiencing "taste blindness" you may find you want spicier foods, such as this Chinese Beef Tomato. Serve it over boiled rice or soft noodles for extra calories.

1 lb. beef, top round or flank
1 piece ginger*, crushed
1 clove garlic*, crushed
1 medium onion
1 green pepper
2 stalks celery
2 tomatoes, cut in wedges
2 stalks green onion

Seasonings
3 tablespoons soy sauce
1/2 teaspoon sugar
1 tablespoon sherry
1 tablespoon cornstarch

Gravy
1/2 teaspoon salt
1 cup water or broth
1/4 teaspoon MSG
1 teaspoon cornstarch

Slice beef thin and soak in seasonings for 15 minutes. Cut all vegetables into 1-inch lengths. Heat 1 tablespoon oil in pan and brown ginger and garlic lightly. Add beef, stirring quickly, and cook to medium rareness. Remove from pan. Add 1 tablespoon oil in pan and fry onions, green pepper, and celery for 10 minutes. Add beef and tomatoes and stir for another 1 minute. Combine gravy ingredients, add to beef, and bring to boil. Add green onion. Serves 4.

200 calories, 25 grams protein per serving

*May be irritating.

Mongolian Beef

This is a spicy recipe you may especially enjoy if you are experiencing "taste blindness."

1 lb. flank, sirloin, T-bone or top round steak, 1-inch thick, scored and pounded

1/2 cup green onions, sliced

2 garlic cloves*, crushed

1/4 cup parsley, chopped

1 cup water

1/2 cup soy sauce

1 tablespoon sugar

Marinate steak in remaining ingredients for 30 minutes and broil. Serves 4.

163 calories, 24 grams protein per serving

Yummy Meatloaf

1 can cream of mushroom soup

1/2 cup 100% bran cereal, crushed with rolling pin

1/3 cup chopped onion

1 egg, beaten

1 teaspoon salt

2 lbs. ground beef

1/3 cup water

Mix ingredients in a bowl. Shape into loaf in 8" × 4" loaf pan. Bake at 375 degrees for 1 hour/15 minutes. Makes six servings.

400 calories, 45 grams protein per serving

*May be irritating.

Creamed Chicken

This is also a quick-and-easy way to prepare cut-up meat or seafood.

3/4 cup canned white sauce
1/2 lb. finely chopped cooked chicken
1/2 cup milk
Salt and pepper to taste

In a saucepan, mix together white sauce and milk and heat. Stir in chicken, salt, and pepper and heat to desired temperature. Serve over rice, noodles, or toast. Serves 4.

110 calories, 6 grams protein per serving

Easy Honey-Glazed Chicken

Honey and butter add extra calories and flavor to this easy recipe.

1 store-bought cooked, barbecued chicken, quartered
1/4 cup honey
1/2 cup butter

Put chicken in baking pan, top with pats of butter and drizzle honey over all. Bake at 350 degrees until chicken is glazed, about 15 minutes. Serves 4.

581 calories, 23 grams protein per serving

Cantonese Chicken

Serve this spicy recipe with boiled rice for extra calories.

3 pounds chicken thighs
1/4 cup lemon juice
1/4 cup honey
1/4 cup soy sauce
1/2 cup catsup
1/4 teaspoon ginger*
1/4 teaspoon salt

Place chicken thighs in baking pan. Combine remaining ingredients and pour over chicken. Bake at 350 degrees until brown. If desired, chicken may be pre-salted. Serves 6.

284 calories, 31 grams protein per serving

*May be irritating.

Chicken Tofu

Tofu (soybean curd) is a soft, bland protein food that assumes the flavor of the foods it is cooked with.

4 pieces chicken
1 tablespoon oil
2-1/2 tablespoons sugar
1 teaspoon salt
2 cups water
1/4 cup soy sauce
1 bunch green onions, cut in 1-1/2-inch lengths
1 block tofu, cut in 1-inch squares

Brown chicken with 1 tablespoon oil. Add sugar, salt, water, and soy sauce and simmer until chicken is tender. Add green onions and tofu. Flip the pot in upward movement to mix. Stirrings will break up the tofu. Serves 4.

175 calories, 26 grams protein per serving

Hot Chicken Casserole

2 cups chopped chicken
2 cups chopped celery
1/2 cup blanched almonds
1/3 cup chopped green pepper
2 tablespoons chopped pimiento
2 tablespoons chopped onion
1/2 teaspoon salt
2 tablespoons lemon juice
1/3 cup mayonnaise
1/3 cup grated Swiss cheese
2 cups 100% bran cereal

Mix all ingredients except cheese and cereal. Spoon into 13" × 7" casserole dish and top with cereal and cheese. Bake at 350 degrees for 25 minutes or microwave 5 minutes. Serves 6.

262 calories, 11 grams protein per 1/2-cup serving

Oyako Donburi

The following recipe covers rice with a soft chicken and egg topping. Soy sauce and green onions spice an otherwise bland dish. Their amounts may be decreased if you desire.

1-1/2 cups chicken, sliced thin
1 tablespoon oil
1-1/2 cups chicken bouillon
4 tablespoons soy sauce
2 tablespoons sugar
1/2 teaspoon salt
1/2 teaspoon MSG
1 cup green onions, chopped
5 eggs
3 cups cooked rice

Saute chicken in oil. Add bouillon and cook until chicken is tender. Add seasonings and green onions. Beat eggs slightly and pour evenly over chicken. Cook over low heat until eggs are coddled. Fill individual serving bowls 2/3 full with cooked rice. Cover with the chicken-egg mixture and pour sauce from cooking pan over all. Serves 6.

284 calories, 17 grams protein per serving

Tortillas with Chicken

1 onion, chopped
1 can boneless chicken
1 can diced green chilis*
1/2 cup milk
8 or 10 flour tortillas
2 tablespoons margarine
1 can cream of chicken soup
1/4 cup white wine
1 cup shredded Monterey Jack cheese

Saute onion in margarine, add all ingredients, except tortillas, and stir to mix. Layer the mix and the tortillas in greased ovenproof pan. Bake about 45 minutes at 350 degrees. Serves 8.

235 calories, 11 grams protein per serving

*May be irritating.

Easy Tuna Casserole

1 can cream of mushroom soup
1/4 cup milk
1 7-oz. can tuna, drained
2 hard-boiled eggs, sliced
1 cup green peas, cooked
1/2 cup crumbled potato chips

Mix soup and milk together in a 1-quart casserole. Stir in tuna, eggs, and peas. Bake 25 minutes at 350 degrees. Top with crumbled chips and bake 5 minutes more. Serves 4.

Variation: Shrimp or diced chicken may be substituted for tuna.

200 calories, 18 grams protein per serving

Tuna Tofu Patties

Tofu (soybean curd) is a soft, bland protein food that assumes the flavor of the foods it is cooked with.

1/2 cup chopped mushrooms
1 block tofu
2 7-oz. cans tuna, drained
4 eggs
1 small carrot, finely chopped
1 stalk green onion, finely chopped
3/4 teaspoon salt
2 tablespoons sugar
1/2 teaspoon MSG
2-1/2 tablespoons soy sauce

Squeeze excess water from tofu well and crumble. Add remaining ingredients and mix thoroughly. Drop by spoonfuls onto a greased frying pan. Brown on both sides. Serves 8.

173 calories, 14 grams protein per serving

Tuna Loaf

8 slices bread
1 can condensed cream of mushroom soup
1 cup milk
1/2 teaspoon salt
1/4 teaspoon paprika*
2 eggs
1 7-oz. can flaked tuna, drained

Tear bread into crumbs and mix with tuna. Mix together soup, milk, salt, paprika, and eggs and add to bread and tuna. Bake in greased loaf pan for 45 minutes at 350 degrees. Serve with cream sauce or condensed cream of mushroom soup diluted with cream to sauce consistency. Serves 6.

314 calories, 22 grams protein per serving

Fish Fillets Baked in Cream

1 lb. fish fillets (sole, flounder, etc.)
Salted flour
1-1/2 cups cream
Seasonings to taste

Dip fish fillets in salted flour and arrange in a shallow baking dish. Cover with cream and bake 15 minutes at 450 degrees. Transfer fish to plates and season cream to taste with salt, pepper, chopped parsley, or a dissolved chicken bouillon cube. Pour sauce over fish. Serves 3.

458 calories, 11 grams protein per serving

*May be irritating.

Creamed Fish

1 cup cream sauce* or concentrated cream of mushroom soup diluted with cream to sauce consistency

1/2 cup cooked fish or canned tuna or salmon

Flake cooked fish, removing bones and skin, or use canned tuna or salmon. Add to cream sauce and heat in double-boiler. Season to taste. Serve on toast or with rice, noodles, or mashed potatoes. Serves 1

Variations: Add a raw egg yolk to the sauce just before serving. Add sauteed mushrooms, chopped hard-cooked eggs, or green peas. Instead of heating in a double-boiler, put mixture in casserole, top with buttered breadcrumbs and bake at 350 degrees until crumbs are brown.

580 calories, 34 grams protein per serving

Pineapple Shrimp

This deep-fried shrimp dish is served with a pineapple sauce.

1 lb. shrimp (medium or large size is best)

1 can pineapple tidbits or chunks (reserve 1/2 cup juice)

2 tablespoons sesame seeds,* toasted

Batter

1 cup flour

1 egg, beaten

1/2 teaspoon salt

1/8 teaspoon MSG

3/4 cup water

Sauce

3 tablespoons brown sugar

1 tablespoon cornstarch

2 tablespoons vinegar

1/2 cup pineapple juice

1/4 cup water

Clean and devein shrimp. Combine ingredients for batter. Dip shrimp in batter and deep-fry in fat a few at a time until golden brown. Combine sauce ingredients and bring to a boil. Simmer for 1 minute. Place drained pineapple tidbits or chunks on shrimp. Cover with sauce and garnish with sesame seeds. Serves 6.

191 calories, 13 grams protein per serving

*May be irritating.

Vegetables

The recipes found here will give you new cooking ideas to liven up your vegetable dishes, especially if you are experiencing "taste blindness." If you boil your vegetables in water you will lose much of the valuable vitamins and minerals found in them. To retain these nutrients, save the water you used to boil the vegetables and use it in recipes calling for water.

Breaded Eggplant

1 medium eggplant, peeled and sliced thin
1 egg
1/2 cup breadcrumbs
1/2 cup 100% bran cereal crumbs
1 flavor packet from Ramen Pride Oriental Noodles®

Mix dry ingredients (crumbs and noodles flavor packet) together. Beat the egg. Dip each slice of eggplant in the beaten egg, then the crumbs. Fry in small amount of margarine at a very low temperature (to avoid burning) for about 20 minutes. Makes 12 slices.

40 calories, 2 grams protein per slice

Italian Eggplant

1 eggplant, peeled and sliced into 3/8-inch rounds
olive oil
1 diced onion, fried limp
1/2 teaspoon garlic salt
1 cup grated yellow cheese
1 small can stewed tomatoes
1/2 large can garbanzos
1/2 teaspoon basil

Brush eggplant with olive oil. Broil until golden brown, turn, brush and broil again. Combine onion, garlic salt, tomatoes, garbanzos and basil in pan; simmer 20 minutes into a sauce. Layer eggplant and sauce in a baking dish or casserole, ending with a cheese topping. Sprinkle with additional Parmesan cheese, if desired. Bake at 350 degrees for 45 minutes. Serves 6.

190 calories, 6 grams protein per serving

Asparagus Parmesan Cheese Casserole

1 can asparagus

1/4 cup dry breadcrumbs

1/4 cup margarine or butter

1/4 cup Parmesan cheese

Drain and arrange asparagus in baking dish, sprinkle top with mixture of margarine or butter, dry breadcrumbs, and Parmesan cheese. Bake at 375 degrees for 10 to 12 minutes. Serves 4.

105 calories, 3.5 grams protein per serving

Hot Artichoke-Cheese Bars

2 tablespoons oil

1 clove garlic, minced*

1 14-oz. can artichoke hearts, drained

2 tablespoons minced parsley

1/4 teaspoon oregano

1/3 cup finely chopped onion

4 eggs

1/4 cup dry breadcrumbs

8 oz. Swiss or cheddar cheese, shredded

Salt and pepper to taste

Grease an 11" × 7" baking dish. Preheat oven to 350 degrees. In small skillet heat oil and saute onion and garlic until limp. Beat eggs to a froth in mixing bowl. Chop artichokes into small pieces and add to bowl. Stir in onion and garlic, breadcrumbs, cheese, parsley, and seasonings. Turn into baking pan and bake at 325 degrees for 25 to 30 minutes, until set when touched lightly. Let cool a bit before cutting into bars. Serves 12.

150 calories, 9 grams protein per serving

*May be irritating.

Broccoli Casserole

1 20-oz. package frozen broccoli, lightly cooked
1 16 oz. container cottage cheese
1 tablespoon flour
1 can green chilis,* diced
3 beaten eggs
1 cup grated cheddar cheese

Mix and bake at 325 degrees for 20 to 30 minutes. Serves 8.

123 calories, 10.3 grams protein per serving

Carrots Baked

1 package thin, tender carrots, pared
1/2 cup butter or margarine
1 tablespoon lemon juice
2 tablespoons water
1/2 cup packed brown sugar
1 teaspoon salt
Pepper

Boil carrots in water for 10 minutes and drain. Melt margarine in saucepan. Add lemon juice, water, sugar, salt and pepper to create sauce. Place carrots in ovenproof dish and top with sauce. Cover and bake for 30 minutes at 375 degrees. Serves 6.

180 calories, 2 grams protein per serving

*May be irritating.

Carrots Elegante

2 lbs. carrots
2 teaspoons salt
1/4 teaspoon cardamon
2 teaspoons sugar
1/2 cup butter or margarine
1/2 cup orange juice

Coarsely grate carrots. Melt butter, stir in carrots, sugar, and spices, cover and cook for 10 minutes stirring occasionally. Add orange juice and cook 5 more minutes until crisply tender. Spoon into heated bowl and garnish with wedges of orange and parsley. Serves 10.

135 calories, 2 grams protein per serving

Marinated Carrots

2 pounds of carrots, pared and sliced in 1/8-inch rounds
1 can tomato soup
3/4 cup sugar
1 teaspoon salt
1 onion, chopped
1 green pepper, chopped
1/2 cup salad oil
1/2 cup vinegar

Cook carrots until al dente, about 5 minutes. Set aside in covered dish. Heat remaining ingredients in sauce pan until sugar dissolves. Pour over vegetables and marinate overnight or longer. Drain to serve. Serves 10.

100 calories, 1 gram protein per serving

Green Bean Casserole

3 packages frozen cut green beans
1/2 cup butter or margarine
2 cups milk
3/4 lbs. sharp cheddar cheese, grated
2 teaspoons soy sauce
1 large can mushrooms
1 chopped onion
1/4 cup flour
1 cup light cream
1 can water chestnuts
1/8 teaspoon tobasco
1/2 teaspoon pepper
1/2 cup slivered almonds

Cook beans lightly. In microwave or double-boiler, melt together butter, milk, soy sauce, cream, tobasco and cheese. Saute mushrooms and onion in butter. Stir in flour and pepper. Toss beans, cheese sauce, mushrooms, water chestnuts and almonds together. Bake at 375 degrees for 25 minutes. Serves 10.

150 calories, 7.3 grams protein per serving

Rice Pilaf

2 tablespoons butter
1 cup rice
2 cups chicken stock
1/2 teaspoon salt
4 tablespoons melted butter (optional)
Optional: Pepper

Melt butter and when foam subsides, add rice and stir for 3 minutes until evenly coated. Do not brown. Add seasoned stock, stir and bring to a boil. Lower heat to lowest point and simmer for 20 minutes until liquid is absorbed. Toss rice with 4 additional tablespoons of butter (if desired) and let stand covered for 15 minutes. Serves 6.

Variation: Wild rice may be prepared this way also. **Additives:** Limp fried onions, peppers, tomatoes or sliced mushrooms.

147 calories, 3 grams protein per serving

Spinach and Artichokes Au Gratin

2 6-oz. jars marinated artichoke hearts, drained
3 3-oz. packages cream cheese
1/3 cup Parmesan cheese, grated
Pepper (to taste)
3 10-oz. packages chopped spinach, thawed
4 tablespoons margarine, softened
6 tablespoons milk

Distribute artichokes over 1-1/2-quart casserole dish. Squeeze moisture from spinach and layer over artichokes. Blend cream cheese, margarine, milk and pepper until smooth and spread over spinach. Dust with Parmesan cheese. Cover and refrigerate at least 1 hour. Bake uncovered at 375 degrees for 45 minutes. Serves 10.

110 calories, 5 grams protein per serving

Spinach and Zucchini

1 10-oz. package chopped spinach, thawed
1 lb. sliced zucchini
1 small chopped onion
1 egg, lightly beaten
2 tablespoons margarine
1 can mushrooms
Parmesan cheese
1 clove garlic, minced
3 soda crackers, crushed
Pepper (to taste)
1/2 teaspoon salt

Cook spinach and zucchini for 5 minutes in boiling water. Saute onion and garlic in margarine. Combine spinach mixture, onion mixture, mushrooms and egg in buttered casserole dish. Top with Parmesan and crushed crackers. Bake at 350 degrees for 35 minutes. Serves 6.

75 calories, 4 grams protein per serving

Spinach Pie

2 10-oz. packages chopped spinach, thawed
3 tablespoons oil
2 cups grated cheddar cheese
1/4 cup grated onion
2 eggs, lightly beaten
1/2 teaspoon salt
Pepper (to taste)
1 frozen or homemade pie pastry

Cook spinach as directed and drain well. Add other ingredients, reserving a small amount of oil. Make (or thaw frozen) pie pastry and roll thin into a rectangle shape. Brush with oil and enclose the spinach mixture, tucking in the ends. Bake on cookie sheet at 350 degrees for 30 minutes until brown. Serves 8.

320 calories, 12 grams protein per serving

Spinach with White Sauce

1 10-oz. package spinach, cooked and well-drained
1/2 cup white sauce (recipe below)
1 teaspoon lemon juice
1/2 onion, diced and fried limp
1/4 teaspoon nutmeg*
Salt and pepper to taste

Add ingredients to cooked spinach and heat thoroughly. Serves 4.

White Sauce
2 tablespoons butter
1/2 cup milk
2 tablespoons flour
Optional: 2 tablespoons white wine

Heat butter until foamy stage. Blend in flour; slowly add milk and continue stirring. If desired, add 2 tablespoons white wine. Do not boil sauce.

120 calories, 3.25 grams protein per serving

*May be irritating.

Squash Bake

1 acorn, butternut or banana squash

Sauce

1/4 cup honey

1/4 cup white wine

1/4 teaspoon paprika*

Salt and pepper

Halve squash lengthwise, scrape out seeds and strings, and place cut side up in an ovenproof pan with 1/4-inch water. Wisk together a sauce from the honey, wine and seasonings. Pour the sauce over the squash. Bake covered at 350 degrees for 45 minutes, or until the squash is soft. Serves 4.

120 calories, 1 gram protein per serving

Sweet Potato

4 peeled and cooked sweet potatoes

1/2 cup packed brown sugar

1 jar sliced, spiced apples (**save juice**)

2 eggs

1/2 cup orange juice

1 teaspoon salt

1 cup marshmallows, miniature

Mix potatoes, brown sugar, eggs, orange juice and salt in a mixer, adding as much of the spiced apple juice as needed for the potatoes to be good and moist, but not runny. Place sliced apples in ovenproof pan, top with potatoes. Sprinkle the marshmallows on top. Bake at 350 degrees for 45 minutes. Serves 10.

NOTE: Spiced apples can be hard to find, but are easy to make. Core 2 or 3 apples and slice in 1/4-inch slices. Cover with water and 1/2 cup sugar and 1/4 cup red hot candies. Boil to soft/firm stage; cloves and ginger may be added.

175 calories, 2.4 grams protein per serving

*May be irritating.

Salads

You will find these nutritious salads cool and refreshing, especially if you need soft, moist foods or if you are finding the aroma of cooked foods difficult to tolerate.

Chinese Chicken Salad

1 chicken breast, steamed and shredded
1/3 head iceberg lettuce, shredded
4 green onions, finely chopped
1/3 cup cashews*, chopped
Handful Chinese parsley, chopped

Dressing
1/4 cup chicken juice from steaming, or canned chicken broth
Salt and pepper to taste
1/2 teaspoon dry mustard*
1 teaspoon sesame oil

Toss chicken, lettuce, green onions, nuts and parsley in dressing. Serves 1.

450 calories, 33 grams protein

Chicken Salad

1 cup cooked and diced chicken
1 stalk celery, diced
1 tablespoon lemon juice
2 to 4 tablespoons mayonnaise
Salt and pepper to taste

Mix chicken and celery in bowl. Sprinkle with lemon juice. Add enough mayonnaise to bind. Add salt and pepper to taste. Serves 1.

500 calories, 40 grams protein

*May be irritating.

Shrimp and Avocado Salad

Avocados are high in calories and also have a high fat content.

1/2 cup cooked shrimp
1/2 cup diced avocado
1 stalk celery, diced
2 to 4 tablespoons mayonnaise
Catsup
Lemon juice

Mix shrimp, avocado, and celery. Add mayonnaise as desired. Add catsup and lemon juice to taste. Serves 1.

400 calories, 16 grams protein

Cottage Cheese and Fruit Salad

1 cup cottage cheese
Mixed fruit: sliced peaches, fresh strawberries, grapes, melon balls, sliced bananas

Place a scoop of cottage cheese in the center of a plate and surround with your favorite fruits. Serves 1.

340 calories, 32 grams protein

Cucumbers in Sour Cream**

2 medium cucumbers, peeled, thinly sliced
1 cup sour cream
1 tablespoon sugar
2 tablespoons vinegar
5 green onions, chopped (including greens)
1 teaspoon salt
Paprika* (garnish)

Mix sour cream, sugar, salt and vinegar until well blended. Pour over cucumbers and onions. Cover and refrigerate at least 2 hours before serving. Serve in individual salad plates. Sprinkle top with paprika. Serves 4 to 6.

115 calories, 2 grams protein

*May be irritating.

**May cause gas.

Yogurt and Fruit Salad

1 cup yogurt, plain or fruit

Mixed fruit: sliced peaches, fresh strawberries, grapes, melon balls, sliced bananas

Fill a bowl with sliced fruit and top with your favorite yogurt. Serves 1.

340 calories, 12 grams protein

Cranberry Salad

1 small package cherry Jell-O®

1 cup sugar

1 cup drained crushed pineapple (**save juice**)

1 orange, chopped

1/2 cup pecans,* chopped

1 cut hot water

1 tablespoon lemon juice

1 cup raw ground cranberries (**save juice**)

1 cut celery, chopped

Dissolve Jell-O® in hot water. Add sugar and all juices, then all other remaining ingredients. Chill in oiled pan. Serves 6.

340 calories, 4.6 grams protein

*May be irritating.

Salad Dressings

Basic Mayonnaise, and Mayonnaise with Sour Cream Blue Cheese Variation

Mayonnaise

1 egg
1/2 teaspoon dry mustard*
2 tablespoons lemon juice
3/4 teaspoon salt
1/4 teaspoon paprika*
1 cup salad oil

Put the egg, lemon juice, spices, and 1/4 of oil in a blender, cover and process at "High." Immediately remove feeder cap and pour remaining oil in a steady stream. All the oil should be added in less than 30 seconds. Makes 1-1/4 cups.

100, 1 gram protein per tablespoon

Sour Cream Blue Cheese Variation

1 cup sour cream
1/2 teaspoon garlic salt
1/2 teaspoon Worcestershire
1 cup crumbled blue cheese (less for milder flavor)

Add all ingredients except the cheese to mayonnaise, cover and process at "High" until smooth. Stop blender and add cheese, cover and process at "High" only until cheese is mixed throughout. For a smoother dressing process longer. Makes 3 cups.

75 calories, 1 gram protein per tablespoon

*May be irritating.

Fruit Dressing

1/2 cup sugar
1 teaspoon paprika*
1/4 cup vinegar
1 teaspoon onion juice
1 cup salad oil
1 teaspoon dry mustard*
1 teaspoon salt
1 teaspoon poppy seed or celery seed

Combine all ingredients except oil in small mixer bowl. Add oil 2 teaspoons at a time while beating. If the oil is added slowly the dressing will remain mixed and thick for several weeks. Very good over fresh fruits, and can be used on vegetable salads. Makes1-1/2 cups.

70 calories, 1 gram protein per tablespoon

Omar's Dressing

2 eggs
1 teaspoon salt
1/2 teaspoon dry mustard*
1/2 cup catsup
1/2 cup vinegar
1 tablespoon sugar
1/2 teaspoon paprika*
1 teaspoon Worcestershire sauce
2 cups salad oil
2/3 cup warm water
1 clove garlic, mashed

Mix all ingredients except oil, vinegar and water in mixing bowl that has been rubbed with garlic clove. Stir them into a smooth paste. Add oil slowly, alternating with vinegar. Beat with electric mixer into a thick dressing; add the warm water slowly. Keep refrigerated. Excellent on spinach salad—spinach, red onion slices and sliced mushrooms. Makes slightly more than 1 quart.

75 calories, 1 gram protein per tablespoon

*May be irritating.

Poppy Seed Dressing

3/4 cup sugar
1 teaspoon salt
1 tablespoon instant minced onions
1 teaspoon dry mustard*
1/3 cup red wine vinegar
1 cup corn oil
1 teaspoon poppy seed
1 teaspoon sesame seed

Blend sugar, salt, onion, mustard and vinegar thoroughly in blender or food processor. Add oil, 1/3 cup at a time, blending well after each addition of oil. Lastly, blend in seeds. Chill. Good on salad, fruits or slaw. Makes 1-1/2 cups.

85 calories, 1 gram protein per tablespoon

Sweet-and-Sour Dressing

1 egg
1/4 cup honey
1/2 teaspoon garlic salt
3/4 cup apple cider vinegar*
1/4 cup salad oil

Beat egg white until stiff. Add beaten egg yolk. Beat separately or shake remaining ingredients. Add to egg and beat until well mixed. Makes 1-1/4 cups.

35 calories, 1 gram protein per tablespoon

*May be irritating.

Soups

Often when you don't feel like eating solid food, but want to eat something substantial, you will find that soup is a good answer.

Creamy Vegetable Soup

This is an easy and delicious way to digest your favorite vegetables, hot or cold.

1 lb. spinach, asparagus, broccoli, zucchini, or any other favorite vegetable

1 10-oz. can chicken broth

1 10-oz. can water

1 scallion

Tarragon to taste

Parsley to taste

1/2 cup cream or sour cream

Put all ingredients except cream in a pot and cook until vegetables are done. Pour into blender and puree until smooth. Add cream and blend. Serves 1.

350 calories, 17 grams protein

Easy Cream of Vegetable Soup

1 jar pureed baby vegetables, such as creamed spinach, creamed corn, or peas

1 cup milk or cream

Mix and heat. Serves 1.

250 calories, 11 grams protein

Japanese Noodle Soup

Take any one of the packaged Japanese instant noodle soups (such as Top Ramen®) that cook up in 3 minutes. Garnish with leftover cooked chicken, ham, chopped hard-boiled egg, or anything else that appeals to your taste. Serves 1.

250 calories, 11 grams protein

Chicken Soup with Matzo Balls

1 large fryer (almost 4 lbs.)
3 quarts water
2 large onions, cut in half
3 to 4 carrots, cut up
4 to 5 celery stalks and tops
2 chicken bouillon cubes
Salt and pepper to taste

Cut up chicken into quarters, place in large pot, and add 3 quarts water. Add vegetables, bouillon cubes, salt, and pepper. Bring to a boil, cut to medium heat, then to low heat, and simmer about 2 hours. Strain and add matzo balls. Serves 4.

188 calories, 12 grams protein per serving (3 matzo balls)

Matzo Balls

2 eggs
2 tablespoons melted fat
1 teaspoon salt
1/2 cup matzo meal
2 tablespoons chicken broth

Beat eggs and add melted fat. Mix salt with matzo meal and pour into egg mixture. Mix thoroughly. Add soup and mix once more. Refrigerate at least 1 hour. Form into 12 balls the size of walnuts and place in 4 quarts salted boiling water. Cover and cook 1 hour over medium heat. Drain and use in soup or stew.

48 calories, 2 grams protein per ball

Egg Drop Soup

3 cups chicken broth

1 teaspoon salt

1 scallion, finely chopped

1 tablespoon cornstarch dissolved in 2 tablespoons cold water

1 egg, slightly beaten

Bring chicken broth to a boil in saucepan and add salt. Add cornstarch mixture to pan, stirring until broth thickens and becomes clear. Slowly pour in egg and stir once gently. Remove from heat. Spoon into soup bowls and garnish with chopped scallions. Serves 2.

103 calories, 8 grams protein per serving

Easy Tofu Soup

Tofu (soybean curd) is a good source of protein. It is soft and bland and easy to digest.

1 cup prepared beef bouillon

2 oz. tofu, diced

Add diced tofu to bouillon and heat. Serve in a bowl, garnished with chopped green onion, if desired. Serves 1.

Variation: Add diced or shredded leftover meat or raw vegetables.

70 calories, 9 grams protein

Easy Cream of Corn Soup

2 cans corn, drained

2 tablespoons dried onion

Salt and pepper to taste

4 cups milk

2 or 3 slices bread

Cut crust off bread and pulverize in blender. Remove. Put drained corn and 1 cup milk in blender, cover and blend on medium speed. Place corn, bread, salt, pepper, onion and rest of milk in saucepan. Heat and serve. Serves 4.

185 calories, 7.25 grams protein per serving

Shrimp Bisque

1 10-oz. can frozen cream of shrimp soup
1 cup cream or milk
1 ripe avocado, diced
1 teaspoon lemon juice
1/2 teaspoon salt
Dash nutmeg*
1 4-1/2-oz. can shrimp

In saucepan cook everything but canned shrimp until bubbling. Drain and rinse shrimp and add just before serving. Can also be served cold. Serves 2.

550 calories, 26 grams protein per serving

Iced Curry Soup

1 10-oz. can cream of chicken soup
1 cup cream
1 tablespoon lemon juice
1/2 to 1 teaspoon curry powder*
Leftover chicken, diced

Blend everything but leftover chicken in blender. Remove from blender and stir in chicken. Chill before serving. Serves 2.

500 calories, 5 grams protein per serving

*Cold Cucumber Soup***

1 10-3/4-oz. can cream of celery soup
1/4 cup cottage cheese
1 tablespoon onion, coarsely chopped
1 cup milk
1/2 cup cucumber, peeled and coarsely chopped

Combine all ingredients in the container of electric blender. Process until smooth. Chill. Sprinkle with chopped parsley or chopped chives. Makes 4 servings.

130 calories, 5.5 grams protein per serving

*May be irritating.

**May cause gas.

Chilled Cucumber Soup *

3 medium cucumbers, chopped (about 4 cups)
3 tablespoons margarine
2 13-3/4-oz. cans chicken broth
1 teaspoon dill weed or 1 tablespoon snipped fresh dill
2/3 cup sliced scallions or green onions
3 tablespoons flour
1 teaspoon salt (taste first)
1/8 teaspoon ground black pepper
1-1/2 cups buttermilk
1 tablespoon lemon juice
Cheese Parmesan snack crackers
Dill sprigs, optional

Saute the chopped cucumbers and scallions or green onions in margarine until soft; stir in flour. Gradually add chicken broth, stirring constantly until mixture thickens slightly and comes to a boil. Add salt, pepper and dill weed. Simmer, covered for 10 minutes. Chill thoroughly. (May be prepared up to this point and refrigerated overnight.) Puree in blender. Stir in buttermilk and lemon juice. Garnish with dill sprigs, if desired. Serve with Parmesan cheese crackers. Makes 6 1-cup servings.

160 calories, 4 grams protein per serving

*May cause gas.

Cold Green Bean Soup

1 medium onion, chopped
4 to 5 cups green beans, cut into small pieces
Salt and pepper to taste
1/4 cup slivered almonds (toasted or sauteed until golden)
1 clove garlic,* minced
3 cups chicken bouillon (strong)
1/4 teaspoon savory leaves
Sour cream

Saute onion and garlic in 2 tablespoons butter or margarine until limp. Stir in beans and bouillon, cover, and simmer about 10 minutes, or until beans are tender. Put mixture into blender container and whirl until smooth. Add salt, pepper and savory. Chill well. To serve, pour into mugs and garnish with a dollop of sour cream and a sprinkling of almonds. Makes 6 servings.

60 calories, 4.2 grams protein per serving

New England Clam Chowder

3 strips bacon, diced
1 can cream of potato soup
1 teaspoon minced parsley
Pinch of rosemary
1/3 cup milk
1 medium onion, chopped
1 8-oz. can minced clams
1 teaspoon thyme
Salt and pepper
1/2 cup sour cream

Brown bacon, add onion, then soup. Drain clams. Add juice only. Blend and simmer briefly. Add clams and seasonings. Simmer two minutes. Just before serving, add milk and sour cream. Heat to boiling and stir. Serve hot. Makes 4 servings.

170 calories, 6.25 grams protein per serving

*May be irritating.

Sauces

Sauces add calories and are a good way to moisten meat, vegetables, noodles, and rice to make swallowing easier.

Basic White Sauce

Use this sauce as a base for creamed meats and vegetables.

2 tablespoons flour

Salt and pepper (preferably white) to taste

2 tablespoons butter

1 to 1-1/2 cups milk

Melt butter in a 1-quart saucepan over medium heat, being careful not to let it burn. Add flour and immediately start stirring. Add milk all at once, stirring rapidly. Add salt and pepper to taste. Cook over medium heat, stirring frequently, about 5 minutes. Makes 1 to 1-1/2 cups.

465 calories, 12 grams protein

Variations:

Cheese Sauce: To basic white sauce, add 4 oz. shredded cheddar cheese. Makes 1-1/2 cups.

900 calories, 40 grams protein

Egg Sauce: To basic white sauce, add 2 finely chopped, hard-cooked eggs. Makes 1-1/2 cups.

615 calories, 24 grams protein

Quick Cheese Sauce

Serve this sauce over cooked vegetables.

1 can condensed cheddar cheese soup

1/4 to 1/3 cup milk

Mix and heat. Makes 1-1/2 cups.

350 calories, 8 grams protein

Yogurt Hollandaise Sauce

Serve this sauce over cooked vegetables or over a poached egg on toast.

1 cup plain yogurt
4 egg yolks, beaten
1 tablespoon lemon juice
Dash of hot pepper sauce
1/2 teaspoon salt

Mix all ingredients in top of double-boiler. Stir vigorously over simmering water until smooth and thickened. Makes 1-1/2 cups.

485 calories, 27 grams protein

Quick Tomato Sauce

1 can condensed tomato soup
2 tablespoons milk or cream

Mix and heat. Makes 1-1/4 cups.

240 calories, 3 grams protein

Korean Barbecue Sauce

This spicy sauce may be irritating and should be used with care.

1 cup soy sauce
1/2 cup salad oil
1/2 cup dark brown sugar
5 stalks green onion, chopped fine
1/4 cup bourbon whiskey
3 large cloves garlic, crushed
1/2 cup sesame oil
1 teaspoon black pepper

Combine all ingredients in a quart-size jar and shake well.

2,277 calories, 13 grams protein

Tart B-B-Q Sauce

1 small onion, chopped
2 tablespoons vinegar
1/4 cup lemon juice
3 tablespoons Worcestershire sauce
Pinch salt
2 tablespoons oil
2 tablespoons brown sugar
1 cup tomato catsup
1/2 teaspoon prepared mustard
1/2 cup water
Dash cayenne

Brown onion in oil. Add remaining ingredients. Simmer for 30 minutes. For less tangy sauce, add more catsup. Makes 2 cups.

80 calories, 1 gram protein per 4-tablespoon serving

Teriyaki Marinade

1 cup pineapple juice
1/2 cup brown sugar
2 teaspoons ginger*
1 cup soy sauce
2 cloves garlic
2 bay leaves

Combine and marinate any meat in a large bowl for 2 hours or overnight. Especially good with flank steak to be barbecued. Makes 2 cups.

680 calories, 25 grams protein

*May be irritating.

Homemade Steak Sauce

1 tablespoon Kitchen Bouquet®
1 teaspoon Worcestershire sauce
2 tablespoons wine vinegar
1/2 cup catsup
1 teaspoon Angostura bitters
1/2 teaspoon garlic powder

Mix all ingredients in a bottle and shake well. Refrigerate. (This is a considerable saving over commercial steak sauces.) Makes 3/4 cup.

18 calories, trace grams protein per tablespoon

Never-Fail Quick Spaghetti Sauce

1 lb. ground beef
3 cups water
1 can sliced mushrooms
12 oz. tomato paste
1 package onion soup mix
1 to 1-1/2 tablespoons Italian seasonings

In a large skillet, brown ground beef. Drain. Add tomato paste and water and stir in well. Add onion soup mix and stir well until dissolved. Add mushrooms and seasonings and simmer 1 hour. Serve over spaghetti. Serves 4.

330 calories, 19 grams protein per serving

Sauce for Vegetables

1 cup mayonnaise
2 tablespoons hot water
1/4 to 1/2 teaspoon curry powder*
1 bouillon cube
1 cup sour cream

Dissolve bouillon cube in hot water, and mix with mayonnaise, sour cream and curry powder. This is delicious served over cooked asparagus, broccoli, green beans or spinach. It can be stored in the refrigerator in a closed glass jar. Makes 2 cups.

48 calories, 1 gram protein per 1 tablespoon

Fruit with Sauce

2 cups fruit salad
4 tablespoons brown sugar
3 tablespoons butter
1 teaspoon cinnamon*
1/2 cup cognac
3 teaspoons cornstarch
2 bananas, sliced
Optional: whipped cream or ice cream for topping

Drain fruit, reserve juice and set aside. In sauce pan, combine juice, brown sugar, butter, cinnamon, cognac and corn starch. Heat. Garnish fruit salad with banana slices. Pour warm sauce over fruit. Serve with dab of whipped cream or ice cream. Serves 6.

160 calories, 1.4 grams protein per serving

*May be irritating.

Desserts

Dessert Toppings

Use your imagination to add extra calories with your favorite dessert toppings:

Add cinnamon*, nutmeg*, vanilla, or other flavored extracts to whipped cream.

Make fruit sauces from fruit canned in heavy syrup or from thawed frozen fruit.

Use sundae toppings on ice cream and other desserts as well.

Serve heavy cream over fruit, puddings, and cake.

Crunchy Topping for Desserts

1/3 cup brown sugar (packed)
1/3 cup margarine
1 cup 100% bran cereal
1 cup Grape-nuts® cereal
1 cup chopped nuts

Mix ingredients together in 10-inch skillet. Cook over medium heat stirring constantly for 6 minutes. Spread on cookie sheet to cool. Store in covered container in refrigerator. This topping is delicious on ice cream, pudding or yogurt. Makes 3 cups.

100 calories, 1 gram protein per 3 tablespoons

Custard Pie

4 cups milk
2 cups sugar
8 eggs
2 tablespoons cornstarch
Unbaked pie shell

Scald milk and beat in sugar, eggs, and cornstarch. Pour into unbaked pie shell and bake 30 to 40 minutes at 300 degrees. Serves 8.

460 calories, 12 grams protein per serving

*May be irritating.

Egg Custard

3 eggs
1/4 cup sugar
1 teaspoon vanilla
Dash of salt
2-1/2 cups scalded milk

Blend eggs, sugar, salt, and vanilla. Gradually add scalded milk. Pour into 6 custard cups. Place cups in pan of hot water 1/2-inch deep. Bake at 350 degrees until set, approximately 45 minutes. Serves 6.

Variation: Make a caramel sauce by putting a tablespoon of brown sugar at the bottom of each cup before filling.

140 calories, 6 grams protein per serving

Lemon Sponge Pudding

1-1/2 cups sugar
1/2 cup flour
1/2 teaspoon baking powder
1/4 teaspoon salt
3 eggs, separated
2 teaspoons grated lemon rind
1/4 cup lemon juice
2 tablespoons melted butter
1-1/2 cups milk

Sift together 1 cup of the sugar with the flour, baking powder, and salt. Beat egg whites until stiff, then beat in gradually the remaining 1/2 cup sugar. Beat egg yolks until light and add the lemon rind, lemon juice, melted butter, and milk. Stir into flour mixture until smooth. Gently fold in beaten egg whites and pour into buttered 2-quart baking dish. Set in a pan of hot water 1/2-inch deep and bake 45 minutes at 350 degrees. Chill one hour before serving. Serves 6.

335 calories, 6 grams protein per serving

Pistacchio Dessert

Crust

1-1/2 sticks butter

2 tablespoons sugar

1-1/2 cups flour

1 cup chopped nuts

Mix ingredients and press into 9" × 13" pan and bake for 20 minutes at 350 degrees. Cool partially.

Next Layer

1/2 large carton Cool Whip®

1 cup powdered sugar

8 oz. cream cheese, softened

Beat until smooth and spread over crust.

Next Layer

2 packages instant Pistachio pudding

1-1/4 cups cold milk

1/2 carton Cool Whip®

Chopped nuts (for garnish)

Beat pudding mix and milk together and pour over cheese layer. Top with remaining Cool Whip® and sprinkle with chopped nuts. Cut into 24 squares.

200 calories, 4 grams protein per square

Rice Pudding

4 cups milk

2/3 cup sugar

1/4 cup uncooked rice

1/2 teaspoon salt

1 teaspoon vanilla or a dash of nutmeg*

1/2 cup raisins

Combine ingredients in a casserole and bake, uncovered, for 3 hours at 300 degrees. Stir several times during the first hour to keep rice from settling to bottom. Serves 8.

180 calories, 5 grams protein per serving

*May be irritating.

Flan De Queso (Cheese Flan)

1 cup sugar
1 8-oz. package cream cheese
1 can condensed milk
4 eggs
1 13-oz. can evaporated milk
1/2 teaspoon vanilla

Caramelize sugar by melting it in a small 9-inch skillet, stirring constantly. Pour into a 2 to 2-1/2-quart well-buttered mold and cover sides and bottom with caramel mixture. Set aside. Place eggs, cream cheese, milks and vanilla in a blender. Mix well until liquefied and pour into caramelized bowl. Place in a pan of water in a preheated 350-degree oven for 1 hour or until knife comes out clean. When cooled, place in refrigerator until ready to serve. This can be made up to 3 days ahead. When ready to serve, run a knife around the border and unmold onto a plate. Serves 8 to 10.

Variation: If desired, substitute 3 bananas for the cream cheese, and you will have a banana flan, or if desired, 1 can of Coco Lopez can be substituted to have a coconut flavor.

320 calories, 8.1 grams protein per serving

Tapioca

1 egg
2 tablespoons tapioca
1/4 cup sugar
1/4 teaspoon salt
2 cups milk
1/2 teaspoon vanilla

Break egg into saucepan and beat slightly with fork. Add remaining ingredients except vanilla. Cook and stir over medium heat until pudding boils. Let stand 15 minutes and stir in vanilla. Serve warm or chilled, plain or topped with whipped cream, a spoonful of jam or fruit. Serves 4.

165 calories, 6 grams protein per serving

Bread Pudding

1/2 cup sugar
1/2 teaspoon cinnamon*
1/4 teaspoon salt
2 eggs
4 cups milk
1 teaspoon vanilla
8 slices bread, cut in cubes
1/2 cup raisins, *optional*
2 tablespoons melted butter

Mix sugar, cinnamon, and salt in a bowl. Beat in eggs. Add milk and vanilla. Stir in bread, raisins, and butter. Pour into 9-inch square baking dish and bake for 1 hour at 350 degrees. Serves 9.

230 calories, 7 grams protein per serving

Zabaglione

6 egg yolks
2 tablespoons sugar
3/4 cup Marsala wine

Beat egg yolks with sugar until very light and thick. Heat Marsala wine. Put egg mixture in top of double-boiler over hot water; add Marsala gradually, beating constantly with a rotary beater. Cook, beating until thick and hot (to avoid curdling, don't allow water to boil). Pour into heated sherbet or wine glasses and serve at once. Serves 4.

173 calories, 3 grams protein per serving

*May be irritating.

Raisin Pudding

Pudding Mixture

1-1/3 cups flour

3/4 cup sugar

1-2/3 tablespoons melted butter

3/4 cup milk

3/4 teaspoon nutmeg*

1-1/2 teaspoons baking powder

3/4 teaspoon baking soda

3/4 teaspoon vanilla

1-1/2 cups raisins

Caramel Sauce

4 tablespoons butter

3-1/2 cups water

1-1/2 cups brown sugar

Whipped cream as garnish

Combine all pudding mixture ingredients and place in a well-buttered 2-1/2-quart casserole. Combine caramel sauce ingredients in a saucepan, bring to a boil and pour over pudding mixture. Bake in a preheated 350 degree oven for 30 minutes. Serve warm or cold with dollops of whipped cream. Serves 6 to 8.

255 calories, 3.5 grams protein per serving

With sauce: 455 calories, 3.5 grams protein per serving

Almond Jewel

1 envelope unflavored gelatin

1-1/2 cups water

1/2 cup evaporated milk

1/2 cup sugar

2 teaspoons almond extract

Dissolve gelatin in 1/2 cup hot water. Heat evaporated milk, 1 cup water, and sugar to just below boiling point. Add gelatin and stir until completely mixed. Cool and add almond extract. Pour into rectangular pan and refrigerate to set. Cut into cubes and serve with fruit. Serves 4.

140 calories, 4 grams protein per serving

Frozen Fruit Slush

The slushy consistency of this dessert makes it easy to swallow.

1 6-oz. can frozen fruit juice concentrate

4 tablespoons sugar

3 cups crushed ice

Put all ingredients in blender and blend to desired consistency. Spoon into dishes and serve. Serves 4.

130 calories, 1 gram protein per serving

Cheesecake Squares

1/2 cup margarine
1/3 cup brown sugar
1 cup flour
1/2 cup finely chopped walnuts*
1/4 cup honey
8 oz. cream cheese, softened
1 egg
1 cup milk
1 tablespoon lemon juice
1 tablespoon lemon peel
1 teaspoon vanilla extract

Blend margarine, brown sugar, and flour together with fork until crumbly, then add finely chopped walnuts. Save 1/2 cup for topping and press remainder into bottom of greased 8-inch square pan. Bake 12 to 15 minutes at 350 degrees. Blend together well the soft cream cheese, honey, egg, milk, lemon juice, lemon peel, and vanilla. Spread over baked crust and sprinkle with remaining 1/2 cup of flour mixture. Bake 25 minutes at 350 degrees. Cool and cut into squares. Makes 16 2-inch squares.

195 calories, 3 grams protein per square

*May be irritating.

Pound Cake

4 cups cake flour
1 teaspoon salt
2 teaspoons baking powder
1 lb. butter
3 cups sugar
8 eggs
1 cup milk
2 teaspoons vanilla

Have all ingredients at room temperature. Sift and measure cake flour, and then resift with salt and baking powder. Cream butter well, then add sugar and continue creaming until light and fluffy. Add eggs one at a time, beating well after each addition. Add the flour alternately with the milk and vanilla and stir only until just blended. Bake in 2 greased 9"×9" cake pans or in 2 loaf pans lined with greased brown paper. Bake 45 to 50 minutes at 350 degrees. Makes 24 slices.

120 calories, 2 grams protein per slice

Old World Noodle Ring

1/2 lb. broad noodles
1/2 teaspoon salt
1 tablespoon oil
Maraschino or glazed cherries
1/2 cup brown sugar
1/4 cup white or brown sugar
1 lb. cottage cheese
2 teaspoons vanilla
3 tablespoons sour cream
2 eggs, beaten

Cook noodles until tender in boiling water with salt and oil. Rinse in cool water and drain. Grease a ring mold well. On bottom alternate cherries and 1/2 cup brown sugar. Mix noodles with remaining ingredients and place in ring mold. Bake 45 minutes to 1 hour at 350 degrees. Run knife around edge of pan and invert on plate. Serves 10.

245 calories, 11 grams protein per serving

Fiber Bran Cake

1 cup 100% bran cereal
1 cup flour
1 cup sugar
2 teaspoons baking powder
1/4 teaspoon salt
1 teaspoon cinnamon
1/2 cup shortening
2 eggs
1/2 cup milk
1 cup shredded carrots
1 cup coarsely chopped nuts

Mix dry ingredients, except bran cereal and sugar. Cream sugar and shortening. Add eggs. Mix until creamy. Stir in dry ingredients, alternately with milk. Add carrots, bran and nuts. Mix well, but don't overmix. Pour into greased, floured, 9-inch square pan. Bake at 350 degrees, 30 to 35 minutes. Makes 9 3-inch squares.

375 calories, 7 grams protein per square

Raisin Bran Bars

1-1/4 cup 100% bran cereal
1 cup milk
2 eggs
1 teaspoon vanilla
1/2 cup flour
1 cup nuts
1 cup raisins
3/4 cup shredded coconut

Mix together first 4 ingredients. In a separate bowl, mix together next 4 ingredients. Combine the 2 mixtures. Spread on a cookie sheet with sides. Bake at 325 degrees for 25 minutes. Makes 2 dozen.

90 calories, 3 grams protein per bar

Raisin Nut Bars (Microwave)

1 cup raisins
1/2 cup apple juice
2 tablespoons natural sweetener or Equal® (2 packets)
1 teaspoon all-purpose flour
1/2 cup chopped nuts, divided
1/2 cup + 2 tablespoons margarine
1/4 cup brown sugar
1 teaspoon vanilla
1 teaspoon baking powder
3/4 cup flour
1-1/2 cups 100% bran cereal

Combine raisins, apple juice, sweetener, and the 1 teaspoon flour in a 4-cup glass measure. Cover with plastic wrap. Cook in microwave on "High" 5 to 6 minutes or until thickened, stirring once during cooking time. Stir in 1/4 cup nuts and set aside. In mixing bowl, cream margarine, brown sugar and vanilla. Mix baking powder with 3/4 cup flour; add to creamed mixture. Stir in bran and remaining nuts. Press 1/2 of the flour mixture into loaf pan (microwave dish). Cook on "High" 3 to 4 minutes or until surface is no longer moist. Spread raisin mixture over top. Spoon remaining flour mixture over raisin filling; press lightly. Cook on "high" 7 to 8 minutes. Let stand on heat-resistant countertop or breadboard until cool. Cut into bars. Makes 12 bars.

Variation: Use dates; substitute dried papaya and dry fruit for part of raisin allocation.

225 calories, 3 grams protein per bar

Fudge Brownies

1 package Fudge Brownie Mix
1/2 cup crushed 100% bran cereal

Prepare as directed on package **except** add bran cereal and increase water by 2 tablespoons. Bake as directed. (May have to increase time due to added bran and water.) Makes 24 bars.

70 calories, 1 gram protein per bar

No-Bake Chocolate Cookies

3 cups of **Instant** Oats (**Not** Quick Oats)
6 tablespoons cocoa
8 tablespoons milk
2 cups sugar
1 tablespoon margarine
3/4 teaspoon vanilla
1 cup chopped nuts
1 cup 100% bran cereal

Measure the oats and set aside, blended dry with the cereal. Boil cocoa, milk and sugar for 1 whole minute. Drop in the margarine and the vanilla and stir until well mixed. At once add nuts and blended oatmeal and cereal. Stir until well blended. Drop by teaspoonfuls on greased cookie sheet or waxed paper. Put in refrigerator to set and to store. Makes 4 dozen cookies.

65 calories, 1 gram protein per cookie

Snacks

The following nutritious snacks are high in protein and calories. Most are of a soft consistency that you will find easy to swallow and digest.

Cottage Cheese Dip

Cottage cheese is an excellent source of protein and easy to eat. Use it as a base for your favorite dip.

1 cup creamed cottage cheese
1 envelope dry onion soup mix
1/4 cup milk

Blend all ingredients in blender until smooth. Serve with crackers or chips.

Variation: Blend cottage cheese with 1/4 to 1/2 cup barbecue sauce instead of onion soup mix. This is a zesty dip for those who want more flavor.

280 calories, 32 grams protein

Czechoslovakian Cheese Spread

Hungarian paprika, obtainable at supermarkets, has a sweeter, richer taste and enhances the spread more than other kinds. However, any type of paprika may prove irritating.

8 oz. cottage cheese, small curd

3 teaspoons Hungarian paprika*

2 teaspoons chopped capers

2 teaspoons finely chopped onion, *optional*

Blend all ingredients in blender or with a wooden spoon. Spread on bread or crackers.

Variations: To the above ingredients add any leftover bits of meat, very finely chopped. The amount of paprika should be decreased (or omitted) according to your taste. However, chicken and veal are always enhanced by this kind of seasoning.

240 calories, 30 grams protein

Sour Cream Dip

Sour cream contains more calories than cottage cheese, but less protein. If you are on a milk-free diet, IMO®, can be used in place of sour cream.

1/3 cup sour cream

1/3 cup mayonnaise

1 tablespoon dry onion soup mix

Mix all ingredients together well. Serve with crackers or chips.

685 calories, 3 grams protein

Variations: Mix 1-1/2 cups sour cream, 1 cup (4 oz.) shredded cheddar cheese and 1 to 2 tablespoons milk together.

980 calories, 39 grams protein.

Mix 1 can (4-1/2 oz.) deviled ham with 1/4 cup sour cream. Can be spread on crackers or bread.

560 calories, 20 grams protein.

*May be irritating.

Avocado Spread

Avocados are very high in calories and also have a high fat content. This toned-down version of guacamole can be used on bland diets.

1 mashed avocado
1 tablespoon lemon juice
2 hard-boiled eggs, chopped
1 tablespoon mayonnaise
1 tablespoon catsup
Salt to taste

Combine all ingredients. Serve on crackers or bread.

650 calories, 12 grams protein

Chopped Liver

1 lb. chicken livers
2 large onions
2 hard-boiled eggs
Salt and pepper to taste

Chop onions and saute in oil or margarine. Remove onions from pan and saute chicken livers until done. Cool. Grind all ingredients in a grinder or chop very fine. Add salt and pepper to taste. Serve on crackers, bread, or anything you like.

823 calories, 102 grams protein

Liverwurst Pate

The following ingredients can be mixed in quantities to your taste.

Liverwurst
Cream cheese
Mayonnaise
Dry sherry
Salt and pepper
Worcestershire sauce
Curry powder*
Chopped parsley

Mash, mix, and chill. Serve on crackers or pumpernickel bread.

*May be irritating.

Deviled Egg

Because it is moist, a deviled egg is much easier to eat than a plain, hard-cooked egg if you have a dry mouth or some swallowing difficulties.

6 hard-cooked eggs, peeled
1/2 teaspoon dry mustard* or curry powder*
1/2 teaspoon salt
1/4 teaspoon pepper
3 tablespoons mayonnaise

Cut eggs in half lengthwise. Slip out yolks and mash with fork. Mix in rest of ingredients. Fill whites with egg yolk mixture.

Variations: You can make a deviled egg spread by chopping up eggs and combining with other ingredients. Serve spread on crackers or bread.

142 calories, 6 grams protein per 2 filled halves

Croque Monsieur

"Croque" means "crusty." This is a delicious French version of a grilled ham and cheese sandwich.

1 egg
1 to 2 tablespoons milk
2 slices bread
1 slice ham
1 slice cheese (your favorite kind)
Butter

Beat egg and milk. Make sandwich of bread, ham, and cheese. Dip sandwich into egg mixture and saute in hot butter until golden brown on both sides. If desired, spread cheese with prepared mustard* before covering with bread. Serves 1.

450 calories, 22 grams protein

*May be irritating.

Hamburger Toast

1 slice bread

1/4 cup ground beef

Toast bread on one side. Spread untoasted side with ground beef and sprinkle with seasoning of your choice (salt, pepper, garlic salt, onion salt, seasoning salt). Put under broiler for about 5 minutes or until done to your taste. Top with your choice of catsup, a tomato slice, mayonnaise, or sour cream. Serves 1.

Variation: When hamburger is done, top with a slice of cheese and return to broiler until cheese is melted.

214 calories, 12 grams protein per serving

With cheese: 297 calories, 16 grams protein per serving

Apple-Cheese Sandwich

1 slice whole wheat bread

Diced apple

Peanuts*

Muenster cheese

Butter

Cinnamon*

Butter bread. Sprinkle diced apple and peanuts on bread. Cover with muenster cheese and dust with cinnamon. Bake in oven or toaster oven until cheese melts. Serves 1.

235 calories, 8 grams protein

Hot Peanut Butter Sandwich

1 slice whole wheat bread

1/2 tablespoon butter

1 tablespoon peanut butter

Honey

Spread slice of whole wheat bread with butter. Then spread with peanut butter, drizzle a little bit of honey on it, and broil. Serves 1.

206 calories, 7 grams protein

*May be irritating.

Fancy Cream Cheese Sandwich

1 tablespoon honey
3 oz. cream cheese
1/3 cup chopped dates
1/4 cup chopped walnuts*
2 slices raisin or whole wheat bread
1 apple, sliced

Mix room-temperature cream cheese with honey, dates, and walnuts. Spread on raisin or whole wheat bread and garnish with slices of apple. Serves 1.

926 calories, 18 grams protein

Cream Cheese and Fruit

Whole-grain bread
Cream cheese
Honey
Fresh fruit

Spread whole-grain bread with cream cheese and honey and top with fresh fruit.

175 calories, 5 grams protein per slice

Cream Cheese and Jam

Whole-grain crackers or bread
Cream cheese
Honey
Jam

Spread whole-grain crackers or bread with cream cheese and honey. Top with jam.

175 calories, 5 grams protein per slice

*May be irritating.

Cream Cheese and Nut Bread

Banana nut bread
Cream cheese
Honey

Spread banana nut bread with cream cheese and drizzle with honey.

125 calories, 2 grams protein per slice

Cinnamon Milk Toast

1 slice toast
1 cup milk
Sugar and cinnamon* to taste

Heat milk and pour over toasted bread in a bowl. Sprinkle with sugar and cinnamon. Serves 1.

246 calories, 10 grams protein

High-Protein Munch Mix

Keep on-hand a mixture of any of the following, according to your taste.

Dry-roasted soybeans*
Sunflower seeds*
Walnuts*
Peanuts*
Cashews*
Raisins

Note: You can coarsely chop this mix to make it easier to chew.

160 calories, 6 grams protein per ounce

*May be irritating.

Peanut Butter Balls

1/4 cup peanut butter
2 tablespoons honey
1/4 cup non-fat dry milk powder
1/3 cup chopped raw cashews*
4 teaspoons sesame seeds* (toasted or non-toasted)

Mix together peanut butter, honey, and milk powder until evenly blended. Add cashews; if mixture is too stiff add 1 teaspoon hot water. Taking 1 teaspoonful at a time, form into 1" balls; roll in sesame seeds to coat. Makes 10 balls.

80 calories, 3 grams protein each

Sesame Rolls

1/4 cup sesame paste (tahini)
3 tablespoons honey
1/2 cup wheat germ
1/4 cup sunflower seeds, ground in blender or food processor

Combine all ingredients and, when thoroughly blended, form into a roll 1" in diameter and 12" long. Wrap in foil or waxed paper and store in refrigerator.

78 calories, 3 grams protein per 1" slice

Easy High-Protein Snack Suggestions

Breakfast bars
Cereal and milk
Cottage cheese with canned fruit or baby fruit
Dried fruits
Granola*
Granola bars*
Ice cream
Mixed cheese platter
Nuts*
Peanut butter on crackers, celery, or apple wedges
Yogurt

*May be irritating.

Cooking with Commercial Supplements

These recipes use commercial high-protein and high-calorie supplements for added nutritional value. Ensure®** adds both protein and calories. It is lactose-free and therefore can be used even if you have milk (lactose) intolerance. Polycose®** is a tasteless and odorless source of calories; it can be added to foods and beverages without significantly changing their natural flavors or volume. Vivonex T.E.N.®** is used to fortify clear liquid diets. Ask the dietitian member of your healthcare team if you have questions about them or have difficulty locating them in stores.

Cocoa Diablo

1 tablespoon sugar
1 tablespoon cocoa
1 tablespoon instant coffee granules
Dash cinnamon*
Dash salt
1/4 cup water
3/4 cup vanilla Ensure®

Combine dry ingredients with water and stir until dissolved. Stir in Ensure® and heat to serving temperature, stirring frequently. Serves 1.

280 calories, 8 grams protein per serving

*May be irritating.

**Ensure® and Polycose® recipes from "Nutrition: A Helpful Ally in Cancer Therapy," courtesy of Ross Laboratories. Vivonex T.E.N.® recipes courtesy of Eaton Laboratories.

Ensure® Pancakes

1 cup flour
1 tablespoon baking powder
1/2 teaspoon salt
1 teaspoon cinnamon*
1 slightly beaten egg
1-1/4 cups vanilla Ensure®
2 tablespoons salad oil
1/2 cup finely chopped apple

Combine flour, baking powder, salt, and cinnamon. Mix egg, Ensure® and oil in bowl. Add this mixture, along with chopped apple, to dry ingredients. Stir only until moistened. Fry pancakes on hot griddle. Serves 2.

429 calories, 10 grams protein per serving

Ensure® Imitation Ice Cream

3 tablespoons sugar
1-1/2 teaspoons unflavored gelatin
2 tablespoons cold water
2 tablespoons light corn syrup
1-1/2 cups vanilla Ensure®
2 tablespoons plus 1 teaspoon corn oil
1 teaspoon vanilla extract

Mix sugar, gelatin, cold water, and corn syrup in saucepan. Heat slowly until dissolved. Combine Ensure®, corn oil, and the gelatin mixture. Mix well and put into blender. Blenderize until thick and creamy. Add vanilla extract and blend well. Pour blended mix into an ice cube tray and freeze until firm. Serves 8.

Variation: Omit vanilla and add pureed fruits, such as strawberries or peaches to taste.

114 calories, 2 grams protein per serving

*May be irritating.

Ensure® Shake

1/2 cup vanilla Ensure®
1/2 cup frozen vanilla Ensure®
1/2 cup powdered coffee creamer
6-1/2 tablespoons Polycose® powder

Combine all ingredients in a blender and blend to desired consistency. Serves 1.

Variation: For additional flavor and color, add 2 tablespoons sundae topping (*50 calories*).

756 calories, 11 grams protein

Polycose® Shake

1-1/2 cups ice cream
1/4 cup whole milk
2 tablespoons sundae topping
6-1/2 tablespoons Polycose® powder

Combine all ingredients in a blender and blend to desired consistency. Serves 2.

358 calories, 6 grams protein per serving

Fruit Eggnog

1 cup Polycose® powder
1/4 cup sugar
1/8 teaspoon salt
4-1/2 oz. strained peaches
1 egg
1 teaspoon fresh lemon juice
1-1/2 cups whole milk

Combine all ingredients in a blender and blend until smooth and creamy. Chill before serving. Serves 3.

363 calories, 7 grams protein per serving

Fortified Fruit Juice

1/2 cup fruit juice
1/4 cup Polycose® liquid

Mix the two ingredients together. Serves 1.

180 calories, 1 gram protein

Fortified Coffee

1/2 cup hot water (not boiling)
1 teaspoon instant coffee
1/4 cup Polycose® liquid

Mix all ingredients together well. Serves 1.

120 calories, 0 grams protein

Fortified Ice Tea

1/2 cup water
1/2 cup Polycose® liquid
2 teaspoons instant tea
2 teaspoons sugar
1/4 teaspoon lemon juice

Mix water and Polycose® liquid. Add tea, sugar, lemon juice, and mix well. Chill before serving. Serves 1.

162 calories, 0 grams protein

Polycose® Gelatin

1 tablespoon + 2-1/4 teaspoons flavored gelatin
1/4 cup water
1/4 cup Polycose® liquid

Dissolve gelatin in 1/4 cup boiling water. Add Polycose® liquid and refrigerate until set. Serves 1.

205 calories, 2 grams protein

High-Calorie Chocolate Pudding

1 cup Polycose® powder
2 cups half-and-half
1 cup chocolate syrup
1 cup heavy whipping cream
9 tablespoons chocolate pudding powder
11 tablespoons non-fat dry milk powder

Mix Polycose® powder, pudding powder and milk powder with half-and-half in a saucepan. Add chocolate syrup. Heat until thick and creamy, stirring frequently. Cool. Beat whipping cream and fold into completely cooled pudding. Chill before serving. Serves 8.

365 calories, 6 grams protein per serving

High-Protein Rice Pudding

2/3 cup Polycose® powder
1/4 cup non-fat dry milk powder
1/4 cup hot water
2-1/2 cups whole milk
3 tablespoons sugar
1/4 cup cooked rice
2 tablespoons margarine
Dash salt

Mix Polycose® powder and non-fat dry milk powder with hot water. Add to milk and mix. Add remaining ingredients and cook in top of double-boiler until thick and creamy, stirring frequently. Pudding may also be baked in a casserole for 2 to 2-1/2 hours at 275 degrees. Serves 3.

439 calories, 11 grams protein per serving

Cream of Wheat® with Polycose®

1 cup milk (use 1-1/3 cups for thinner cereal)
1/8 teaspoon salt
Sugar to taste
8 tablespoons Polycose® powder

Bring milk and salt to a rapid boil. Lower heat and slowly sprinkle in cereal and Polycose® powder, stirring constantly. Return to a boil, then lower heat and cook for 5 minutes or until thickened, stirring constantly. Add sugar to taste. Serves 1.

Variation: Water may be substituted for milk.

505 calories, 12 grams protein

Macaroni and Cheese

1/2 cup Polycose® powder
1/2 cup milk
1 tablespoon margarine
1 tablespoon flour
1/2 cup grated cheddar cheese
Salt and pepper to taste
1/2 cup macaroni

Mix Polycose® powder with 1 to 2 tablespoons of milk and set aside. Melt margarine and blend in flour. Add remaining milk and cook until thickened, stirring constantly. Remove from heat and add cheese, salt, and pepper. Return to heat, stirring until cheese is melted. Remove from heat and beat in Polycose® solution. Cook 1/2 cup of macaroni in boiling salted water until tender. Drain. Mix cheese sauce with macaroni and place in a casserole. Sprinkle with additional grated cheese, if desired. Bake 30 minutes at 350 degrees. Serves 1.

742 calories, 16 grams protein

Vivonex® Grapefruit Drink

8-1/2 oz. water
1 package Vivonex T.E.N.®
4 tablespoons grapefruit Tang®

Mix in a blender and serve over crushed ice. Sip slowly. Serves 1.

300 calories, 6 grams protein

Vivonex® Jell-O®

1 package Vivonex T.E.N.®

1/2 cup Jell-O® powder (any flavor)

1 cup hot water

3/4 cup cold water

Pour cold water into blender. Add hot water plus Vivonex® and blend until dissolved. Add Jell-O® powder and blend until well-mixed. Pour into 4 dessert cups and chill.

75 calories, 4 grams protein per serving

Vivonex® Beef Broth

8-1/2 oz. hot (**not boiling**) beef broth

1 Vivonex® beef flavor packet

1 package Vivonex T.E.N.®

Mix in a blender and serve. Sip slowly. Serves 1.

320 calories, 9 grams protein

---

*Swallowing Training Program Recipes**

Stiff-Jelled Consistency

Stiff-Jelled Fruit

2 jars baby fruit, any kind

1 package (1 tablespoon) Knox® plain unflavored gelatin

2 tablespoons dry Jell-O® powder, any flavor

1/2 cup hot water

Combine Knox® gelatin, Jell-O® powder, and 1/2 cup hot water by whipping. Heat mixture until boiling. Add baby fruit and whip lightly until thoroughly mixed. Refrigerate. Serves 4.

85 calories, 2 grams protein per serving

*These recipes were developed by Caroline Cassens, R.D., Clinical Dietitian, Rose Medical Center, Denver, Colorado, formerly Clinical Dietitian, Leon S. Peters Rehabilitation Center, Fresno Community Hospital, Fresno, California and by Gaylee Amend, M.A., C.C.C., Senior Speech Pathologist, Leon S. Peters Rehabilitation Center, Fresno Community Hospital, Fresno, California.

Stiff-Jelled Yogurt

1 cup plain unflavored yogurt

4 tablespoons dry Jell-O® powder, any flavor

1 package (1 tablespoon) Knox® plain unflavored gelatin

1/2 cup hot water

Combine Knox® gelatin, Jell-O® powder, and 1/2 cup hot water by whipping. Heat mixture until boiling. Add yogurt and whip lightly until thoroughly mixed. Refrigerate. Serves 4.

89 calories, 5 grams protein per serving

Stiff-Jelled Cottage Cheese

1 cup cottage cheese

1 cup orange juice

2 packages (3 tablespoons) Knox® unflavored gelatin

Combine orange juice and gelatin by whipping. Heat mixture until boiling. Pour into a blender and add cottage cheese. Puree until liquid. Strain liquid to remove lumps. Refrigerate. Serves 3.

137 calories, 14 grams protein per serving

Stiff-Jelled Meat

2 jars baby meat, any kind

2 packages (2 tablespoons) Knox® unflavored gelatin

1-1/2 cups evaporated milk

Seasoning as desired

Heat meat in double-boiler. Combine gelatin with cold evaporated milk by whipping and heat until hot. Add meat and mix thoroughly. Add seasoning if desired. Refrigerate. Serves 5.

151 calories, 13 grams protein per serving

Stiff-Jelled Casserole

1 jar baby meat

1 jar baby vegetables

1/2 cup mashed potatoes

1 package (1 tablespoon) Knox® plain unflavored gelatin

1/4 cup hot water

Seasoning

Heat baby meat, baby vegetables, and potatoes together in double-boiler. Combine gelatin and water. Add meat mixture to heated gelatin mixture, whipping constantly. Add seasoning if desired. Refrigerate. Serves 4.

64 calories, 6 grams protein per serving

Stiff-Jelled Vegetables

2 jars baby vegetables

1/2 cup hot water

4 tablespoons Knox® unflavored gelatin

Combine gelatin and water by whipping. Heat mixture until boiling. Add vegetables and whip lightly until thoroughly mixed. Refrigerate. Serves 4.

33 calories, 3 grams protein per serving

Stiff-Jelled Tomato Aspic

2 cups tomato juice

3 tablespoons vinegar

1/2 teaspoon Worcestershire sauce

1/2 teaspoon onion salt

2 packages (2 tablespoons) Knox® plain unflavored gelatin

Combine gelatin and tomato juice by whipping. Add onion salt, vinegar, and Worcestershire sauce and heat until boiling. Refrigerate. Serves 4.

35 calories, 3-1/2 grams protein per serving

Standard-Jelled Consistency

Standard-Jelled Fruit

2 jars baby fruit, any kind

1/2 teaspoon Knox® plain unflavored gelatin

4 tablespoons dry Jell-O® powder, any flavor

1/2 cup hot water

Combine Knox® gelatin, Jell-O® powder and 1/2 cup hot water by whipping. Heat mixture until boiling. Add baby fruit and whip lightly until thoroughly mixed. Refrigerate. Serves 4.

106 calories, 2 grams protein per serving

Standard-Jelled Yogurt

1 cup plain unflavored yogurt

1/2 cup hot water

3 tablespoons dry Jell-O® powder, any flavor

Combine Jell-O® powder and 1/2 cup hot water by whipping. Heat mixture until boiling. Add yogurt and whip lightly until thoroughly mixed. Refrigerate. Serves 4.

70 calories, 3 grams protein per serving

Standard-Jelled Cottage Cheese

1 cup cottage cheese

1 cup orange juice

2 teaspoons Knox® plain unflavored gelatin

Combine orange juice and gelatin by whipping. Heat mixture until boiling. Pour into a blender and add cottage cheese. Puree until liquid. Strain liquid to remove lumps. Refrigerate. Serves 3.

125 calories, 11 grams protein per serving

Standard-Jelled Meat

2 jars baby meat, any kind

3 teaspoons Knox® unflavored gelatin

1-1/2 cups evaporated milk

Seasonings as desired

Heat meat in double-boiler. Combine gelatin in cold evaporated milk by whipping and heat until hot. Add meat and mix thoroughly. Add seasoning if desired. Refrigerate. Serves 5.

146 calories, 11 grams protein per serving

Standard-Jelled Vegetables

2 jars baby vegetables

1/2 cup water

3 teaspoons Knox® unflavored gelatin

Combine gelatin and water by whipping. Heat mixture until boiling. Add vegetables and whip lightly until thoroughly mixed. Refrigerate. Serves 4.

30 calories, 2-1/2 grams protein per serving

Standard-Jelled Tomato Aspic

2 cups tomato juice

4 teaspoons Knox® unflavored gelatin

1/2 teaspoon onion salt

1/2 teaspoon Worcestershire sauce

3 tablespoons vinegar

Combine gelatin and tomato juice by whipping. Add onion salt, vinegar, and Worcestershire sauce and heat until boiling. Refrigerate. Serves 4.

30 calories, 2-1/2 grams protein per serving

Other Foods that may be Served

Regular Jell-O®
Custard
Danish pudding
Baked winter squash

Applesauce Consistency

Thickened Cream Soup

1/2 cup strained cream soup
8 squares saltine crackers, finely crumbled

Stir finely crumbled crackers into soup. Allow thickened soup to stand a few minutes before serving. Serves 1.

125 calories, 3 grams protein per serving

Finely Ground Meat

Grind cooked meat using fine attachment of a meat grinder. If no fine attachment is available, meat may be ground twice using regular attachment. Serve with hot broth or gravy if desired.

NOTE: A meat grinder is required to produce proper consistency. A blender will not produce correct consistency.

Thick Mashed Potatoes

Serve well-mashed but very thick mashed potatoes.

Riced Vegetables

Using a spoon, mash cooked vegetables through coarse sieve or ricer.

NOTE: Carrots, beets, wax beans, green beans, or turnips are the only vegetables that will produce the desired consistency using this recipe. No other vegetables should be used.

Riced Fruit

Pears

Using a spoon, mash pears through a coarse sieve or ricer.

Bananas

Using a fork, mash a banana very finely. May be served covered with a small amount of orange juice.

Applesauce

Canned applesauce may be served with no special preparation.

NOTE: These are the only fruits that will produce the desired consistency. No other fruit should be used.

Blenderized Cottage Cheese and Fruit

1/2 cup cottage cheese

1 jar baby fruit

Blenderize cottage cheese and fruit together until mixture has applesauce consistency. Mixture should not be smooth. Serves 1.

222 calories, 15 grams protein per serving

Other Foods that May be Served

Very thick refined cereal (e.g., Cream of Wheat®, Cream of Rice®, Malt-O-Meal®, Farina).

Plain tapioca pudding.

Thick-Soup Consistency

Thickened Cream Soup

Combine equal amount of strained cream soup and well-mashed potatoes. Mix well. Strain through sieve before serving.

Thick-Soup-Like Pureed Meat

Combine 1/4 cup baby pureed meat or osterized cooked meat and 1/4 cup well-mashed potatoes. Add 2 tablespoons broth. Mix well. Strain through sieve before serving.

Thick-Soup-Like Mashed Potatoes

Combine 1/3 cup mashed potatoes with 1/4 cup warm milk. Mix well. Strain through sieve before serving.

Thick-Soup-Like Pureed Vegetables

Combine 1 jar baby pureed vegetables or osterized cooked vegetables with 1/4 cup strained cream soup or broth. Mix well. Strain through sieve before serving.

Thick-Soup-Like Pureed Fruit

Combine 1 jar baby fruit or osterized canned fruit with 1/4 cup strained fruit juice or strained fruit (such as nectar or apple juice). Mix well. Strain through sieve before serving.

Other Foods that May be Served

Smooth yogurt (plain or without pieces of fruit).
Smooth pudding.

Nectar Consistency

Thin Pureed Meat

Use baby meat or osterized cooked meat. Add broth to the pureed meat until mixture is consistency of nectar. Mixture should pour freely. Strain through sieve before serving.

Thin Mashed Potatoes

Add warm milk to well-mashed potatoes until mixture is consistency of nectar. Mixture should pour freely. Strain through sieve before serving.

Thin Pureed Vegetables

Use baby vegetables or osterized cooked vegetables. Add broth or strained cream soup to pureed vegetables until mixture is consistency of a nectar. Strain through sieve before serving.

Thin Pureed Fruit

Use baby fruit or osterized canned fruits. Add strained fruit juice (such as nectar or apple juice) to pureed fruit until mixture is consistency of a nectar. Strain through sieve before serving.

Other Foods that May be Served

Nectar, any kind.
Tomato juice.
Strained cream soup.
Refined cereal with cream (e.g., Cream of Wheat®, Cream of Rice®, Malt-O-Meal®, or Farina).

Table 1

Protein and Calorie Contents of Common Foods

The following list of the protein and calorie contents of common foods will help you determine your daily protein and calorie intake. It will also help you choose foods high in protein and calories if you need to add more protein and calories to your diet in order to gain weight.

Again, it is important to remember that the need for protein and calories has been emphasized because cancer patients have special needs for them. This is not the case generally; the need for many nutrients in balance (including protein) is the guiding principle for good nutrition. Ask your physician or dietitian for good sources of information.

Protein and calorie contents are calculated for an average serving of the foods listed. You may approximate the protein and calorie contents of foods not listed from similar foods on the list (for instance, all breads will have approximately the same protein and calorie counts; all cheese will have approximately the same counts, etc.).

Description	*Protein*	*Calories*
Beverages		
Beer (12 oz.)	1	151
Coca Cola (12 oz.)	0	144
Coffee (1 cup)	0	3
Eggnog (1 cup whole milk, 1 egg, 3 teaspoons sugar)	15	286
Ginger ale (12 oz.)	0	113
Tea (1 cup)	0	2
Dry Wine (3 oz.)	0	88
Breads and Cereals		
All Bran®, Kellog's (1/2 cup)	3	64
Bagel (1 whole)	4	150
Biscuit, baking powder (2" diameter)	2	129
Bread (1 slice)	2	62
Cornflakes (1 cup)	2	112
Cream of Wheat®, regular (1 cup, cooked)	5	133
Doughnut, plain cake	1	125
Grape-nuts® (1/4 cup)	3	104
Oatmeal, cooked (1 cup)	5	148
Pancake (4" diameter)	3	104
Puffed Rice (1 cup)	1	160
Cereal Products		
Macaroni, cooked (1 cup)	5	151
Noodles, cooked (1 cup)	7	200
Popcorn, plain, popped (1 cup)	2	54
Rice, brown, cooked (1 cup)	4	200
Rice, white, cooked (1 cup)	3	164
Spaghetti, cooked, plain (1 cup)	5	166
Dairy Products		
Butter (1 tablespoon)	0	100
Cheese, American (1 oz., 1 piece)	7	112
Cheese, cottage, creamed (1 cup)	31	240

Description	*Protein*	*Calories*
Cheese, cream (1 oz., 2 tablespoons)	2	105
Cream, half-and-half (1 cup)	8	325
Cream, heavy whipping (1 cup)	5	838
Cream, sour (2 tablespoons)	1	50
Ice cream (3/4 cup)	4	174
Milk, non-fat, fluid (1 cup)	8	88
Milk, non-fat, dry solids (1/4 cup)	10	103
Milk, whole (1 cup)	8	161
Yogurt, plain, made from skim milk (1 cup)	8	122
Desserts		
Cake, angel food (1/12 of cake)	3	140
Cake, pound (1 slice, 3" × 3" × 1/2")	2	123
Cake, white, with icing (1/16 of 10" layer cake)	3	375
Cookie, chocolate chip	1	52
Cookie, oatmeal with raisins	1	50
Cream puff (1 average with cream filling)	4	296
Custard, baked (1/2 cup)	9	205
Jell-O®, plain (1/2 cup)	1	65
Pie, apple (1/6 of 9" pie)	4	404
Pie, Boston cream (1/12 of 8" pie)	3	208
Pudding, chocolate (1/2 cup)	4	219
Pudding, rice with raisins (3/4 cup)	5	212
Pudding, tapioca (1/2 cup)	6	174
Fruits and Fruit Juices		
Apple, raw (1 medium)	0	87
Apple juice (1/2 cup)	0	60
Applesauce (1/2 cup)	0	119
Apricot, canned (4 medium halves)	1	105
Apricot, raw (1)	0	18
Apricot nectar (1/2 cup)	0	65
Avocado (1 half)	2	167

Description	*Protein*	*Calories*
Banana, raw (1 small)	1	185
Grape juice (1/2 cup)	0	100
Grapefruit (1 medium)	1	82
Grapefruit juice (1/2 cup)	1	50
Orange (1 medium)	1	73
Orange juice (1/2 cup)	1	60
Peach, canned (2 medium halves)	1	191
Peach, raw (1 medium)	1	38
Peach nectar (1/2 cup)	1	70
Pineapple, canned (1 large slice)	0	90
Pineapple juice (1/2 cup)	0	60
Prune, stewed (1 cup)	2	300
Prune juice (1/2 cup)	0	100
Raisins (1/2 cup)	2	205
Strawberries, fresh (1 cup)	1	53
Watermelon, balls or cubes (1 cup)	1	42
Protein Foods		
Bacon, broiled or fried (1 strip)	2	48
Beef, ground, broiled (3 oz.)	21	243
Beef, roast, lean (3 oz.)	24	204
Bologna (1 slice)	4	66
Chicken, breast, broiled (3 oz.)	21	110
Egg (1 large)	6	81
Frankfurt, all-beef (1)	7	124
Ham (3 oz.)	15	159
Lamb, loin chop (2.3 oz. trimmed, without bone)	36	230
Sausage, pork (1 link)	4	94
Sole (3 oz.)	14	67
Tofu (soybean curd) (4 oz.)	8	75
Tuna, oil-pack, drained (3-1/2 oz.)	22	147
Turkey, roast (3 oz.)	32	176
Salad Dressings		
Blue cheese, Roquefort (1 tablespoon)	1	71

Description	*Protein*	*Calories*
French (1 tablespoon)	0	57
Italian (1 tablespoon)	0	77
Mayonnaise (1 tablespoon)	0	101
Salad oil (1 tablespoon)	0	100
Thousand Island (1 tablespoon)	0	70
Salads		
Carrot and raisin (1/4 cup)	2	153
Chicken and celery (1/4 cup)	16	185
Coleslaw (1/2 cup)	1	108
Gelatin with chopped vegetables (1 square)	2	115
Lettuce and tomato (4 leaves lettuce, 3 slices tomato)	2	139
Macaroni (1/2 cup)	3	203
Potato (1/2 cup)	2	178
Snack Foods and Sweets		
Almonds (9 to 10 nuts)	2	60
Caramels (1 medium)	0	42
Carrot sticks (3 sticks, 3" × 3/8")	0	13
Cashews, roasted (4 to 5 nuts)	2	56
Chocolate bar (1 oz.)	2	152
Grape jelly (1 tablespoon)	0	50
Jelly beans (10 beans)	0	66
Onion dip, sour cream (3 teaspoons)	1	31
Peanut butter (1 tablespoon)	5	115
Peanuts, roasted (20 to 22 nuts)	5	114
Potato chips (5 chips)	1	54
Pretzel sticks (10 sticks)	0	10
Sugar, white (1 teaspoon)	0	16
Soups		
Asparagus, cream of, Campbell (1 cup)	2	80
Beef broth, Campbell (1 cup)	4	23
Chicken, cream of, Campbell (1 cup)	6	146
Chicken, with matzo balls (1 cup)	3	60

Description	Protein	Calories
Chicken bouillon cubes (1 cube)	1	10
Chicken broth, diluted (1 cup)	2	11
Chicken noodle, Campbell (1 cup)	3	62
Clam chowder, New England, Campbell (1 cup)	8	157
Mushroom, cream of, Campbell (1 cup)	2	131
Onion, Campbell (1 cup)	4	52
Tomato, Campbell (1 cup)	2	79
Vegetable, Campbell (1 cup)	3	64
Vegetables and Vegetable Juices		
Asparagus, cooked (1/2 cup)	2	15
Beans, green, cooked (1/2 cup)	1	16
Beans, lima, cooked (1/2 cup)	6	94
Beets, cooked (1/2 cup)	1	33
Brussels Sprouts, cooked (1/2 cup)	3	30
Cabbage, raw (1 cup shredded)	1	10
Carrots, cooked (1/2 cup)	1	25
Corn, canned (1/2 cup)	3	88
Kale, cooked (1/2 cup)	2	15
Lettuce (1 cup)	1	10
Onions, chopped raw (1/2 cup)	1	33
Peas, black-eyed, cooked (1/2 cup)	8	111
Peas, green, cooked (1/2 cup)	4	58
Pepper, green, raw (1 medium)	1	13
Pickle, dill (1 large)	1	11
Pickle, sweet or mixed (1 pickle)	1	146
Potato, boiled in skin (1 medium)	2	76
Potato, french fried (10 pieces)	2	137
Potato, mashed (1/2 cup)	2	70
Sauerkraut (1/2 cup)	1	15
Soybeans, cooked (1/2 cup)	11	130
Spinach, fresh, cooked (1/2 cup)	3	21
Squash, summer, cooked (1/2 cup)	1	19
Squash, winter, cooked (1/2 cup)	1	50

Description	*Protein*	*Calories*
Sweet potato, baked in skin (1 small)	1	141
Tomato, raw (1 large)	2	33
Tomato juice (1/2 cup)	1	19
Turnip greens, cooked (1/2 cup)	3	28
Vegetable juice cocktail (1/2 cup)	1	17

Table 2
High-Protein Supplements

Product: Citrotein® (Sandoz)
*Calories per liter:** 660
*Protein grams per liter:** 39.9
Powder; mix with water; egg protein derivative; low-residue; lactose-free; orange flavor

Product: Ensure® Ross
*Calories per liter:** 1,060
*Protein grams per liter:** 37.0
Liquid; soy-protein derivative; lactose-free; strawberry, cherry, pecan, orange, lemon flavors, black walnut, chocolate, vanilla, eggnog

Product: Ensure Plus® (Ross)
*Calories per liter:** 1,420
*Protein grams per liter:** 55.0
Liquid; soy-protein drivative; lactose-free; strawberry, cherry, pecan, orange, lemon flavors, chocolate, vanilla

Product: Instant Breakfast (Carnation or Lucerne)
*Calories per liter:** 1,055 (With Whole Milk)
*Protein grams per liter:** 57.0
Powder; mix with milk, milk-protein derivative; chocolate, strawberry, vanilla flavors

*1.1 quart

Product: Meritene® (Sandoz)
*Calories per liter:** 1,000
*Protein grams per liter:** 60.0 (Liquid); 69.0 (Powder with Whole Milk)

Liquid; or powder to be mixed with milk; milk-protein derivative; plain, eggnog, chocolate flavors

Product: Nutri-1000® (Syntex)
*Calories per liter:** 1,000
*Protein grams per liter:** 32.5

Liquid; milk-protein derivative; low-sodium; chocolate and vanilla flavors

Product: Sustacal® (Mead Johnson)
*Calories per liter:** 1,000
*Protein grams per liter:** 61.0

Liquid; milk and soy-protein derivative; high-sodium; chocolate and vanilla flavors

Product: Suscatal HC (Mead Johnson)
*Calories per liter:** 1,500
*Protein grams per liter:** 61.0

Liquid; milk and soy-protein derivative; high-sodium; chocolate and vanilla flavors

Product: Sustagen® (Mead Johnson)
*Calories per liter:** 1,850
*Protein grams per liter:** 113.0

Powder; mix with water; milk-protein derivative; chocolate and vanilla flavors

Product: Osmolite® (Ross)
*Calories per liter:** 1,060
*Protein grams per liter:** 37.0

Liquid; soy-protein derivative; MCT and soy oil; lactose-free, unsweet taste

*1.1 quart

Product: Magnacal® (Sherwood Medical)
*Calories per liter:** 2,000
*Protein grams per liter:** 70.0
Liquid; contains sucrose, caseinates, as protein source, vanilla flavor

Product: Resource® (Sandoz Nutrition)
*Calories per liter:** 1,060
*Protein grams per liter:** 37.0
Liquid; or powder; mix with water or milk in blender; soy-protein derivative; contains sucrose; chocolate and vanilla flavors

Product: Isocal® (Mead Johnson)
*Calories per liter:** 1,060
*Protein grams per liter:** 37.0
Liquid; soy-protein derivative; MCT and soy oil; lactose-free, unsweet taste

---

Table 3
High-Calorie Supplements

Product: Polycose® (Ross)
Calories per tablespoon: 32
*Protein grams per liter:** 0
Liquid; or powder to mix with any food; cornstarch derivative; relatively tasteless

Product: Contolyte® (Sandoz)
Calories per tablespoon: 35
*Protein grams per liter:** 0
Powder; mix with juices; cornstarch derivative

Product: Medium-Chain Triglycerides® (Mead Johnson)
Calories per tablespoon: 115
*Protein grams per liter:** 0
Oil; mix with juices or sauces; for individuals with fat intolerance; given as 1 tablespoon 3 to 4 times per day; recipes available

*1.1 quart

Product: Nutrisource® (Sandoz Nutrition)
Calories per tablespoon: 30
*Protein grams per liter:** 0
Oil; mix with soups or put on vegetables

Table 4
Elemental Diets

Product: Flexical® (Mead Johnson)
*Calories per liter:** 1,000
*Protein grams per liter:** 27.0
Powder; mix with water; casin derivative; very low-residue; lactose-free

Product: Vivonex® (Eaton)
*Calories per liter:** 1,000
*Protein grams per liter:** 20.0
Powder; mix with water; amino-acid derivative; low-residue; lactose-free

Product: Vivonex T.E.N.® (Eaton)
*Calories per liter:** 1,000
*Protein grams per liter:** 41.6
Unflavored highly unpalatable (recommended as tube feeding only); flavored packets available

*1.1 quart

Part II

Advising the Chemotherapy Patient—The Medical Perspective

Introduction to Part II
Nutrition and the Chemotherapy Patient

The Importance of Nutrition

Food preparation and the circumstances of eating are as much psychological as physiological in nature. In fact, food itself can be more beneficial than simply eating, often serving as an expression of love and caring. In this way, food becomes a vehicle of concern, and a medium of expression for cancer patients' caregivers.

On the other hand, inattention to food and feeding means passing over fruitful opportunities for giving aid and comfort. And it is vital that the patient be neither harassed nor manipulated by food. The point is to help the patient keep eating, in whatever way possible, choosing foods that serve critical nutritional needs, and eliminating those that cause discomfort.

Most discussion of nutrition for the cancer patient has addressed the nutritional and metabolic problems that cancer itself causes. Discussion of treatment-related problems usually focuses on nutrition problems related to surgery (which are not necessarily unique to cancer surgery) and, to a lesser extent, radiotherapy.

Detailed material on nutrition and chemotherapy is still relatively scarce, despite its obvious importance—since chemotherapy drugs can influence both dietary intake and the body's use and elimination of nutrients. The converse of this relationship—how the patient's nutritional status can influence the therapeutic benefits of the chemotherapy and the likelihood of developing drug toxicities—has also, up to now, gone relatively untreated.

This book represents an effort to fill both gaps in the clinical literature. It will also provide the practical information about food and eating the patient on chemotherapy needs in order to apply the basic principles.

The Healthcare Team

The specific dietary recommendations and recipes in this book will show directly that many drug side effects can be reduced or controlled by dietary means. Clearly, nutrition can play a central role in the care of the patient on chemotherapy.

But who should make the nutritional assessment, offer dietary advice, and oversee the shaping of the diet to meet the patient's specific needs? Ideally, a qualified dietitian should be working with the attending oncologist, but where no dietitian is available, nutritional assessment, counseling, and diet planning fall to nurse or physician. This book is designed to assist the practitioner in guiding patients on chemotherapy and those involved in their meal-planning to best choose and tolerate foods that will make the chemotherapy treatment as successful as possible.

Prescribing for the Patient

It is recommended that the medical practitioner read the parts of Part II that pertain to a particular patient, and create a specific nutrition plan, using the "Nutrition Prescription" forms provided in the Appendix. Patients and their caregivers will then use the recommendations of their medical advisors to select the portions of Part I that are of greatest importance to them.

Nutritional Assessment

In clinical practice as in the literature, nutrition is often neglected. The assessment of nutritional status, not only of patients about to begin chemotherapy, but of most cancer patients, is generally quite casual. Often, patients are judged "well-developed," "well-nourished," or "poorly-nourished" on the basis of a quick glance, a mental estimate of body fat stores, and data on possible recent weight loss or dehydration.

What is usually missed with such a "once-over" approach is that beneath the layer of body fat that may contribute to a well-nourished appearance, the patient may have lost significant lean-body mass. Further, where there are no overt signs of vitamin deficiency, such as cheilosis, glossitis, or hyperkeratosis, the physician making the quick assessment usually assumes the vitamin status to be normal. In fact, the patient's vitamin status (particularly in the case of an elderly patient) is often marginal at best.

In addition to influencing dietary intake, drugs can affect the assimilation of nutrients in a wide variety of ways—altering, for example, intestinal absorption, plasma binding and transport, peripheral utilization, transport across membranes, intercellular reactions, storage in tissues, and turnover rates in the liver.

The Importance of Patient Involvement

Of great if not equal importance for nutritional well-being is the opportunity here for involving the patient in his or her own care through nutritional counseling and education. The short-term goal is to enhance the patient's ability to tolerate and respond to the medical treatment; but the ultimate objective is to enhance recovery, reduce convalescent time, and generally to improve chances of a long and healthy life.

The patient should be made aware that when chemotherapy is successful (e.g., partial or complete remission has been achieved), the physical effects of the disease are usually reduced or disappear, and that ultimately the goal of physical and nutritional support is to permit the body to repair itself. Thus ideally, the patient's commitment to sound nutrition will be a permanent one.

Personal Considerations and Treatment

All individualized nutrition care plans must address several factors:

- The patient's energy (calorie) and nutrient requirements determined by age, sex, usual weight, and baseline nutritional status prior to the commencement of chemotherapy, plus the anticipated type and duration of drug treatment.
- The patient's food tolerance as determined by his or her sense of taste and ability to ingest, absorb, and utilize the required nutrients and calories.
- The administration route,* and attendant nutritional considerations required by the particular type of cancer involved and the patient's clinical condition.

*The physician or dietitian's decision to use parenteral vs. enteral administration routes is subject to change and requires frequent reevaluation. Parenteral routes are expensive and generally should be used *only* when the outcome for remission, cure, and high quality of life is deemed good. Other considerations are capability of gut to digest and absorb nutrients, food particle size introduced via enteral route, and the nutrient balance. With both enteral and parenteral materials, the risk of complications, such as overhydration, dehydration, and infection must also be addressed. This book does not address parenteral routes of administration; for detailed discussions see, for example, S. Klein, et al. "Total Parenteral Nutrition and Cancer Trials," *Cancer* 58:1378-86, 1986; M.F. Brennan. "Total Parenteral Nutrition in the Cancer Patient," *New Eng. J. Med.* 305:373, 1981; P.N. Benotti, A. Bothe, Jr., J.O.B. Miller, et al. "Safe Cannulation of the Int. jugular vein for long-term hyperalimentation," *Surg, Gynecol. Obstet.* 144:574-576, 1977; Ang. S. and Daly, J.M. "Potential Complications and Monitoring of Patients Receiving Vital Parenteral Nutrition" in Ranbean, J. and Caldwell, R.: *Parenteral Nutrition*, Philadelphia, W.B. Saunders, 331-343, 1986.

These factors will all affect the patient's willingness and/or ability to eat the amounts and types of foods needed. To ensure that they are addressed, the customized diet plans will reflect the patient's particular caloric and nutrient requirements, particular food tolerances, clinical condition, and prognosis.

Energy and Protein Needs

Both the disease and the circumstances of treatment may be causing metabolic and/or mechanical problems for the cancer patient facing chemotherapy. For example, the patient might still be recovering from surgery or might be recovering from or receiving radiotherapy when the chemotherapy treatments begin.

Whatever the attendant circumstances, however, all cancer patients are under psychological and physiological stress. In most cases their energy and nutrient needs are greater than normal.

A healthy adult generally requires 25 to 30 kilocalories per kilogram of body weight per day. However, the average cancer patient under stress may need 35 to 45 kilocalories per kilogram per day.

The stress of chemotherapy also may increase protein requirements to greater-than-normal levels, of perhaps 1.5 grams to 2 grams of protein per kilogram of body weight per day.

Serum albumin measurement can provide a helpful index of protein status.[1] A major protein synthesized by the liver, albumin has a half-life of 17 days and an exchangeable pool of 4 gm to 5 gm per kg of body weight. When stressed, a person's extravascular albumin is utilized first, preserving intravascular albumin levels until late in the depletion phase. (Normal serum albumin is 3.5 gm/dl.) Hence, a low albumin reflects a *chronic* not short-term, protein-deficiency.[2] Generally, a serum albumin of 2.8 gm/dl to 3.2 gm/dl reflects mild visceral protein depletion, and a concentration of less than 2.1 gm/dl demonstrates severe depletion (exhibited by a wasting of extremities and skin).

Transferrin, a globulin, transports plasma iron. It may be measured to assess short-term protein changes, since it has a half-life of 8 to 10 days and a plasma pool of only 5.2 gm (normal serum transferrin is 200 mg/dl to 400 mg/dl).[3] A transferrin level of 150 mg/dl to 200 mg/dl reflects mild visceral depletion and less than 100 mg/dl shows a severe deficit.

An important index of nutrition-protein status—metabolic rate, or resting energy expenditure—may be measured via oxygen consumption. Oxygen consumption declines with lean body mass losses in a linear fashion.[4] Oxygen consumption may vary somewhat with stress,[5] exhibited by an increase of about 30% in O_2 consumption, and of about 55% in CO_2 production. When measured with albumin and transferrin, oxygen consumption can provide good information about protein and calorie requirements.

Cancer patients under stress also have difficulty maintaining a positive nitrogen balance. Encouraging high protein intakes during chemotherapy treatment may help preserve nitrogen balance and support lean body mass. (However, some loss of lean body mass is inevitable.)

Nutrient Composition of the Diet

Although the approach in this book is to customize diet plans to meet patients' individual needs, it is possible to generalize to some degree about the nutritional composition of a diet suitable for cancer patients facing chemotherapy. For example 50% to 60% or more of the total calories should come from carbohydrates, particularly when, as is often the case, fat is poorly tolerated.

Ample carbohydrate generates energy while allowing protein to be spared for the synthesis of tissue—daily protein consumption should reach 1.5 grams to 2.0 grams per kilogram of body weight per day (assuming normal renal function), providing 15% to 20% of the total calories from protein sources.

In some cases, simple sugars may be the best carbohydrate source, since they require less digestion than the complex carbohydrates. As an alternative, where chemotherapy is distorting the taste of foods and "over or under-sweetening" them, a glucose polymer (Polycose BR) added to foods or liquids can serve as an acceptable alternative to simple sugars in the diet.

Dietary fats should compose 20% to 30% of total caloric intake, with saturated, monounsaturated, and polyunsaturated fat present in approximately equal amounts. If fat is tolerated, the concentrated energy provided by this source offers a ready supply of additional calories for underweight, underfat patients. (If the patient does not tolerate long-chain triglycerides well—that is, if steatorrhea is present—medium-chain triglycerides may be substituted.)

Source	*Percent of Total Calories*	*Food Choices*
Carbohydrates	50–60	Grains, cereals, fruits, vegetables, sugars
Protein	15–20	Meat, poultry, fish, eggs, dairy products
Fat	20–30	Oil, butter, margarine, gravies, etc.

Under normal circumstances, a variety of nutrient-dense foods provides ample vitamins and minerals, without the need for supplements. However, some cancer patients may require more than the Recommended Dietary Allowance of specific micronutrients (see Chapter 2, General Dietary Guidelines 3 and 4, pp. 45–57), especially if they are borderline nutrient-deficient.

During convalescence especially, the diet should emphasize vitamin balance and replacement of vitamins and minerals lost as a result of treatment side effects, such as vomiting and diarrhea. But vitamin and mineral supplements must be prescribed with great care, especially as to amount, timing and frequency of intake, to protect against potential toxicities and interference with the effectiveness of the chemotherapy.

Hydration

Too often dehydration is overlooked during chemotherapy. Losses of fluids owing to vomiting and diarrhea can increase fluid requirements to 3 liters or more per day. Increased fluids can help prevent urinary tract infections, hemorrhagic cystitis, and the renal lithiasis that can result from treatment with some drugs (e.g., Cis-Platinum® or Cytoxan®).

Oncologists are aware of, and responsive to the patient's need for ample hydration during chemotherapy, but all those involved in the patient's dietary planning and preparation need to be concerned with the increased fluid requirements as well. The patients themselves need education and encouragement in this area, since it is they who must consume the extra fluids.

Nutrient Drug Interrelationships and Drug Toxicities

Many chemotherapy drugs directly or indirectly affect the appetite, taste, or other factors relating to the perception of hunger. In a physiological context, the term *hunger* is understood to be a composite signal sent by the body to the brain when energy intake is needed. *Appetite*, on the other hand, is the psychological desire to eat, and it can override the body's hunger signals. Appetite remains a very complex and poorly understood subject.

Anorexia, as the term is used with respect to cancer, refers to a decreased desire for and intake of food. In this context, it is usually attributable to a lack of appetite, but it may have physiological components as well. Anorexia among cancer patients has been studied in detail, but its causes have still not been fully identified. Some theories suggest an aberration of gluco-receptor binding in the hunger and satiety centers of the hypothalamus, or defective or blocked signals in the appetite center of the brain.[4] Altered levels of lactate or blood amino acids may also contribute to anorexia.[5]

In this book, *anorexia* will be used to mean a decreased food intake, irrespective of whether the cause is psychological, physiological, or a combination of both. *Appetite* will simply refer to a desire for food.

In addition to cancer itself, some chemotherapy drugs have been associated with otherwise unexplained anorexia—examples are methotrexate, 5-fluorouracil (5-FU), and cyclophosphamide (Cytoxan®). Estrogens may also reduce appetite. On the other hand, androgens (which are anabolic), corticosteroids (which are catabolic), and progestins (which are usually neither) may stimulate appetite.

Chemotherapy-induced stomatitis (ulceration in and around the mouth) may lead to anorexia. Many of the drugs—for example 5-FU, methotrexate, chlorambucil (Leukeran®), nitrogen mustard or dactinomycin—induce stomatitis and mucositis, making swallowing difficult and painful. Others, such as steroids, cause dry mouth or dysphagia (difficulty in swallowing), and many, for example, dactinomycin, 5-FU, and methotrexate, cause malabsorption and early satiety, all of which lead to reduced food intake. Also there are times where anorexia is protracted and depression seems to play a role, where antidepressants may help the patient eat more, and increase his or her food intake.

Almost all drugs used in cancer chemotherapy can eventually lead to weight loss because of reduced food intake, enhanced nutrient turnover, and nutrient loss. But some drugs, particularly the steroids, can mask weight loss by causing edema. Therefore, in monitoring the effects of the drugs, you should not use weight or appearance as the only parameters. Again, measuring albumin, transferrin, and oxygen consumption, and simple anthropometrics—using Harbendon skinfold calipers—are all useful in assessing lean-fat body mass changes.

There are other common physiologic changes to look for: most chemotherapy drugs are toxic to the bone marrow and cause temporary marrow hypoplasia; methotrexate may cause megablastic anemia by interrupting folate and vitamin B_{12} function, particularly for the patient who is marginally nourished initially; and the steroids and other drugs may cause iron deficiency anemia owing to gastrointestinal bleeding. (Some, though not all of these anemias can be influenced by nutritional intervention.)

Parameters for Assessing Nutritional Status

Weight
Weight change
Percent of usual body weight
Serum albumin
Serum transferrin
Oxygen consumption (resting energy expenditure)
Anthropometric measurements

Nutritional Assessments

It is important to convey the fact that **not all patients necessarily experience all, or even any, of the common side effects** associated with the chemotherapy drugs. Nor should the oncologist, nurse, or dietitian assume that such problems will arise. Still, on-going evaluations are necessary, beginning with a thorough nutritional assessment before chemotherapy begins.

If the patient has nutritional problems going into chemotherapy, chemotherapy can be expected to compound these problems; but even if a patient's status is good, the medical team should emphasize the importance of maintaining a healthful, well-balanced diet. And once chemotherapy has begun, if the patient develops signs and symptoms of nutritional problems or cannot eat adequately, therapeutic dietary interventions become essential.

The specifics of these interventions are found in the related nutritional recommendations in Chapters One and Two, but in general the goal is to meet the patient's increased calorie and protein requirements (for the adult, 35 to 45 kilocalories and 1.5 grams to 2.0 grams of protein per kilogram of body weight per day). This means encouraging the patient to eat nutrient-dense (high nutrient/calorie ratio), high-calorie, high-protein foods.

References

1. Arbeit, J.M., et al. "Resting Energy Expenditure in Controls and Cancer Patients With Localized and Diffuse Disease." *Ann. Surg*, 199:292-297, 1984.
2. Blackburn, G.L., et al. "Nutritional and Metabolic Assessment of the Hospitalized Patient." *JPEN*, 1:11-22, 1977.
3. Bradley, J., Nass, S. Nutrition of the Cancer Patient: Knowing the Four Major Food Groups is Not Enough. Nutritional Research Consultants, Publisher, 1988.
4. Brennan, M.F. Total parenteral nutrition in the cancer patient. *New Engl. J. Med.* 305:373, 1981.
5. Brennan, M.F. Uncomplicated starvation versus cancer cachexia. *Cancer Res.* 37:2359, 1977.
6. Brinson, R., Kolts, B. "Hypoalbuminemia as an indicator of diarrheal incidence in critically ill patients." *Crit. Care Med.* 15(5):506-509, 1987.
7. Burt, M.E., Gorschboth, C., Brennan, M.F. A controlled prospective randomized trial evaluating the metabolic effects of enteral and parenteral nutrition in the cancer patient. *Cancer* 49:1249, 1982.
8. Council on Scientific Affairs. "Vitamin Preparations as Dietary Supplements and as Therapeutic Agents." *JAMA*, 257:1929-1936, 1987.
9. Dairy Council Digest. "Nutrition and the Immune Response." Vol. 56, No. 2, March/April 1985.
10. DeWys, W.D., Berg, C., Lavin, P.T., et al. Prognostic effect of weight loss prior to chemotherapy in cancer patients. *Am. J. Med.* 69:491, 1980.
11. Dodd, M. Managing Side effects of Chemotherapy and Radiation Therapy: A Guide for Nurses and Patients. Appleton and Lange, 1987.
12. Heber, D. "Malnutrition in Cancer." *Nutrition and the M.D.* 15(7):1-5, 1989.

13. Ingenbleck, Y., et al. "Albumin, Transferrin and the Thyroxin Binding Prealbumin, Retinol Binding Protein Complex in Assessment of Malnutrition." *Clin. Chim. Acta* 61:673, 1975.

14. Klein, S., et al. Total parenteral nutrition and cancer clinical trials. *Cancer* 58:1378-86, 1986.

15. Long, C.L., et al. "Metabolic Response to Injury and Illness: Estimation of Energy and Protein Needs from Indirect Calorimetry and Nitrogen Balance." *JPEN* 3:452, 1979.

16. Mann, S., et al. "Measured and Predicted Caloric Expenditure in the Acutely Ill." *Crit. Care Med.* 13:173, 1985.

17. National Cancer Institute, the National Library of Medicine, cancer information, supportive care (anticipatory nausea and vomiting, constipation, oral complication of cancer therapy, and radiation enteritis).

18. NIH Consensus, Development Conference. "Oral Complications of Cancer Therapies—Diagnosis, Prevention, and Treatment," pp. 17-19, 1989.

19. PDQ. Physician Data Query, 1990.

20. Rothchild, M.A., Oratz, M., and Schreiber, S.S. "Albumin Metabolism." *Gastroenterology* 64:326, 1973.

21. Shatzkin, A., et al. "The Dietary Fat—Breast Cancer Hypothesis is Alive." *JAMA* 261(22):3284-3287, 1989.

22. Shaw, J. "Influence of stress, depletion, and/or malignant disease or the responsiveness of surgical patients to total parenteral nutrition." *Am. J. Clin. Nut.* 98:144-147, 1988.

23. Shetty, P.S., et al. "Rapid Turnover Transport Proteins: An Index of Subclinical Protein-Energy Malnutrition." *Lancet* 2:230, 1979.

24. Shike, M., Berner, Y.N., Gerdes, H., et al. Percutaneous endoscopic gastrostomy and jejunostomy for long-term enteral feeding in patients with cancer of the head and neck. *Otolaryngology-Head and Neck Surg.*, 1989.

25. Shike, M., Brennan, M.F. "Nutritional Support," in *Cancer: Principles and Practice of Oncology 3rd Edition*, eds V.T. DeVita, Jr., S. Hellman, S. Rosenberg. J.B. Lippincott & Co., Philadelphia, pp. 2029-2044, 1989.

26. Shike, M., Russell, D., McR, Detsky, A.S., et al. Changes in body composition in patients with small-cell lung cancer: The effect of TPN as an adjunct for chemotherapy. *Ann Intern Med.* 101:303, 1984.

27. Shike, M., Schroy, P., Ritchie, M.A., et al. Percutaneous endoscopic jejunostomy in cancer patients with previous gastric resection. *Gastrointestinal Endoscopy* 33:372-374, 1987.

28. Shils, M.E. Effects of nutrition on surgery of the liver, pancreas and genourinary tract. *Cancer Res.* 37:2387, 1977.

29. Silberman, H., Eisenberg, D. Parenteral and Enteral Nutrition in the Hospitalized Patient. Appleton-Century-Crofts, Norwalk, Connecticut, 1982.

30. Silver, C. "Elemental Diet and TPN as Treatment Against Radiation Injury of the Bowel." *Nutritional Support Services* 8(1):36-40, 1988.

31. Taber's Cyclopedic Medical Dictionary, 15th Edition. F.A. Davis Company, Philadelphia, 1985.

Chapter Four

Description of Chemotherapeutic Drugs

Robert J. Ignoffo, Pharm.D.
Janet L. Ramstack, Dr.P.H.
Ernest H. Rosenbaum, M.D.

Adrenocorticosteroids
Allopurinol
Aminoglutethimide
Androgens
Asparaginase
Bleomycin
Busulfan
Carboplatin
Carmustine
Chlorambucil
Cisplatin
Cyclophosphamide
Cytarbine
Dacarbazine
Dactinomycin
Daunorubicin
Doxorubicin
Dronabinol
Estramustine
Estrogens
Etoposide
Fluourouracil/ Floxuridine
Flutamide
Hydroxurea
Ifosfamide
Interferon
Leucovorin
Lomustine
Leuprolide
Mechlorethamine
Melphalan
Mercaptopurine
Mesna
Methotrexate
Mitomycin C
Mitotane
Mitoxantrone
Octreotide
Plicamycin
Procarbazine
Progestins
Streptozocin
Tamoxifen
Thioguanine
Triethylenethio-phosphoramide
Vinblastine
Vincristine

- **Adrenocorticosteroid**
- **Prednisone**
- **Prednisolone**
- **Dexamethasone** (Burroughs Wellcome)

Nutritionally Significant Side Effects

Peptic ulceration
Altered taste and smell
Abdominal discomfort
Hypocalcemia
Electrolyte imbalance
Edema
Protein catabolism
Nausea and vomiting
Esophagitis
Diabetes
Pancreatitis
Increased appetite
Hypertension

Properties and Use in Treatment

The adrenocorticosteroids have both anti-inflammatory (glucocorticoid), salt-retaining (mineralocorticoid) and antiproliferative properties. The synthetic steroid compounds, such as prednisone, prednisolone, and dexamethasone, are used primarily in cancer patients for their anti-proliferative effects.

Prednisone and prednisolone are given orally in the treatment of acute or chronic lymphocytic leukemia, breast cancer, multiple myeloma, Hodgkin's disease, and non-Hodgkin's lymphomas. Dexamethasone has been administered orally, intramuscularly, or intravenously for the treatment of multiple myeloma or brain tumors, and also as an antinausea drug.

General Toxicities

Large doses of hydrocortisone or cortisone can cause sodium retention, resulting in edema, heart failure, and hypertension; potassium loss, which may produce muscle weakness; and reduced glucose tolerance, which may result in steroid-induced diabetes mellitus. These effects are less likely to occur with the synthetic derivatives, except when used in large doses. The sodium-retaining effects of dexamethasone are minimal.

Abrupt discontinuation of corticosteroid after prolonged therapy (greater than 2 weeks) can result in a withdrawal syndrome consisting of fever, hypotension, malaise, hyperkalemia, and weakness. Other symptoms may include such nutritional effects as anorexia, nausea, vomiting, diarrhea, and weight loss. Fatigue, weakness, dizziness, and low blood sugar can also be experienced.

Interactions with Other Drugs

Numerous drug interactions can occur, including enhanced potassium depletion caused by amphotericin-B, ethacrynic acid, furosemide, and thiazide diuretics. Additionally, the corticosteroid may increase circulating glucose levels, necessitating the dose adjustment of oral hypoglycemic agents. Several agents, including barbiturates, phenytoin, and rifampin can increase the metabolism of corticosteroid which can require an increase in corticosteroid dosage.

Food-Drug Interactions

It is recommended that corticosteroid be given with antacids one hour before or two to three hours after a full meal or during fasting. If antacids are contraindicated, the drug can be given with a moderate amount of starchy food, such as bread or crackers, that will quickly clear the stomach and not interfere with drug absorption.The drug should be given at the same time each day, during daytime hours, though some regimens call for alternative-day dosing to minimize adrenal insufficiency. Most programs favor administration in the morning, to imitate the body's own production time for hormones.

Notes on Nutritional Side Effects

Peptic ulceration—The cause-and-effect relationship between peptic ulceration and glucocorticoid therapy is unclear. However, physicians routinely prescribe antacids or H2-antagonists prophylactically with these drugs. However, some antacids have a high sodium content and may also cause hypophosphatemia (low phosphate levels). Magnesium containing antacids may cause diarrhea.

Altered taste and smell—Corticosteriod may cause altered taste or smell sensation which leads to decreased threshold to bitterness and sweetness. Dietary means are available to help cope with this problem.

Nausea and vomiting—Corticosteroids may cause gastric dyspepsia through stimulation of acid secretion in the stomach leading to nausea and vomiting. Relief may sometimes be obtained from the prophylactic administration of antiemetic drugs.

Esophagitis—This is rare, but when it occurs it can be severe enough to cause bleeding and ulceration, with resultant iron loss. Swallowing may become difficult. A soft, blenderized diet may be needed.

Abdominal discomfort—If the problem is severe enough to interfere with nutritional intake, a low residue diet may be warranted.

Diabetes—These drugs can increase the needs of diabetics for insulin or oral hypoglycemic agents or induce overt diabetes in prediabetic or subclinical patients. Blood glucose levels should be monitored routinely.

Hypocalcemia (low blood calcium)—Prolonged use of corticosteroid can lead to reduced calcium absorption, which may contribute to osteoporosis. Supplementation with calcium and vitamin D_3 may be necessary in some instances. On the other hand, the generally mild hypocalcemic effect of glucocorticoid can sometimes be used to control hypercalcemia from cancer metastases.

Pancreatitis, electrolyte imbalance, increased appetite, weight gain, edema, hypertension—Such symptoms require routine monitoring of levels. Dietary sodium restriction and potassium supplementation may be necessary.

Protein catabolism—Because corticosteroids are catabolic, they may lead to loss of muscle tissue. A liberal protein intake is essential during prolonged corticosteroid therapy.

Refer patients, as needed, to:

Chapter One: How to Deal with Specific Problems
Problem 1—Loss of Appetite, page 4
Problem 2—Nausea and Vomiting, page 8
Problem 3—Taste Changes, page 12
Problem 4—Sore or Ulcerated Mouth and Throat (Stomatitis/Mucositis), page 14
Problem 7—Protecting the Gastrointestinal Tract (Enteritis), page 22
Problem 9—Dehydration, page 26

Chapter Two: General Dietary Guidelines
Guideline 1—Basic Nutrition for the Cancer Patient, page 30
Guideline 2—A High-Protein/High-Calorie Diet, page 38
Guideline 3—Food Sources of Minerals, page 45
Guideline 4—Food Sources of Vitamins, page 52
Guideline 5—The Fiber and Residue Contents of Foods, page 58
Guideline 11—Transient Glucose Intolerance/Diabetic Diet, page 76
Guideline 12—A Sodium-Restricted Diet, page 79
Guideline 14—A Soft-Food/Pureed-Food Diet, page 86

- **Allopurinol**
- **Allopurinol tablets** (Barr, Danbury, Geneva, Lederle, Par)
- **Lopurin** (Boots)
- **Zyloprim®** (Burroughs Wellcome)

Nutritionally Significant Side Effects

Anorexia
Nausea and vomiting

Properties and Use in Treatment

Allopurinol is not an antineoplastic (cancer) drug although it was originally synthesized as one. It was found to lack antimetabolite activity. As a structural analogue of hypoxanthine, a natural purine base, allopurinol inhibits the terminal steps in the biosynthesis of uric acid. This drug is very commonly prescribed for the prevention and treatment of hyperuricemia secondary to antineoplastic therapy. Allopurinol is administered orally and is 90 percent absorbed from the gastrointestinal tract.

Hyperuricemia secondary to antineoplastic therapy is caused by the rapid destruction of cells by the chemotherapeutic drugs. The high uric acid levels can result in gout, a disease characterized by the deposition of urate in the tissues, particularly the joints and kidneys. Allopurinol works by inhibiting the formation of uric acid, resulting in a decrease in both the serum and urinary uric acid levels.

Allopurinol is not an innocuous drug, and its use should be discontinued after the potential for the overproduction of uric acid is abated. However, use of allopurinol is generally preferable to the alternative of prescribing a low-protein diet for the patient in cancer treatment.

General Toxicities

The initial use of allopurinol may result in an acute attack of gout in less than 1 percent of patients. This may require concomitant administration of colchicine or an antiinflammatory agent. It is important to maintain a fluid intake sufficient to yield a daily urinary output of at least two liters with a neutral or slightly alkaline urine to prevent uric acid kidney stones. It is highly recommended that the patient with symptoms of gout be counseled and monitored throughout allopurinol therapy by an oncology nutritionist or dietitian familiar with the needs of the cancer patient and the treatment of hyperuricemia. An alkaline ash diet may be necessary.

The most frequent adverse reaction to allopurinol (occurring in fewer than 1 percent of patients) is skin rash. Skin reactions can be severe and sometimes fatal. Treatment with allopurinol should be discontinued immediately if a rash develops.

Other possible side effects causally related to allopurinol therapy and occurring in 1 to 3 percent of patients include ecchymosis, fever, headache, necrotizing angiitis, vasculitis, hepatic necrosis, granulomatous hepatitis, hepatomegaly, hyperbilirubinemia, cholestatic jaundice, intermittent abdominal pain, gastritis, dyspepsia, thrombocytopenia, eosinophilia, leukocytosis, leukopenia, myopathy, arthralgias, peripheral neuropathy, neuritis, paresthesia, somnolence, epistaxis, erythema multiform exudativum (Stevens-Johnson syndrome), toxic epidermal neurolysis (Lyell's syndrome), hypersensitivity vasculitis, purpura, vesicular bullous dermatitis, exfoliative dermatitis, eczematoid dermatitis, pruritus, urticaria, alopecia, onycholysis, lichen panus, taste loss or perversion, renal failure, and uremia.

Adverse reactions of which the causal relationships are unknown and occurring in fewer than 1 percent of patients, include general malaise, pericarditis, peripheral vascular disease, thrombophlebitis, bradycardia vasodilation, infertility (male), hypercalcemia, gynecomastia (male), hemorrhagic pancreatitis, gastrointestinal bleeding, salivary gland swelling, hyperlipidemia, tongue edema, aplastic anemia, agranulocytosis, eosinophilic fibrohistiocytic lesion of bone marrow, pancytopenia, prothrombin decrease, anemia, hemolytic anemia, reticulocytosis, lymphadenopathy, lymphocytosis, myalgia, optic neuritis, confusion, dizziness, vertigo, food drop, decrease in libido, depression, amnesia, tinnitus, asthenia, insomnia, bronchospasm, asthma, pharyngitis, rhinitis, furunculosis, facial edema, sweating, skin edema, cataracts, macular retinitis, iritis, conjunctivitis, amblyopia, nephritis, impotence, primary hematuria, and albuminuria.

Interactions with Other Drugs

The pharmacologic effects of oral mercaptopurine (e.g., 6-mercaptopurine) are increased by allopurinol. Bone-marrow depression (leukopenia, thrombocytopenia, and anemia) may occur. The onset is delayed and the severity is major. The dose of mercaptopurine should be decreased by 75 percent of the usual dose.

The bone-marrow toxicity of cyclophosphamide may also be increased by allopurinol. The onset is delayed and the severity is moderate.

Certain risks may be associated with the concomitant use of allopurinol and dicumarol, sulfinpyrazone, mercaptopurine, azathioprine, ampicillin, amoxicillin, and thiazide diuretics.

Notes on Nutritional Side Effects

Anorexia—Anorexia has been noted as a side effect of this drug, resulting in reduced food intake. Dietary measures can help to increase appetite.

Nausea and vomiting—Nausea and vomiting occur in fewer than 1 percent of patients and may be ameliorated by antiemetic agents. Starchy foods taken with the drug may minimize nausea, and other dietary measures can mitigate the aftereffects of vomiting and lessen residual nausea.

If nausea and vomiting are a problem, favorite foods should not be ingested prior to the administration of allopurinol because a conditioned food aversion may result.

Refer patients, as needed, to:

Chapter One: How to Deal with Specific Problems
Problem 1—Loss of Appetite, page 4
Problem 2—Nausea and Vomiting, page 8
Problem 9—Dehydration, page 26

Chapter Two: General Dietary Guidelines

- **Aminoglutethimide**
- **Cytadren®** (CIBA)

Nutritionally Significant Side Effects

Anorexia
Nausea and vomiting
Constipation

Properties and Use in Treatment

Aminoglutethimide is an inhibitor of steroid synthesis and is indicated for the suppression of adrenal function in selected patients with Cushing's syndrome. Because the drug does not affect the underlying disease process, it is primarily used as an interim measure until more definitive therapy, such as surgery, can be undertaken or in cases where such therapy is inappropriate. It is administered orally.

Aminoglutethimide inhibits the aromatase enzyme involved in steroidogenesis, essentially causing a reversible chemical "adrenalectomy." The drug blocks synthesis of all steroid hormones and interferes with the conversion of androgens to estrogens. Consequently, replacement corticosteroid (hydrocortisone 20-30 mg daily by mouth) is required. It is primarily used to treat metastatic breast and prostate carcinoma and unresponsive adrenal carcinoma.

General Toxicities

The most common side effect of aminoglutethimide is a self-limiting rash. If the rash is severe, steroids, benadryl and drug discontinuation may be necessary. Transient lethargy—found most often in the elderly—is an acute toxicity and includes severe somnolence, visual blurring, and dizziness. Hypothyroidism, with goiter, may occur and is indicated by obesity, sluggishness, dry skin and hair, and constipation.

Less common side effects include anemia; adrenal insufficiency, masculinization and hirsutism in females; precocious sexual development in males; headache; hypotension; tachycardia; pruritus; fever; and myalgia. Neutropenia, leukopenia, pancytopenia, agranulocytosis, reduced hemoglobin levels and hematocrit, and hepatotoxicity have been known to occur rarely.

Interactions with Other Drugs

The metabolism of dexamethasone is increased by aminoglutethimide, necessitating the use of supraphysiologic doses of dexamethasone (usually 3 mg daily). No interaction has been observed with hydrocortisone. Aminoglutethimide also reduces the effect of coumarin and warfarin, requiring dose adjustment and close monitoring of prothrombin time.

Food-Drug Interactions

Full meals may delay and change the absorption of this orally administered drug with respect to both the rate of absorption and peak serum concentrations. Complete absorption by the oral route is particularly questionable if the patient is concurrently receiving drugs that are toxic to the gastrointestinal tract.

To promote maximal absorption, aminoglutethimide should not be taken with full meals or with fatty foods that delay absorption. It is recommended that the drug be administered one hour before or two to three hours after a full meal. Taking the drug on an empty stomach may engender nausea and other stomach disturbances. It should be taken along with a starchy food, such as bread or crackers, in order to clear the stomach quickly and not interfere with drug absorption. The drug should be taken at the same time(s) each day.

Notes on Nutritional Side Effects

Anorexia—Loss of appetite is an infrequent side effect of this drug. The cause is not clear, but the result is reduced food intake. Dietary measures can help increase appetite.

Nausea and vomiting—Mild nausea and vomiting occur infrequently and may be ameliorated by antiemetic agents. Starchy foods taken with the drug may minimize nausea, and other dietary measures can mitigate the aftereffects of vomiting and lessen residual nausea.

If nausea and vomiting are a problem, favorite foods should not be ingested prior to the administration of aminoglutethimide because a conditioned food aversion may result.

Constipation—Aminoglutethimide-induced hypothyroidism may lead to constipation which often does not respond to standard bowel stimulants. Laxatives such as mineral oil may cause nutritional depletion and may be habit forming. Laxatives are discouraged because they prevent the absorption of fat-soluble vitamins in the gut. Constipation is probably best treated by dietary measures when these are not contraindicated.

Refer patients, as needed, to:

Chapter One: How to Deal with Specific Problems
Problem 1—Loss of Appetite, page 4
Problem 2—Nausea and Vomiting, page 8
Problem 8—Constipation, page 24

Chapter Two: General Dietary Guidelines
Guideline 1—Basic Nutrition for the Cancer Patient, page 30
Guideline 2—A High-Protein/High-Calorie Diet, page 38
Guideline 3—Food Sources of Minerals, page 45
Guideline 4—Food Sources of Vitamins, page 52
Guideline 5—The Fiber and Residue Contents of Foods, page 58

- **Androgens** (Testosterone®)
- **Fluoxymesterone** (Halotestin®, Upjohn)
- **Methyltestosterone** (Android-5,Brown)

Nutritionally Significant Side Effects

Fluid and electrolyte disturbances
Nausea and gastrointestinal upset

Properties and Use in Treatment

Fluoxymesterone and methyltestosterone are synthetic derivatives of testosterone. They are used primarily to palliate androgen-responsive metastatic (especially skeletal) breast cancer in women who are more than one year, but less than five years, postmenopausal or women proven to have a hormone-dependent tumor as shown by previous beneficial response to oophorectomy. Administration is oral or buccal.

Fluoxymesterone and methyltestosterone have predominant anabolic and minor androgenic activities. Androgens increase protein anabolism, but nitrogen balance is improved only with sufficient concurrent intake of protein and calories. Androgens are primarily used to treat breast cancer and insufficient testosterone production in men.

General Toxicities

The most common side effects of androgen therapy for women are amenorrhea and other menstrual irregularities; inhibition of gonadotropin secretion; and virilization, including hirsutism, deepening of the voice, acne, and clitoral enlargement. The latter is usually not reversible after androgens are discontinued.

Other toxicities may include hematologic side effects (suppression of clotting factors II, V, VII, and X; bleeding with patients on concomitant anticoagulant therapy; and polycythemia); nervous system side effects (increased or decreased libido, headache, anxiety, depression, and generalized paresthesia); and allergic reactions (hypersensitivity, including skin manifestations and anaphylactoid reactions).

Hypercalcemia may occur in immobilized patients and in patients with metastatic breast cancer, in which case therapy must be discontinued.

Cholestatic hepatitis and jaundice, with significant elevations of serum bilirubin (especially direct), may occur with 17-alpha-alkyl-androgens and require discontinuation of drug therapy. These conditions are reversible with cessation of therapy.

Edema, with or without congestive heart failure, may be a serious complication for patients with preexisting cardiac, renal, or hepatic disease.

It is essential to closely monitor diabetics and patients with family histories of diabetes because blood glucose may be reduced and insulin or oral hypoglycemic agent requirements may change.

Interactions with Other Drugs

Androgens may increase sensitivity to oral anticoagulants, requiring reduced dosage of the anticoagulant to maintain satisfactory therapeutic hypoprothrombinemia.

Concurrent administration of oxyphenbutazone and androgens may result in elevated serum levels of oxyphenbutazone. In diabetic patients, the metabolic effects of androgens may decrease blood glucose and therefore, insulin requirements.

Food-Drug Interactions

Full meals accompanying the drug may delay and reduce its absorption. Complete absorption by the oral route is particularly questionable if the patient is concurrently receiving drugs that are toxic to the gastrointestinal tract.

It is recommended that the drug be ingested one hour before or two to three hours after a full meal. For maximal absorption, androgens should not be taken with full meals or fatty foods that delay absorption. Taking androgens on an empty stomach may cause nausea or other stomach disturbances. The drug should be taken together with a starchy food, such as bread or crackers, in order to clear the stomach quickly and not interfere with drug absorption.

If the administration of the androgen is via a buccal tablet, the patient must understand that the tablet should be allowed to dissolve between the gum and the cheek or under the tongue and not be swallowed. Eating, drinking, and smoking should be avoided while the tablet is in place.

Notes on Nutritional Side Effects

Fluid and electrolyte disturbances—Fluid and electrolyte disturbances have been described with androgen use; notably the retention of sodium, chloride, water, potassium, calcium, and inorganic phosphates. Appropriate dietary measures, such as a sodium-restricted and increased fluid intake diet may be necessary. With hypercalcemia, it is highly unlikely that restriction of dietary calcium will make any difference; thus medical treatment may be indicated.

Nausea and gastrointestinal upset—Androgens can cause nausea which may be ameliorated by antiemetic agents. Starchy foods taken with the drug may minimize nausea and gastrointestinal upset. Other dietary measures may lessen residual nausea.

If nausea is a problem, favorite foods should not be ingested prior to the administration of androgens because a conditioned food aversion may result.

Refer patients, as needed, to:

Chapter One: How to Deal with Specific Problems
Problem 2—Nausea and Vomiting, page 8

Chapter Two: General Dietary Guidelines
Guideline 1—Basic Nutrition for the Cancer Patient, page 30
Guideline 2—A High-Protein/High-Calorie Diet, page 38
Guideline 3—Food Sources of Minerals, page 45
Guideline 4—Foods Sources of Vitamins, page 52
Guideline 9—A Cholesterol and Fat-Restricted Diet, page 71
Guideline 11—Transient Glucose Intolerance/Diabetic Diet, page 76
Guideline 12—A Sodium-Restricted Diet, page 79

• L-Asparaginase
• Elspar® (Merck Sharp & Dohme)

Nutritionally Significant Side Effects

Anorexia
Nausea and vomiting
Abdominal discomfort
Malabsorption

Properties and Use in Treatment

L-Asparaginase is an enzyme that hydrolizes serum asparagine to nonfunctional aspartic acid and ammonia in tumor cells but not normal cells. Thus, tumor growth is blocked by the interruption of asparagine-dependent protein synthesis. The action of asparaginase is cell-cycle specific for postmitotic G_1 phase. Asparaginase may be given intravenously or intramuscularly in the treatment of acute lymphocytic leukemia. It is used primarily to treat acute lymphoblastic leukemia and lymphomas.

General Toxicities

Toxicities unrelated to nutritional status include hepatoxicity (biochemical evidence of dysfunction is present in more than 50 percent of treated adults); allergic reactions, including chills, urticaria, fever, and anaphylactic shock; blood coagulation defects (usually subclinical, associated with reduced synthesis of clotting factors); azotemia, usually prerenal (frequent); impaired sensorium; coma; lethargy; somnolence; depression; and psychosis. NOTE: A rise in serum urea nitrogen and ammonia is due to action of the enzyme and is not evidence of toxicity.

Other side effects may include difficulty in breathing, puffy face, skin rash or itching, seizures, sore throat, headache (mild to severe), flank or stomach pain, joint pain, inability to move an arm or leg, pain in lower legs, swelling of feet or lower legs, unusual bleeding or bruising, unusually frequent urination, unusual thirst, yellowing of eyes and skin, tiredness, nervousness, confusion, and hallucinations.

Interactions with Other Drugs

The combination of cytarabine and asparaginase may be synergistic. When administered after methotrexate, asparaginase may antagonize the effects of methotrexate. The effect of warfarin may be enhanced necessitating that prothrombin time be closely monitored.

Notes on Nutritional Side Effects

Anorexia—Unexplained anorexia has been noted as a side effect of this drug, reducing food intake. Dietary measures may help increase appetite.

Nausea and vomiting—Nausea and vomiting are uncommon but if present may be relieved by antiemetics. Starchy foods taken with the drug may minimize nausea, and other dietary measures can mitigate the aftereffects of vomiting and lessen residual nausea.

If nausea and vomiting are a problem, favorite foods should not be ingested prior to the administration of asparaginase because a conditioned aversion to foods taken immediately beforehand may result.

Abdominal discomfort—Asparaginase may cause vague abdominal discomfort, which may be aggravated by a full or distended gut. A low-fiber, residue-restricted diet may be necessary if the discomfort is severe enough to interfere with food intake.

Malabsorbtion—There has been malabsorbtion reported.

Refer patients, as needed, to:

Chapter One: How to Deal with Specific Problems
Problem 1—Loss of Appetite, page 4
Problem 2—Nausea and Vomiting, page 8
Problem 9—Dehydration, page 26

Chapter Two: General Dietary Guidelines
Guideline 1—Basic Nutrition for the Cancer Patient, page 30
Guideline 2—A High-Protein/High-Calorie Diet, page 38
Guideline 3—Food Sources of Minerals, page 45
Guideline 4—Food Sources of Vitamins, page 52
Guideline 5—The Fiber and Residue Contents of Foods, page 58
Guideline 6—A Lactose-Free/Lactose-Restricted Diet, page 61
Guiideline 11—A Transient Glucose Intolerance/Diabetic Diet, page 76

• Bleomycin Sulfate
• Blenoxane® (Bristol)

Nutritionally Significant Side Effects

Anorexia
Nausea and vomiting
Stomatitis and mucositis
Weight loss
Mechanical eating difficulties

Properties and Use in Treatment

Bleomycin sulfate is a mixture of cytotoxic glycopeptide antibiotics isolated from a strain of Streptomyces verticillus. The exact mechanism by which bleomycin acts is unknown but its main function appears to be the inhibition of DNA synthesis and to a lesser extent RNA and protein synthesis. Bleomycin is cell-cycle specific and is most active in the G_2 phase. It is also active in the late G_1, early S_1, and M phases.

Bleomycin is used primarily to treat squamous cell carcinoma of the head and neck, Hodgkin's disease, non-Hodgkin's lymphomas, testicular, anus, vulva and uterine cervix carcinomas. The drug is given intravenously, subcutaneously or intramuscularly and as a sclerosing agent in malignant hydrothorax (pleural effusion).

General Toxicities

The most significant dose-limiting toxicity is pulmonary dysfunction. Caution is recommended in patients with impairment of pulmonary function. Patients with preexisting pulmonary impairment may not be able to tolerate the full dose of bleomycin. Renal failure will impair the excretion of bleomycin; the dosage of bleomycin should be decreased in proportion to a decrease in creatinine clearance. Nonnutritional side effects include fever (up to 40°C) and chills, often within three to six hours after receiving a dose, as well as faintness, confusion, sweating, and wheezing. Cough, shortness of breath, and sores on the lips, mouth and sometimes in the axilla have been noted. Darkening or thickened skin, itching, rash, and colored lesions on the fingertips and elbows have been noted as has palm and skin redness or tenderness and swelling of the fingers with edema.

Interactions with Other Drugs

Nephrotoxic drugs such as amphotericin B and cisplatin have been reported to delay the renal clearance of bleomycin. There have been two case reports describing bleomycin pulmonary toxicity in patients pretreated with cisplatin.

Notes on Nutritional Side Effects

Anorexia—Anorexia is an uncommon side effect of this drug. If it does occur, dietary measures may help increase appetite.

Nausea and vomiting—Nausea and vomiting are uncommon with this drug. If experienced, prophylactic administration of antiemetic drugs may provide relief. Starchy foods taken with the drug may minimize nausea, and other dietary measures can mitigate the aftereffects of vomiting and lessen residual nausea.

If nausea and vomiting are a problem, favorite foods should not be ingested prior to the administration of bleomycin because a conditioned food aversion may result.

Stomatitis and mucositis—This drug can be directly toxic to the rapidly replicating mucosal cells in and around the mouth and throughout the digestive tract. Prophylactic administration of enhanced nutrition, with an emphasis on the B vitamins may mitigate or prevent this problem. Once the problem does exist, appropriate dietary restrictions may be necessary to keep the patient eating. A prescribed mouth care program may also help reduce toxic symptoms.

Weight loss—Unexplained weight loss has been described with the administration of this drug. The patient's dietary intake and nutritional status should be routinely monitored, and caloric intake should be increased where appropriate.

Mechanical eating difficulties—Bleomycin is most commonly used in treating squamous cell carcinoma of the head and neck. Patients with such cancers are likely to have many mechanical eating difficulties, including problems with chewing or swallowing or a dry mouth. Attention to these mechanical nutritional problems is important, as well as to the drug toxicities. Feeding tubes may be needed to maintain optimal nutrition.

Refer patients, as needed, to:

Chapter One: How to Deal with Specific Problems
Problem 1—Loss of Appetite, page 4
Problem 2—Nausea and Vomiting, page 8
Problem 4—Sore or Ulcerated Mouth or Throat (Stomatitis/ Mucositis), page 14
Problem 5—Difficulties in Chewing and Swallowing, page 18 (Dysphagia) and Dry Mouth (Xerostomia), page 18
Problem 9—Dehydration, page 26

Chapter Two: General Dietary Guidelines
Guideline 1—Basic Nutrition for the Cancer Patient, page 30
Guideline 2—A High-Protein/High-Calorie Diet, page 38
Guideline 3—Food Sources of Minerals, page 45
Guideline 4—Food Sources of Vitamins, page 52

- **Busulfan**
- **Myleran®** (Burroughs Wellcome)

Nutritionally Significant Side Effects

Anorexia
Nausea and vomiting
Diarrhea
Dry mouth
Stomatitis and mucositis
Hyperuricemia

Properties and Use in Treatment

Although an alkylating agent, busulfan is not a structural analogue of nitrogen mustard. Alkylation of DNA is felt to be the major biologic mechanism for its cytotoxic effect. Its action is cell-cycle phase non-specific. Busulfan is primarily used in the treatment of chronic myelogenous leukemia and polycythemia vera. In high doses it is used as a preparative regimen for bone marrow transplantation. Busulfan is commercially available in an oral form. Investigationally, it is available in an intravenous injection.

General Toxicities

Myelosuppression is a major dose-limiting effect, occurring approximately ten days after starting busulfan. This may continue to progressive leukopenia, thrombocytopenia, and anemia two weeks after discontinuation. It may take many weeks or months for recovery of the blood counts. A mixed alveolar and interstitial pneumonitis with progressive pulmonary insufficiency is occasionally seen with resultant pulmonary fibrosis and progressive pulmonary insufficiency. Other non-nutritional side effects include skin hyper-pigmentation, gynecomastia, amenorrhea, shortness of breath, cough, fever, bruising, ecchymosis as well as confusion, dizziness, and malaise.

Food-Drug Interactions

Full meals may reduce the absorption of an orally administered drug, affecting both the rate of absorption and peak serum concentrations. Complete absorption by the oral route is a special concern if the patient is concurrently receiving drugs toxic to the gastrointestinal tract.

To promote maximal absorption, busulfan should not be taken with full meals or fatty foods that delay absorption. It is recommended that the drug be administered one hour before or two to three hours after a full meal. Taking the drug on an empty stomach may engender nausea or other stomach disturbances. It should be taken along with a starchy food such as bread or crackers in order to clear the stomach quickly and not interfere with drug absorption.

Notes on Nutritional Side Effects

Anorexia—A clinical syndrome closely resembling adrenal insufficiency may develop with busulfan administration. Characteristics include weakness, severe fatigue, anorexia, weight loss, nausea, vomiting, and melanoderma. Refer to the appropriate Special Problem section for supportive nutritional measures.

Nausea and vomiting—In high doses nausea and vomiting are common with administration of this drug, and may be prevented by antiemetic agents. Starchy foods taken with the drug may minimize nausea, and other dietary measures can mitigate the aftereffects of vomiting and lessen residual nausea.

If nausea and vomiting are a problem, favorite foods should not be ingested prior to the administration of busulfan because a conditioned aversion to foods taken immediately beforehand may result.

Diarrhea—Diarrhea results from the direct toxicity of this drug to the mucosa lining of the gut. The villi and microvilli become flattened, reducing the absorptive surface area and resulting in a "slick gut." Gut lactase is also inhibited. The sum of these effects is that intestinal contents move rapidly through the gut, reducing absorption. Much of the water poured into the gut for digestion is not reabsorbed, and many water-soluble vitamins and minerals are lost.

It is possible to mitigate some of the effects of diarrhea with dietary intervention, for example reducing fiber and residue content of the diet, and/or restricting lactose intake.

Dry mouth—This drug has been noted to cause dry mouth, or xerostomia. The toxicity is to the parasympathetic nervous system, which controls salivary secretions. The thick salivary secretions from the sympathetically controlled glands remain intact, leaving a feeling of "cotton mouth." Specific dietary interventions may be needed to maintain nutritional intake.

Stomatitis and mucositis—This drug can be directly toxic to the rapidly replicating mucosal cells in and around the mouth and throughout the digestive tract. Enhanced nutrition, emphasizing the B vitamins, may mitigate or prevent this problem. Once the problem exists, however, certain dietary measures (e.g., a soft diet) may be needed to keep the patient eating. A prescribed mouth care program is essential.

Hyperuricemia—Busulfan causes rapid cellular destruction, resulting in extensive purine catabolism and hyperuricemia. Renal and joint damage may result from the precipitation of urates. A low-purine diet, the traditional treatment, automatically necessitates a low-protein diet, which is usually contraindicated for cancer patients. For this reason, hyperuricemia should be treated by medical means—that is, by administering a xanthine oxidase inhibitor drug such as allopurinol* without an accompanying low-protein diet.

Supportive dietary measures should include increased hydration (ten to twelve 8-ounce glasses of fluid per day) and an alkaline-ash diet to alkalinize the urine and prevent the precipitation of uric acid stones in the kidney.

Refer patients, as needed, to:

Chapter One: How to Deal with Specific Problems

Problem 1—Loss of Appetite, page 4

Problem 2—Nausea and Vomiting, page 8

Problem 3—Sore or Ulcerated Mouth or Throat (Stomatitis/ Mucositis), page 14

Problem 5—Difficulties in Chewing and Swallowing (Dysphagia) and Dry Mouth (Xerostomia), page 18

*Note: Allopurinol is not without its own nutritional side effects. See the discussion of this drug earlier in this chapter.

Problem 6—Diarrhea, page 20
Problem 9—Dehydration, page 26

Chapter Two: General Dietary Guidelines
Guideline 1—Basic Nutrition for the Cancer Patient, page 30
Guideline 2—A High-Protein/High-Calorie Diet, page 38
Guideline 3—Food Sources of Minerals, page 45
Guideline 4—Food Sources of Vitamins, page 52
Guideline 5—The Fiber and Residue Contents of Foods, page 58
Guideline 6—A Lactose-Free/Lactose-Restricted Diet, page 61
Guideline 10—How to Prevent Kidney Stone Formation (Acid Ash/Alkaline Ash Diet), page 74
Guideline 14—A Soft-Food/Pureed-Food Diet, page 86

• Carboplatin
• Paraplatin® (Bristol)

Nutritionally Significant Side Effects

Nausea and vomiting
Anorexia
Diarrhea
Constipation
Stomatitis and mucositis
Altered taste and smell
Hyperuricemia

Properties and Use in Treatment

Carboplatin is a heavy metal complex, structurally related to cisplatin (Platinol®), with comparable antitumor activity but less renal, gastrointestinal, and neurologic toxicity. Its biochemical properties are similar to those of bifunctional alkylating agents, producing interstrand and intrastrand cross-links in DNA. It is cell-cycle nonspecific.

Carboplatin is active in several cancers, including testicular tumors, cervix, ovarian, small cell lung cancer, head and neck cancer, esophageal mesothelioma and pediatric brain tumors. It is used as a single agent as secondary therapy for patients with metastatic ovarian tumors refractory to standard chemotherapy who have not previously received cisplatin therapy and for patients with transitional cell bladder cancer that is no longer amenable to local treatment. It is also used in treating non-small-cell lung cancer and head neck cancer. The drug is administered by intravenous injection or short infusion.

Carboplatin should be used with caution in patients with preexisting renal impairment, myelosuppression, hearing impairment, or a history of allergic reactions to carboplatin.

Interactions with Other Drugs

Carboplatin produces cumulative nephrotoxicity that may be potentiated by other nephrotoxic agents such as antibiotics, and amphotericin B.

General Toxicities

Dose-related myelosuppression, predominantly thrombocytopenia is common and reversible. Factors associated with an increased risk of myelosupression are age, renal impairment, and concurrent chemotherapy. It is first noted during the second week after a dose and is manifested by elevations in BUN and creatinine, serum uric acid, and/or reduced creatinine clearance. Renal toxicity becomes more prolonged and severe with repeated courses of the drug. Renal function must return to normal before repeating carboplatin dosage.

Ototoxicity has been observed in about 1-5 percent of patients and is manifested by tinnitus and/or hearing loss in the high-frequency range. Ototoxic effects may be more severe with children. Hearing loss tends to become more frequent and severe with repeated doses, and it is unclear whether the loss is reversible.

Increases in serum calcium, magnesium, sodium, and potassium are mild and reversible. Hyperuricemia has been reported to occur at approximately the same frequency as the increases in BUN and serum creatinine.

Neurotoxicity, usually characterized by peripheral neuropathies, has been reported. Optic neuritis, papilledema, and cerebral blindness are reported infrequently.

Anaphylactic-like reactions to carboplatin have been reported in 2 percent of patients and consist of facial edema, wheezing, tachycardia, and hypotension occurring within a few minutes of dose administration. Other allergic reactions include rash, urticaria, erythema, and pruritus. Reactions may be controlled by intravenous epinephrine, corticosteroid, or antihistamines. Reduced serum zinc levels may compromise the host immune system.

Notes on Nutritional Side Effects

Nausea and vomiting—Nausea and vomiting occurs in about 70% of patients and are occasionally dose limiting. In contrast to cisplatin, nausea and vomiting are usually mild and manageable with standard antiemetics and seldom persist longer than twenty-four hours. Standard antiemetic agents should be administered prior to infusion of carboplatin and at regular intervals as needed for at least twenty-four hours. Starchy foods taken with the drug may minimize nausea, and other dietary measures can mitigate the aftereffects of vomiting and lessen residual nausea.

Anorexia—Anorexia occurs infrequently. Where food intake is reduced, dietary measures should be used. Serum zinc deficiency may occur and oral zinc may be added to the diet. Hypozincemia may reduce sense of taste.

Diarrhea—Diarrhea is infrequent. When it occurs it is caused by the direct toxicity of this drug to the mucosa of the gut. The villi and microvilli become flattened, reducing the absorptive surface area and resulting in a "slick gut" and possible lactose intolerance. Intestinal contents move rapidly through the gut, further reducing absorption. Much of the water poured into the gut for digestion is not reabsorbed, and many water-soluble vitamins and minerals are lost. Some of these effects may be mitigated by dietary means.

Constipation—Constipation is also an infrequent side effect of this drug, and may not be readily rectified by an enema or suppository. Commercial laxatives may cause nutritional depletion and are habit forming. Mineral oil is discouraged because it solublizes the fat-soluble vitamins in the gut, preventing their absorption. Constipation is best treated prophylactically with dietary fiber when not contraindicated.

Stomatitis and mucositis—Stomatitis and mucositis have been reported infrequently and are caused by direct toxicity of this drug to the rapidly replicating mucosal cells in and around the mouth and throughout the digestive tract. Enhanced nutrition, with an emphasis on the B vitamins, may mitigate or prevent this problem. Once the problem exists, however, certain dietary measures, such as restriction to a soft diet, may be necessary to keep the patient eating. A prescribed mouth care program may be helpful in reducing toxic symptoms.

Altered taste and smell—Altered taste and smell, or dysgeusia, have occasionally been reported with this drug and can lead to reduced appetite. The most common taste complaints are lowered taste threshold to bitterness and sweetness. Dietary measures can help cope with this problem.

Hyperuricemia—Hyperuricemia is uncommon. Renal and joint damage may result from the precipitation of urates. A low-purine diet, the traditional treatment, automatically necessitates a low-protein diet, which is contraindicated in most cancer patients. Thus, hyperuricemia should be treated by medical means through administration of a xanthine oxidase inhibitor drug such as allopurinol,* without an accompanying low-protein diet. Supportive dietary measures should include increased hydration (ten to twelve 8-ounce glasses of water per day) and an alkaline ash diet to alkanize the urine and prevent the precipitation of uric acid stones in the kidney.

Refer patients, as needed, to:

Chapter One: How to Deal with Specific Problems
Problem 1—Loss of Appetite, page 4
Problem 2—Nausea and Vomiting, page 8
Problem 3—Taste Changes,page 12
Problem 4—Sore or Ulcerated Mouth or Throat (Stomatitis/Mucositis), page 14
Problem 6—Diarrhea, page 20
Problem 8—Constipation, page 24
Problem 9—Dehydration, page 26

Chapter Two: General Dietary Guidelines
Guideline 1—Basic Nutrition for the Cancer Patient, page 30
Guideline 2—A High-Protein/High-Calorie Diet, page 38
Guideline 3—Food Sources of Minerals, page 45
Guideline 4—Food Sources of Vitamins, page 52
Guideline 5—The Fiber and Residue Content of Foods, page 58
Guideline 6—A Lactose-Free/Lactose-Restricted Diet, page 61
Guideline 10—How to Prevent Kidney Stone Formation (Acid Ash/Alkaline Ash Diet), page 74

*Note: Allopurinol is not without its own nutritional side effects. See the discussion of this drug earlier in this chapter.

- **Carmustine** (BCNU)
- **BICNU®** (Bristol)

Nutritionally Significant Side Effects

Nausea and vomiting
Anorexia
Stomatitis and mucositis
Diarrhea
Dysphagia

Properties and Use in Treatment

Carmustine (BCNU) is an alkylating agent used for the treatment of brain tumors, colorectal adenocarcinoma, gastric adenocarcinoma, hepatoma, Hodgkin's disease, non-Hodgkin's lymphomas, malignant melanoma, multiple myeloma, melanoma, lung cancer, and bone marrow transplantation. It is a nitrosourea capable of inhibiting synthesis of DNA, RNA, and protein in a manner similar, but not identical, to that of other alkylating agents. Its action is cell-cycle phase nonspecific. Carmustine is currently available only for intravenous use.

Interactions with Other Drugs

Carmustine may enhance the renal toxicity of aminoglycosides. Amphotericin B and vitamin A may enhance the cytotoxic and toxic effects of carmustine. It is suspected that the bone marrow suppression of carmustine may be increased by cimetidine (Tagamet®). The pharmacologic effects of oral digoxin may be reduced due to reduced gastrointestinal absorption caused by carmustine. The pharmacologic effects of oral hydantoins may be reduced by carmustine due to phenytoin malabsorption.

General Toxicities

The most significant clinical toxicity of BCNU is delayed hematopoietic depression. Toxicities unrelated to nutritional status include hepatotoxicity (usually subclinical), leukopenia (delayed to about four to five weeks after administration), thrombocytopenia (occurring about three to five weeks after administration), cumulative myelosuppression, local venous pain on administration (including isolated reports of optic neuritis following administration), and interstitial pulmonary fibrosis (rare).

Symptoms may include cough, fever, chills, sore throat, flushing of the face, shortness of breath, swelling of the feet or lower legs, bleeding or bruising, decrease in urination, tiredness, weakness, difficulty in walking, discoloration of the skin along the vein of injection, dizziness, skin rash, and itching.

Notes on Nutritional Side Effects

Nausea and vomiting—Dose-related nausea and vomiting are common and usually appear within two hours of injection and last for up to six hours. Nausea and vomiting may be prevented or reduced by administration of antiemetic agents. Taking the drug on an empty stomach may engender nausea or other stomach disturbances. It should be taken along with a starchy food such as bread or crackers in order to clear the stomach quickly and not interfere with drug absorption.

Anorexia—Unexplained anorexia has been noted as a side effect of this drug. It is not known whether the problem is diminished appetite, resulting from nausea and vomiting or physiological. The result is reduced food intake. Dietary and supportive measures can help increase appetite.

Stomatitis and mucositis—This drug can be directly toxic to the rapidly replicating mucosal cells in and around the mouth and throughout the digestive tract. Enhanced nutrition, with an emphasis on the B vitamins, may mitigate or prevent this problem. Once the problem exists, however, certain dietary restrictions may be necessary to keep the patient eating, for example a soft diet. A prescribed mouth care program may be helpful in reducing toxic symptoms.

Diarrhea—Diarrhea results from the direct toxicity of this drug to the mucosa of the gut. The villi and microvilli become flattened, reducing the absorptive surface area and resulting in a "slick gut." Intestinal contents move rapidly through the gut, further reducing absorption. Much of the water poured into the gut for digestion is not reabsorbed, and many water-soluble vitamins and minerals are lost. It is possible to mitigate some of the effects of diarrhea by dietary means.

Dysphagia—Difficulty in chewing and/or swallowing has been described with this drug. Some dietary restrictions may be necessary regarding the consistency of foods.

Refer patients, as needed, to:

Chapter One: How to Deal with Specific Problems
Problem 1—Loss of Appetite, page 4
Problem 2—Nausea and Vomiting, page 8
Problem 4—Sore or Ulcerated Mouth or Throat (Stomatitis/ Mucositis), page 14
Problem 5—Difficulties in Chewing and Swallowing (Dysphagia) and Dry Mouth (Xerostomia), page 18
Problem 6—Diarrhea, page 20
Problem 9—Dehydration, page 26

Chapter Two: General Dietary Guidelines
Guideline 1—Basic Nutrition for the Cancer Patient, page 30
Guideline 2—A High-Protein/High Calorie Diet, page 38
Guideline 3—Food Sources of Minerals, page 45
Guideline 4—Food Sources of Vitamins, page 52
Guideline 5—The Fiber and Residue Contents of Foods, page 58
Guideline 6—A Lactose-Free/Lactose-Restricted Diet, page 61
Guideline 14—A Soft-Food/Pureed-Food Diet, page 86

• Chlorambucil
• Leukeran® (Burroughs Wellcome)

Nutritionally Significant Side Effects

Nausea and vomiting
Hyperuricemia

Properties and Use in Treatment

Chlorambucil is an aromatic derivative of mechlorethamine (nitrogen mustard). It is administered orally, and its action is cell-cycle phase nonspecific. The cytotoxic effects on the bone marrow, lymphoid organs, and epithelial tissues are similar to those observed with nitrogen mustard. It is used primarily to treat chronic lymphocytic leukemia, Hodgkin's, non-Hodgkin's lymphomas, breast, ovarian cancer, and Waldenstrom's macroglobulinemia.

General Toxicities

Chlorambucil is one of the best tolerated of the antineoplastic agents. Myelosuppression is dose related and is generally slow in onset and is reversible with time after discontinuing the drug. Toxicities unrelated to nutrition include occasional rash, alopecia, rarely hepatotoxicity, pulmonary fibrosis, convulsions, amenorrhea, azoospermia and secondary leukemia. Symptoms include cough, fever, chills, sore throat, joint pains, shortness of breath, edema of the lower legs, and ecchymosis and bleeding.

Food-Drug Interactions

Full meals may reduce the absorption of an orally administered drug, affecting both the rate of absorption and peak serum concentrations. Complete absorption by the oral route may be questionable if the patient is concurrently receiving drugs toxic to the gastrointestinal tract.

To promote maximal absorption, chlorambucil should not be taken with full meals or fatty foods that delay absorption. It is recommended that the drug be administered one hour before or two to three hours after a full meal. Taking the drug on an empty stomach may engender nausea or other stomach disturbances. It should be taken along with a starchy food such as bread or crackers in order to clear the stomach quickly and not interfere with drug absorption.

Notes on Nutritional Side Effects

Nausea and vomiting—Nausea and vomiting may result from single oral doses of 20 mg, probably due to the direct stimulation of the stomach and its acid secretion by the physical presence of the drug. These symptoms may sometimes be prevented by the prophylactic administration of antiemetic drugs. Dietary measures cannot prevent this type of nausea and vomiting, but starchy foods taken with the drug may reduce nausea, and other dietary measures can mitigate the aftereffects of vomiting and lessen residual nausea.

If nausea and vomiting are a problem, favorite foods should not be ingested prior to the administration of chlorambucil because a conditioned aversion to foods taken immediately beforehand may result.

Hyperuricemia—This drug may cause rapid cellular destruction, resulting in extensive purine catabolism and hyperuricemia. Renal and joint damage may result from the precipitation of urates. A low-purine diet, the traditional treatment, automatically necessitates a low-protein diet, which may be contraindicated for cancer patients. Thus, hyperuricemia must be treated medically by the administration of a xanthine oxidase inhibitor drug such as allopurinol,* preferably without an accompanying low-protein diet. Supportive dietary measures should include increased hydration (ten to twelve 8-ounce glasses of fluid per day) and an alkaline-ash diet to alkalinize the urine and prevent the precipitation of uric acid stones in the kidney.

*Note: Allopurinol has its own nutritional side effects. See the discussion of this drug earlier in this chapter.

Refer patients, as needed, to:

Chapter One: How to Deal with Specific Problems
Problem 1—Loss of Appetite, page 4
Problem 2—A Nausea and Vomiting, page 8
Problem 9—Dehydration, page 26

Chapter Two: General Dietary Guidelines
Guideline 1—Basic Nutrition for the Cancer Patient, page 30
Guideline 2—A High-Protein/High-Calorie Diet, page 38
Guideline 3—Food Sources of Minerals, page 45
Guideline 4—Food Sources of Vitamins, page 52
Guideline 10—How to Prevent Kidney Stone Formation (Acid Ash/Alkaline Ash Diet), page 74

- **Cisplatin** (CDDP)
- **Platinol®** (Bristol)

Nutritionally Significant Side Effects

Nausea and vomiting
Anorexia
Electrolyte imbalance
Hyperuricemia
Loss of taste

Properties and Use in Treatment

Cisplatin is an inorganic heavy metal coordination complex with biochemical properties similar to the bifunctional alkylating agents. It produces interstrand and intrastrand cross-links in DNA, ultimately affecting cell replication and RNA protein synthesis. It is cell-cycle phase nonspecific. Cisplatin is given intravenously. It is initially rapidly removed from plasma, with only 10% being found after one hour, but a more delayed phase exists with a half-life of about three hours. There is poor central nervous system penetration of the drug. It is primarily eliminated via the kidneys. Cisplatin is used primarily to treat cancers of the testicles, ovary, head and neck, Hodgkin's and non-Hodgkin's lymphoma, sarcomas, bladder, lung, stomach, cervix, myeloma, prostate, breast, melanoma, and mesothelioma.

General Toxicities

Cisplatin may produce an impairment in renal tubular ten to fourteen days after therapy. The dose of cisplatin dosage (creatinine clearance > 50 mg/min) depends upon adequate renal function. Hearing loss, high-frequency tinnitus, and deafness occur as well as a peripheral neuropathy with parasthesias and sensory loss with a glove-and-stocking distribution and muscular weakness. These side effects incease with higher dose and are dose related. Other side effects can include facial swelling, fast heartbeat, wheezing, fever, chills, sore throat, joint pains and swelling of the feet and lower extremities, blurred vision, bleeding, bruising and possible compromise in the host immune system. Renal insufficiency may be reduced by increasing fluid intake and saline and maximizing hydration during therapy.

Interactions with Other Drugs

Concurrent administration of other kidney toxic drugs such as amphotericin-B and aminoglycosides should be avoided. Sodium thiosulfate may decrease the kidney toxicity of cisplatin. Cisplatin may reduce the oral absorption of phenytoin, carbamazepine (Tegretol®) and valproic acid (Depakene®), necessitating dose adjustment. Drug monitoring of these agents should be performed more frequently.

Notes on Nutritional Side Effects

Nausea and vomiting—Nausea and vomiting occur in almost all patients receiving cisplatin. Symptoms may persist up to one week after treatment and may limit drug dosage. In some instances, nausea and vomiting can be prevented by the prophylactic administration of antiemetic drugs. Diet cannot prevent this type of nausea and vomiting, but starchy foods taken with the drug may mitigate the aftereffects of vomiting and lessen residual nausea.

If nausea and vomiting are a problem, favorite foods should not be ingested prior to the administration of cisplatin because a conditioned aversion to foods taken immediately beforehand may result.

Anorexia—Unexplained anorexia has also been noted as a side effect of this drug, resulting in reduced food intake. Decreased serum zinc levels may result in reduced taste. Dietary measures including supplemental zinc may help increase appetite.

Electrolyte imbalance—Electrolyte disturbances have been noted with cisplatin, including hypomagnesemia, hypocalcemia, hypokalemia, and hypophosphatemia, which are probably due to wasting from renal tubular damage. These side effects will require medical management with the administration of supplemental magnesium, potassium, and other electrolytes to restore normal serum levels.

This problem is too severe to be treated by nutritional means, but severe kidney dysfunction may necessitate both a strict renal dietary regimen and intravenous electrolytes as well. Careful evaluation, counseling, and follow-up by a renal dietitian may be needed. Because of the gravity of this condition, the patient with renal dysfunction should be under a renal dietitian's direct supervision.

NOTE: Renal insufficiency will be dose limiting and may mandate cessation of cisplatin therapy.

Hyperuricemia—This drug may cause rapid cellular destruction, resulting in extensive purine catabolism and hyperuricemia. Renal and joint damage may result from the precipitation of urates. A low-purine diet is the traditional treatment, necessitating a low-protein diet, which may be contraindicated in many cancer patients. For this reason, hyperuricemia should be treated by medical means—that is, by administering a xanthine oxidase inhibitor drug such as allopurinol* without an accompanying low-protein diet during periods of acute hyperuricemia. Supportive dietary measures should include increased hydration (ten to twelve 8-ounce glasses of fluid per day) and an alkaline-ash diet to alkalinize the urine and prevent the precipitation of uric acid stones in the kidney.

Loss of taste—Loss of taste (taste blindness) has been seen in many patients receiving Platinol®.

Refer patients, as needed, to:

Chapter One: How to Deal with Specific Problems

Problem 1—Loss of Appetite, page 4

Problem 2—Nausea and Vomiting, page 8

Problem 9—Dehydration, page 26

Chapter Two: General Dietary Guidelines

Guideline 1—Basic Nutrition for the Cancer Patient, page 30

Guideline 2—A High-Protein/High-Calorie Diet, page 38

Guideline 3—Food Sources of Minerals, page 45

Guideline 4—Food Sources of Vitamins, page 52

Guideline 10—How to Prevent Kidney Stone Formation (Acid Ash/Alkaline Ash Diet), page 74

*Note: Allopurinol also has its own nutritional side effects. See the discussion of this drug earlier in this chapter.

- **Cyclophosphamide** (CTX, CPM)
- **Cytoxan®** (Mead Johnson)
- **Neosar®** (Adria)

Nutritionally Significant Side Effects

Alopecia
Anorexia
Nausea and vomiting
Stomatitis and mucositis
Diarrhea
Hyperuricemia
Bleeding and ulceration of the GI tract
Hemorrhagic cystitis

Properties and Use in Treatment:

Cyclophosphamide is a synthetic alklyating agent chemically related to nitrogen mustard. It inhibits DNA synthesis, and though activity is cell-cycle phase nonspecific, it produces more cytotoxicity during the S-phase. Cyclophosphamide becomes biologically active after hepatic metabolism and may be administered orally or intravenously. Active metabolites are excreted via the kidney.

It is used to treat Hodgkin's and non-Hodgkin's lymphoma, multiple myeloma, Burkitt's lymphoma, sarcomas, retinoblastoma, carcinomas of testes, lung, ovary, endometrium, mycosis fungoides and leukemias.

General Toxicities

Severe myelosuppression (bone marrow toxicity) is manifested as leukopenia and anemia. Cyclophosphamide is considered platelet sparing although thrombocytopenia does occur. Bone marrow toxicity occurs by day 10 and recovers by day 21 after drug administration. Amenorrhea, sterility, depression of sperm count, pulmonary fibrosis, and interstital pneumonitis, and respiratory insufficiency, skin hyperpigmentation, and hepatic toxicity may occur.

Interactions with Other Drugs

Allopurinol* may enhance the incidence and degree of myelosuppression. Also, hepatic enzyme inducers such as phenytoin, phenobarbital and chloral hydrate may increase hepatic activation of cyclophosphamide.

Food-Drug Interactions

Complete absorption by the oral route may be affected by concurrently administered drugs toxic to the gastrointestinal tract.

To promote maximal absorption, oral cyclophosphamide should not be taken with full meals or fatty foods that delay absorption. The oral drug should be administered one hour before or two to three hours after a full meal. As taking cyclophosphamide on an empty stomach may engender nausea or other stomach disturbances, the drug should be taken with a starchy snack such as bread or crackers that will clear the stomach quickly and not interfere with drug absorption.

Notes on Nutritional Side Effects

Alopecia—Alopecia is frequent due to the transient effects of the drug on hair follicles. Hair loss cannot be prevented nutritionally, but general good nutrition will promote maximal normal regrowth. New growth begins almost immediately, but its color and texture may be slightly different than before.

Anorexia—Unexplained anorexia has been noted as a side effect of this drug with possible reduced food intake. Dietary measures may help increase appetite.

Nausea and vomiting—Nausea and vomiting are common and in some instances can be prevented by antiemetic agents. Dietary measures cannot prevent this type of nausea and vomiting, but starchy foods taken with the drug may minimize nausea. Other dietary measures can mitigate the aftereffects of vomiting and lessen residual nausea.

If nausea and vomiting are a problem, favorite foods should not be ingested prior to the administration of cyclophosphamide

*Note: Allopurinol is not without its own nutritional side effects. See discussion of this drug earlier in this chapter.

because a conditioned aversion to foods taken immediately beforehand may result.

Stomatitis and mucositis—This drug can be directly toxic to the rapidly replicating mucosal cells in and around the mouth and throughout the digestive tract. Prophylactic administration of enhanced nutrition, emphasizing the B vitamins, may mitigate or prevent this problem. Once the problem exists, dietary restrictions such as a soft diet may be needed to keep the patient eating. A prescribed mouth care program will be helpful in reducing toxic symptoms.

Diarrhea—Diarrhea results from the direct toxicity of this drug to the mucosa lining of the gut. The villi and microvilli become flattened, reducing the absorptive surface area, resulting in a "slick gut." As a result, intestinal contents move rapidly through the gut, reducing absorption. Much of the water poured into the gut for digestion is not reabsorbed, and many water-soluble vitamins and minerals are lost. It is possible to mitigate some of the effects of diarrhea with dietary means.

Hyperuricemia—Cyclophosphamide may cause rapid cellular destruction, resulting in hyperuricemia. Renal and joint damage may result from the precipitation of urates. A low-purine diet, the traditional treatment, necessitates a low-protein diet, which may be contraindicated in many cancer patients. The hyperuricemia should be treated by medical means—that is, by administering a xanthine oxidase inhibitor drug such as allopurinol* without an accompanying low-protein diet. Allopurinol may augment cyclophosphamide toxicity, but clinical significance appears to be small. Supportive dietary measures should include increased hydration (ten to twelve 8-ounce glasses of fluid per day) and an alkaline-ash diet to alkalinize the urine and prevent the precipitation of uric acid stones in the kidney.

Other side effects include potentiation of anthracycline cardiac toxicity, a potent immune suppression, acute water intoxication due to antiduretic effects following IV therapy and secondary malignancies including bladder and acute leukemia.

Hemorrhagic cystitis—Hemorrhagic cystitis is known to occur with this drug and can be severe. It is caused by chemical irritation of

*Note: Allopurinol has its own nutritional side effects. See the discussion of this drug earlier in this chapter.

the urinary bladder mucosa by acrolein, and other reactive metabolites of the drug. Ample fluid intake and frequent voiding is usually preventive. Iron replacement may be necessary if bleeding has occurred. Sulphur-containing nucleophiles such as N-acetylcysteine (Mucomyst®) or Mesna (Mesnex®) can lessen cystitis.

Inappropriate antidiuretic hormone—A syndrome of inappropriate antidiuretic hormone has been associated with high intravenous doses of cyclophosphamide and may produce seizure due to hyponatremia. Treatment includes either water restriction or hypertonic saline. Recovery occurs after several days.

Bleeding and ulceration of the GI tract—The enteritis caused by this drug may be severe enough to result in bleeding and ulceration of the gut. This can lead to a blood loss of iron, loss of many nutrients, and nonreabsorption of bile salts. Dietary means can mitigate some of these side effects.

Refer patients, as needed, to:

Chapter One: How to Deal with Specific Problems
Problem 1—Loss of Appetite, page 4
Problem 2—Nausea and Vomiting, page 8
Problem 7—Protecting the Gastrointestinal Tract (Enteritis), page 22
Problem 9—Dehydration, page 26

Chapter Two: General Dietary Guidelines
Guideline 1—Basic Nutrition for the Cancer Patient, page 30
Guideline 2—A High-Protein/High-Calorie Diet, page 38
Guideline 3—Food Sources of Minerals, page 45
Guideline 4—Food Sources of Vitamins, page 52
Guideline 5—The Fiber and Residue Contents of Foods, page 58
Guideline 6—A Lactose-Free/Lactose-Restricted Diet, page 61
Guideline 10—How to Prevent Kidney Stone Formation (Acid Ash/Alkaline Ash Diet), page 74
Guideline 14—A Soft-Food/Pureed-Food Diet, page 86

- **Cytarabine** (Cytosine Arabinoside, Arabinosyl Cytosine, ARA-C)
- **Cytosar-U®** (Upjohn)

Nutritionally Significant Side Effects

Anorexia
Nausea and vomiting
Stomatitis and mucositis
Dysphagia
Diarrhea
Hyperuricemia

Properties and Use in Treatment

Cytarabine is an antimetabolite which competitively inhibits DNA polymerase. Incorporation of cytarabine into both DNA and RNA may occur as well as inhibition of nucleotide kinases. Its action is S-phase specific, blocking progression of tumor cells from G_1 to S. It is used as first-line treatment of acute granulocytic leukemia and secondary treatment in acute lymphocytic leukemia and lymphomas.

General Toxicities

Hematologic toxicities are dose limiting and include leukopenia (WBC count may continue to fall after the drug is stopped and reach lowest values after drug-free intervals of five to seven days), thrombocytopenia, anemia, and megaloblastosis. Other toxicities unrelated to nutritional status include hepatic dysfunction (uncommon and usually mild and reversible), central nervous system toxicity, and hypersensitivity reactions (rash).

Symptoms may include fever, chills, sore throat, mouth sores, bone or muscle pain, chest pain, cough, fainting spells, flank or stomach pain, general feeling of body discomfort, weakness, heartburn, irregular heartbeat, joint pain, numbness or tingling in fingers or toes or face, pain at place of injection, reddened eyes, shortness of breath, skin rash, swelling of feet or lower legs, tiredness, unusual bleeding or bruising, yellowing of eyes and skin, dizziness, headache, itching of skin, loss of hair, skin freckling, and stomach pain.

Notes on Nutritional Side Effects

Anorexia—Unexplained anorexia has been noted as a side effect of this drug resulting in reduced food intake. Dietary measures can help increase appetite.

Nausea and vomiting—Nausea and vomiting are common, occurring within six hours of administration and may be prevented by antiemetic agents. Starchy foods taken with the drug may minimize nausea, and other dietary measures can mitigate the after effects of vomiting and lessen residual nausea.

If nausea and vomiting are a problem, favorite foods should not be ingested prior to the administration of cytarabine because a conditioned aversion to foods taken immediately beforehand may result.

Stomatitis and mucositis—This drug can be directly toxic to the rapidly dividing mucosal cells in and around the mouth and throughout the digestive tract. Stomatitis and mucositis are common beginning five to seven days after treatment. Enhanced nutrition, emphasizing the B vitamins, may mitigate or prevent this problem. Once the problem exists, however, certain dietary restrictions may be necessary to keep the patient eating, for example a soft or blenderized diet. A prescribed mouth care program is helpful in reducing toxic symptoms.

The enteritis caused by this drug may be severe enough to result in bleeding and ulceration leading to a blood loss of iron, loss of many nutrients, and nonreabsorption of bile salts, with subsequent nutritional effects.

Dysphagia—Difficulty in chewing and/or swallowing has been described with this drug. Some dietary restrictions regarding the consistency of foods, such as a soft or blenderized diet, may be necessary.

Diarrhea—Diarrhea results from the direct toxicity of this drug to the mucosa of the gut. The villi and microvilli become flattened, reducing the absorptive surface area and resulting in a "slick gut." Intestinal contents move rapidly through the gut, further reducing absorption. Much of the water poured into the gut for digestion is not reabsorbed, and many water-soluble vitamins and minerals are lost. It is possible to mitigate some of the effects of diarrhea by dietary means. The ability to manufacture active lactose may be lost. If so, a lactose-restricted diet would become necessary.

Hyperuricemia—This drug may cause rapid cellular destruction resulting in extensive purine catabolism and hyperuricemia. Renal and joint damage may result from the precipitation of urates. A low-purine diet, the traditional treatment, necessitates a low-protein diet, which is usually contraindicated in most cancer patients. The hyperuricemia is best treated by medical means, that is, by administering a xanthine oxidase inhibitor drug such as allopurinol,* without an accompanying low-protein diet. Supportive dietary measures should include increased hydration (ten to twelve 8-ounce glasses of fluid per day) and an alkaline-ash diet to alkalinize the urine and prevent the precipitation of uric acid stones in the kidney.

Refer patients, as needed, to:

Chapter One: How to Deal with Specific Problems

Problem 1—Loss of Appetite, page 4
Problem 2—Nausea and Vomiting, page 8
Problem 4—Sore or Ulcerated Mouth or Throat (Stomatitis/Mucositis), page 14
Problem 5—Difficulties in Chewing and Swallowing (Dysphagia) and Dry Mouth (Xerostomia), page 18
Problem 6—Diarrhea, page 20
Problem 9—Dehydration, page 26

General Dietary Guidelines (Chapter Two)

Guideline 1—Basic Nutrition for the Cancer Patient, page 30
Guideline 2—A High-Protein/High-Calorie Diet, page 38
Guideline 3—Food Sources of Minerals, page 45
Guideline 4—Food Sources of Vitamins, page 52
Guideline 5—The Fiber and Residue Contents of Foods, page 58
Guideline 6—A Lactose-Free/Lactose-Restricted Diet, page 61
Guideline 10—How to Prevent Kidney Stone Formation (Acid Ash/Alkaline Ash Diet), page 74
Guideline 14—A Soft-Food/Pureed-Food Diet, page 86

*Note: Allopurinol has its own nutritional side effects. See the discussion of this drug earlier in this chapter.

• Dacarbazine (Imidazole Carboxamide)
• DTIC-Dome® (Miles)

Nutritionally Significant Side Effects

Anorexia
Nausea and vomiting
Fever
Stomatitis and mucositis

Properties and Use in Treatment

Dacarbazine is an alkylating agent. Its action is cell-cycle phase non-specific and is probably mediated by methylation of DNA. It also has antimetabolite activity as a purine precursor, and interaction with sulfhydral (SH) groups in proteins has been shown. Synthesis of both DNA and RNA is inhibited, and ultimately protein synthesis is also affected.

It is used primarily for Hodgkin's disease, malignant melanoma, sarcomas, carcinoid, islet cell carcinomas, thyroid (medullary carcinoma). Dacarbazine is administered by intravenous injection.

General Toxicities

Non-nutritional side effects include fever, chills, sore throat, mouth and lip sores, and unusual bleeding and bruising. White cell depression and occasional thrombocytopenia are seen, and hepatotoxicity occurs occasionally. Exposure to the sun within one or two days after receiving the drug may produce facial flushing, paresthesia, and light-headedness.

Notes on Nutritional Side Effects

Anorexia—Unexplained anorexia has been noted as a side effect of this drug. It is not known whether the problem is diminished appetite, resulting from nausea and vomiting, or physiological. The result, however, is reduced food intake. Dietary and supportive measures may help increase appetite.

Nausea and vomiting—Nausea and vomiting are severe and require aggressive prophylactic antiemetics. Starchy foods taken with the drug may reduce nausea. Dietary measures can mitigate the after-effects of vomiting and lessen residual nausea.

If nausea and vomiting are a problem, favorite foods should not be ingested prior to the administration of dacarbazine because a conditioned aversion to foods taken immediately beforehand may result.

Fever—Some patients may experience an influenza-like fever to 39° C, myalgias, and malaise lasting for several days. Fever can cause loss of lean body mass as well as fluids and electrolytes. Protein, fluid, and electrolyte losses must be replenished.

Stomatitis and mucositis—This drug can be directly toxic to the rapidly replicating mucosal cells in and around the mouth and throughout the digestive tract. Enhanced nutrition, emphasizing the B vitamins, may mitigate or prevent this problem. Once the problem exists, however, certain dietary restrictions, such as a soft diet may be needed to keep the patient eating. A prescribed mouth care program will help reduce symptoms.

Refer patients, as needed, to:

Chapter One: How to Deal with Specific Problems
Problem 1—Loss of Appetite, page 4
Problem 2—Nausea and Vomiting, page 8
Problem 4—Sore or Ulcerated Mouth or Throat (Stomatitis/Mucositis), page 14
Problem 6—Diarrhea, page 20
Problem 9—Dehydration, page 26

Chapter Two: General Dietary Guidelines
Guideline 1—Basic Nutrition for the Cancer Patient, page 30
Guideline 2—A High-Protein/High-Calorie Diet, page 38
Guideline 3—Food Sources of Minerals, page 45
Guideline 4—Food Sources of Vitamins, page 52
Guideline 5—The Fiber and Residue Contents of Foods, page 58
Guideline 6—A Lactose-Free/Lactose-Restricted Diet, page 61
Guideline 14—A Soft-Food/Pureed-Food Diet, page 86

- **Dactinomycin** (Actinomycin-D, Actinomycin1)
- **Cosmegen®** (Merck Sharpe & Dohme)

Nutritionally Significant Side Effects

Anorexia
Nausea and vomiting
Dysphagia
Stomatitis and mucositis
Diarrhea
Bleeding and ulceration of the GI tract
Abdominal discomfort
Hypocalcemia

Properties and Use in Treatment

Dactinomycin is the principal component of the mixture of the actinomycins produced by *Streptomyces parvullus.* Dactinomycin anchors into a purine pyrimidine (DNA) base pair by intercalation, thereby inhibiting DNA-dependent RNA synthesis. Its action is cell-cycle nonspecific.

Dactinomycin is poorly absorbed orally and must be administered through running IV infusion. It is used principally in the treatment of choriocarcinoma, Ewing's sarcoma, osteogenic sarcoma, rhabdomyosarcoma, sarcomas, testicular carcinoma, and Wilms' tumor. It should be used with special caution in patients with hepatic disease.

General Toxicities

Toxicities unrelated to nutritional status include bone marrow suppression (occurring one to seven days after completion of therapy); thrombocytopenia (often seen first); leukopenia (may be dose limiting); anemia; alopecia; erythema, desquamation, and hyperpigmentation of the skin, especially in areas subjected to irradiation; acne form eruption (reversible after cessation of therapy); and local irritation if the drug is injected subcutaneously.

Other side effects may include fever; chills; sore throat; redness, pain, or swelling at the place of injection; unusual bleeding or bruising; wheezing; black, tarry stools; flank or stomach pain; heartburn; joint pain; swelling of feet or lower legs; yellowing of eyes or skin; feelings of uneasiness; flushing of face; muscle pain; numbness of the face.

Notes on Nutritional Side Effects

Anorexia—Anorexia has been noted as a side effect of this drug, resulting in decreased food intake. Dietary measures can help increase appetite.

Nausea and vomiting—Nausea and vomiting usually begin within a few hours of drug administration and may be ameliorated by antiemetic agents. Starchy foods taken with the drug may minimize nausea, and other dietary measures can mitigate the aftereffects of vomiting and lessen residual nausea.

If nausea and vomiting are a problem, favorite foods should not be ingested prior to the administration of dactinomycin because a conditioned aversion to foods taken immediately beforehand may result.

Dysphagia—Difficulty in chewing and/or swallowing has been described with this drug. Some dietary restrictions may be necessary regarding the consistency of foods.

Stomatitis and mucositis—Stomatitis, cheilitis, glossitis, and directly toxic to the rapidly replicating mucosal cells in and around the mouth and throughout the digestive tract. Enhanced nutrition, with an emphasis on the B vitamins, may mitigate or prevent this problem. Once the problem exists, however, certain dietary restrictions, such as a soft diet, may be necessary to keep the patient eating. A prescribed mouth care program may be helpful in reducing toxic symptoms.

Diarrhea—Diarrhea results from the direct toxicity of this drug to the mucosa of the gut. The villi and microvilli become flattened, reducing the absorptive surface area and resulting in a "slick gut." Intestinal contents move rapidly through the gut, further reducing absorption. Much of the water poured into the gut for digestion is not reabsorbed, and many water-soluble vitamins and minerals are lost. It is possible to mitigate some of the effects of diarrhea by dietary means.

Bleeding and ulceration of the GI tract—The enteritis caused by this drug may be severe enough to result in bleeding and ulceration of the gut. This can lead to a blood loss of iron, loss of many nutrients, and nonreabsorption of bile salts. These side effects may be mitigated by dietary means.

Abdominal discomfort—Dactinomycin may cause vague abdominal discomfort, which may be aggravated by a full or distended gut. A fiber- and residue-restricted diet may be necessary.

Hypocalcemia—Dactinomycin may cause hypocalcemia, but its mechanism has not been explained. Since this drug is often used in the treatment of childhood cancers, it is important for the child to have an adequate intake of calcium. If milk and milk products have been eliminated from the diet because of diarrhea, calcium tablets should be prescribed (1000-1200 mg/day of elemental calcium, in divided doses of 500-600 mg twice a day).

Refer patients, as needed, to:

Chapter One: How to Deal with Specific Problems
Problem 1—Loss of Appetite, page 4
Problem 2—Nausea and Vomiting, page 8
Problem 4—Sore or Ulcerated Mouth or Throat (Stomatitis/ Mucositis), page 14
Problem 5—Difficulties in Chewing and Swallowing(Dysphagia) and Dry Mouth (Xerostomia), page 18
Problem 7—Protecting the Gastrointestinal Tract (Enteritis), page 22
Problem 9—Dehydration, page 26

Chapter Two: General Dietary Guidelines
Guideline 1—Basic Nutrition for the Cancer Patient, page 30
Guideline 2—A High-Protein/High-Calorie Diet, page 38
Guideline 3—Food Sources of Minerals, page 45
Guideline 4—Food Sources of Vitamins, page 52
Guideline 5—The Fiber and Residue Contents of Foods, page 58
Guideline 6—A Lactose-Free/Lactose-Restricted Diet, page 61
Guideline 14—A Soft-Food/Pureed-Food Diet, page 86

• Daunorubicin (Daunomycin, Rubidomycin)
• Cerubidine® (Ives)

Nutritionally Significant Side Effects

Nausea and vomiting
Stomatitis and mucositis
Diarrhea
Hyperuricemia
Iron loss
Lipid peroxidation

Properties and Use in Treatment

Daunorubicin is a cell-cycle nonspecific anthracycline cytotoxic antibiotic which is believed to inhibit RNA synthesis by intercalation between base pairs of DNA.

Daunorubicin is poorly absorbed orally; thus it is given intravenously. It is rapidly metabolized in the liver and excreted in the bile. Daunorubicin can damage cell membranes, which may explain some cytotoxicity. Large, cumulative doses are diffusely damaging to cardiac sarcosomal membranes. This drug should be avoided in patients with heart disease.

Daunorubicin is used primarily in acute lymphoblastic leukemia and myeloblastic leukemia.

General Toxicities

Non-nutritional side effects include myelosuppression, predominantly manifested as leukopenia, thrombocytopenia and anemia and occasionally severe marrow hypoplasia. Other non-nutritional side effects include shortness of breath, swelling of feet and legs, fever, chills, sore throat, lip and mouth sores, joint pains, unusual bleeding and bruising, and skin rash or itching. Daunomycin extravasated outside of the vein may cause serious tissue damage and scarring. Alopecia may occur two to three weeks after treatment; pink or red urine may occur within 24 to 48 hours after administration.

Notes on Nutritional Side Effects

Nausea and vomiting—Nausea and vomiting are usually mild but can be severe in some cases. These symptoms can be prevented by the prophylactic administration of antiemetic drugs. Starchy foods taken before drug administration may minimize nausea. Other dietary measures can be used to mitigate the aftereffects of vomiting and lessen residual nausea.

If nausea and vomiting are a problem, favorite foods should not be ingested prior to the administration of daunorubicin because a conditioned aversion to foods taken immediately beforehand may result.

Stomatitis and mucositis—This drug can be directly toxic to the rapidly replicating mucosal cells in and around the mouth and throughout the digestive tract. Prophylactic administration of enhanced nutrition, emphasizing the B vitamins, may mitigate or prevent this problem. Once the problem exists, however, certain dietary measures such as a soft diet may be needed to keep the patient eating. A prescribed mouth care program is essential.

Diarrhea—Diarrhea results from the direct toxicity of this drug to the mucosa lining of the gut. The villi and microvilli become flattened, reducing the absorptive surface area and resulting in a "slick gut." As a result, intestinal contents then move rapidly through the gut, resulting in further decreased absorption. Much of the water poured into the gut for digestion is not reabsorbed, thus many water-soluble vitamins and minerals may be lost. It is possible to mitigate some of the effects of diarrhea by dietary means.

Hyperuricemia—This drug causes rapid cellular destruction, resulting in extensive purine catabolism and hyperuricemia. Renal and joint damage can result from the precipitation of urates. A low-purine diet, the traditional treatment, necessitates a low-protein diet, which may be contraindicated for a cancer patient. Existing hyperuricemia should be treated primarily by medical means, that is, by administering a xanthine oxidase inhibitor drug such as allopurino,* preferably withoutan accompanying low-protein diet. Supportive dietary measures should include increased hydration (ten to twelve 8-ounce glasses of fluid per day) and an alkaline-ash

*Note: Allopurinol has its own nutritional side effects. See the discussion of this drug earlier in this chapter.

diet to alkalinize the urine and prevent the precipitation of uric acid stones in the kidney.

Iron loss—Anthracyclines have the capacity to chelate iron in the blood. This chelated iron becomes unavailable for later use. However, it is not advisable to administer iron or to promote iron-rich foods at the time of drug administration because iron supplementation may contribute to inactivating the drug. The drug-free interval of the treatment schedule should be used to replace needed iron. Iron taken along with vitamin C-rich foods such as orange juice will be better absorbed.

Cardiac toxicity—Acute and chronic cardiac toxicity, which is dose related, with tachycardia, heart block, and ventricular irritability cardiomyopathy and congestive heart failure may occur. Patients who have received radiation therapy over the heart are more susceptible to cardiac toxicity and failure. Anthracycline drugs are cardiotoxic by virtue of their effect of enhancing lipid peroxidation. The administration of vitamin E may prevent lipid peroxidation in the heart, although the effect has not been proven. Some of the therapeutic action of the drug, however, may be due to the generation of free radicals. Vitamin E prevents free radical form action and could possibly interfere with the efficacy of the drug. For this reason, it is probably advisable not to give vitamin E and daunorubicin concurrently. The drug-free pre-treatment interval should be used to administer supplementary vitamin E, if it is desired. The same advice is pertinent for the ingestion of vitamin C and selenium, which are also antioxidants.

Refer patients, as needed, to:

Chapter One: How to Deal with Specific Problems

Problem 1—Loss of Appetite, page 4
Problem 2—Nausea and Vomiting, page 8
Problem 4—Sore or Ulcerated Mouth or Throat (Stomatitis/ Mucositis), page 14
Problem 6—Diarrhea, page 20
Problem 9—Dehydration, page 26

Chapter Two: General Dietary Guidelines

Guideline 1—Basic Nutrition for the Cancer Patient, page 30
Guideline 2—A High-Protein/High-Calorie Diet, page 38
Guideline 3—Food Sources of Minerals, page 45
Guideline 4—Food Sources of Vitamins, page 52
Guideline 6—A Lactose-Free/Lactose-Restricted Diet, page 61
Guideline 10—How to Prevent Kidney Stone Formation (Acid Ash/Alkaline Ash Diet), page 74
Guideline 14—A Soft-Food/Pureed-Food Diet, page 86

• Doxorubicin
• Adriamycin® (Adria)

Nutritionally Significant Side Effects

Nausea and vomiting
Anorexia
Stomatitis and mucositis
Diarrhea
Iron loss
Lipid peroxidation

Properties and Use in Treatment

Doxorubicin is a cytotoxic anthracycline antibiotic isolated from cultures of *Streptomyces peucetius varcaesius.* The drug's mechanism of action is related to its ability to bind to DNA by intercalation and to inhibit nucleic acid synthesis. It is cell-cycle phase nonspecific, but its efficacy is greater in the S-phase. This class of agent can also cause membrane lipid peroxidation, which can produce cytotoxicity.

Doxorubicin is given intravenously and used in the treatment of most cancers. A slow release from protein binding gives relatively prolonged plasma levels of the drug and its metabolites. Doxorubicin is rapidly metabolized by the liver; *reduced doses should therefore be used with liver insufficiency* or jaundice. The drug is eliminated predominantly in the bile, although small amounts are also excreted in the urine.

It is primarily used to treat cancer of the lung, breast, bladder, prostate, pancreas, stomach, ovary, thyroid, endometrium, sarcomas, leukemias, Hodgkin's and non-Hodgkin's lymphomas, mehothelioma, myelomas, cancer of unknown primary and and Wilm's tumor.

General Toxicities

Doxorubicin has two dose-limiting toxicities—one related to the maximum individual dose and the other related to the total lifetime dose. The first dose-limiting toxicity is myelosuppression, which manifests as leukopenia and thrombocytopenia. This response nadirs at fourteen days and recovers at day twenty-one.

The other dose limiting toxicity is myocardial damage, which manifests as congestive heart failure. The incidence of congestive heart failure is 3 percent at a total cumulative dose of 550 mg/m^2. Risk factors include concurrent cyclophosphamide, mitomycin, and mediastinal radiation therapy. In addition, cardiac arrhythmias are common and may occur within 48 hours of administration but do not preclude further therapy.

Doxorubicin may cause stomatitis about four to seven days after drug administration, which usually recovers by day seventeen to twenty-one. Alopecia is common and accumulates with successive doses. Hair may regrow after discontinuation of therapy. Doxorubicin is a vesicant and can cause severe skin necrosis upon accidental drug extravasation. Less than 10 percent of the drug is excreted in the urine but may cause red or orange discoloration of the urine within twenty-four hours of drug administration.

Interactions with Other Drugs

In vitro interactions have been reported with the following drugs: amphotericin B (increased drug uptake) and phenobarbital (increased aglycone formation). None of these interactions has been reported in patients. Doxorubicin has been reported to exacerbate cyclophosphamide-induced hemorrhagic cystitis and mercaptopurine induced hepatotoxicity.

Notes on Nutritional Side Effects

Nausea and vomiting—Nausea and vomiting are common, mild to moderate in severity, and usually can be prevented by the prophylactic administration of antiemetic agents. Diet usually does not prevent vomiting, but starchy foods taken with the drug may minimize nausea.

If nausea and vomiting are a problem, favorite foods should not be ingested prior to the administration of doxorubicin because a conditioned aversion to foods taken immediately beforehand may result.

Anorexia—Unexplained anorexia has been noted as a side effect of this drug. The result may be decreased food intake. Dietary measures may help increase appetite.

Stomatitis and mucositis—This drug may be directly toxic to the rapidly replicating mucosal cells in and around the mouth and throughout the digestive tract. Prophylactic administration of enhanced nutrition, with an emphasis on the B vitamins, may mitigate or prevent this problem. Once the problem exists, however, certain dietary measures (e.g., a soft diet) may be needed to keep the patient eating. A prescribed mouth care program may be helpful in reducing toxic symptoms.

Diarrhea—Diarrhea results from the direct toxicity of this drug to the mucosa lining of the gut. The villi and microvilli become flattened, reducing the absorptive surface area, resulting in a "slick gut." As a result, intestinal contents move rapidly through the gut, reducing absorption. Much of the water poured into the gut for digestion is not reabsorbed, and many water-soluble vitamins and minerals are lost. It is possible to mitigate some of the effects of diarrhea by dietary means.

Iron loss—Anthracyclines have the capacity to chelate iron in the blood. This chelated iron becomes unavailable for later use. But it is not advisable to administer iron or promote high-iron-containing foods during the time of doxorubicin administration because iron supplementation may contribute to inactivating the drug. The drug-free interval of treatment should be used to replace needed iron. Iron taken along with a vitamin C-containing beverage, such as orange juice, will be better absorbed.

Lipid peroxidation—Anthracycline drugs are cardiotoxic. The administration of vitamin E may prevent lipid peroxidation in the heart, which allegedly causes the cardiac damage. The results of studies, however, are conflicting as to whether vitamin E does indeed provide a protective effect. Some of the cytotoxic action of doxorubicin may be due to the generation of free radicals, which vitamin E would prevent. For this reason, it is probably advisable not to give vitamin E concurrently. The drug-free interval following treatment should be used to administer supplementary vitamin E, if desired.

Refer patients, as needed, to:

Chapter One: How to Deal with Specific Problems
Problem 1—Loss of Appetite, page 4
Problem 2—Nausea and Vomiting, page 8
Problem 4—Sore or Ulcerated Mouth or Throat (Stomatitis/Mucositis), page 14

Chapter Two: General Dietary Guidelines

• Dronabinol
• Marinol® (Roxane)

Nutritionally Significant Side Effects

None

Properties and Use in Treatment

Dronabinol (delta-9-tetrahydrocannabinol) is an antiemetic agent in capsule form for treatment of the nausea and vomiting associated with cancer chemotherapy in patients who have failed to respond adequately to conventional antiemetic treatments. It is a synthetic version of the active substance in marijuana. It has a stimulating effect on appetite.

A substantial proportion of patients treated with Marinol can be expected to experience psychotomimetic reactions not observed with other antiemetic agents. Because it may cause a general increase in central sympathomimetic activity, Marinol should be used with caution in persons with hypertension or heart disease.

Marinol is abusable and is classified as Schedule II of the Controlled Substances Act. Prescriptions should be limited to the amount necessary for a single cycle of chemotherapy (that is, a few days).

General Toxicities

In controlled clinical trials, the most frequently reported adverse reactions involved the central nervous system. In decreasing order of frequency: drowsiness, dizziness, muddled thinking, and brief impairment of coordination, sensory and perceptual functions, easy laughing, elation, and heightened awareness, (often termed a "high") were observed in 24 percent of patients.

Other side effects occurring in more than one percent of patients include anxiety, irritability, depression, weakness, sluggishness, headache, hallucinations, memory lapse, paranoia, depersonalization, disorientation, confusion, dry mouth, paresthesia, visual distortions, tachycardia, and postural hypotension.

Side effects noted in fewer than 1 percent of patients include tinnitus, nightmares, speech difficulty, facial flushing, perspiring, syncope, diarrhea, fecal incontinence, and muscular pains.

Interactions with Other Drugs

Marinol should not be taken with alcohol, sedatives, hypnotics, or other psychotomimetic substances. The effects of this drug on blood ethanol levels are complex. During administration of 60 mg/day for ten days, absorption of ethanol was delayed, resulting in lower and delayed peak blood alcohol levels. Metabolism of ethanol was increased in some subjects and reduced in others. The overall rate of ethanol disappearance was reduced by about 10 percent.

- **Estramustine**
- **Emcyt®** (Pharmacia)

Nutritionally Significant Side Effects

Fluid retention
Nausea and vomiting
Diarrhea

Properties and Use in Treatment

Estramustine phosphate sodium is an oral antineoplastic agent used primarily in the treatment of patients with metastatic and/or progressive carcinoma of the prostate. Estramustine phosphate is a molecule combining estradiol and nor-nitrogen mustard by a carbamate link. The molecule is phosphorylated to make it water soluble. Estramustine phosphate taken orally is readily dephosphorylated during absorption, and the major metabolites in plasma are estramustine, estradiol, and estrone.

General Toxicities

Toxicities unrelated to nutritional status include headache; loss of coordination; pains in chest, groin, or legs (especially calves of legs); shortness of breath; slurred speech; vision changes; fever, chills, or sore throat; skin rash; unusual bleeding or bruising; unusual tiredness or weakness; breast tenderness or enlargement; and swelling of feet or lower legs.

Food-Drug Interactions

Milk, milk products, and calcium-rich foods may impair the absorption of estramustine by binding with the drug. These foods should be avoided at the time estramustine is taken.

Full meals may delay and change the absorption of an orally administered drug with respect to both the rate of absorption and peak serum concentrations. Complete absorption by the oral route is particularly questionable if the patient is concurrently receiving drugs that are toxic to the gastrointestinal tract.

To promote maximal absorption, oral drugs should not be taken with full meals or fatty foods that delay absorption. It is recommended that the drug be administered one hour before or two to three hours after a full meal. Taking the drug on an empty stomach may engender nausea or other stomach disturbances. It should be taken along with a starchy snack, such as bread or crackers, in order to clear the stomach quickly and not interfere with drug absorption.

Notes on Nutritional Side Effects

Fluid retention—Exacerbation of preexisting or incipient peripheral edema or congestive heart disease has been seen in some patients receiving estramustine therapy. Other conditions that might be influenced by fluid retention, such as epilepsy, migraine, or renal dysfunction, require careful observation. A sodium-restricted diet may be necessary. Increased fluid intake may be necessary to help flush out the excess sodium.

Nausea and vomiting—Nausea and vomiting are common and may be ameliorated by antiemetic agents. Starchy foods taken with the drug may minimize nausea, and other dietary measures can mitigate the aftereffects of vomiting and lessen residual nausea.

If nausea and vomiting are a problem, favorite foods should not be ingested prior to taking estramustine because a conditioned food aversion may result.

Diarrhea—Diarrhea results from the direct toxicity of this drug to the mucosa of the gut. The villi and microvilli become flattened, reducing the absorptive surface area, resulting in a "slick gut." Intestinal contents move rapidly through the gut, further decreasing absorption. Much of the water poured into the gut for digestion is not reabsorbed, and many water-soluble vitamins and minerals are lost. Some of these effects may be mitigated by dietary means.

Refer patients, as needed, to:

Chapter One: How to Deal with Specific Problems
Problem 2—Nausea and Vomiting, page 8
Problem 6—Diarrhea, page 20

Chapter Two: General Dietary Guidelines

• Estrogens
• Diethylstilbestrol (DES)

Nutritionally Significant Side Effects

B-vitamin deficiency
Iron deficiency
Gallstones
Glucose intolerance
Sodium retention
Hypercalcemia
Constipation
Anorexia
Nausea and vomiting

Properties and Use in Treatment

Estrogens are used clinically to palliate the symptoms of recurrent and advanced breast cancer in postmenopausal patients and prostate cancer. DES should not be used for pre-menopausal breast cancer patients because it may induce an acute flare of the disease.

The exact mechanism of the antineoplastic action of DES has not yet been clarified.

General Toxicities

When used in higher doses, there is an excessive cardiovascular mortality. Non-nutritional side effects include feminization in males including gynecomastia, testicular atrophy, and loss of libido. Retention with fluid accumulation, gallstones, salt (sodium) and an increase in thromboembolic events are seen. Additional side effects in women include breakthrough vaginal bleeding or hypercalcemia. Estrogens should not be taken by pregnant women, and caution is recommended for women who have had breast cancer at a premenopausal age.

Food-Drug Interactions

Full meals may reduce the absorption of an orally administered drug with respect to both the rate of absorption and peak serum concentrations.

Complete absorption by the oral route is particularly questionable if the patient is concurrently receiving drugs that are toxic to the gastrointestinal tract.

To promote maximal absorption, oral drugs should not be taken with full meals or fatty foods that delay absorption. It is recommended that the drug be administered one hour before or two to three hours after a full meal. Taking the drug on an empty stomach may engender nausea or other stomach disturbances. It should be taken along with a starchy snack such as bread or crackers in order to clear the stomach quickly and not interfere with drug absorption.

Notes on Nutritional Side Effects

Serum vitamin effects—One of the long-term side effects of oral contraceptives use is a reduction in serum levels of water-soluble vitamins. Subclinical vitamin deficiencies may occur, especially in a patient with initial marginal dietary vitamin intake.

Decreased serum folate is common. Other symptoms of folic acid deficiency include glossitis, paresthesia, megaloblastic anemia, leukopenia, and thrombocytopenia. The patient who is suffering from gastrointestinal toxicity from other antineoplastic drugs may develop folic acid malabsorption.

Serum B_{12} is also reduced by chronic intake of oral contraceptives. Whether the defect is in metabolism or absorption remains unknown. Symptoms of B_{12} deficiency include megaloblastic anemia, pallor, weight loss, anorexia, glossitis, nontropical sprue, and nervous degeneration.

The finding of excess metabolites of tryptophan in the urine of women taking steroids is a possible indication of subclinical vitamin B_6 (pyridoxine) deficiency. Features of overt deficiency include seborrheic dermatitis, glossitis, cheilosis, angular stomatitis, peripheral neuropathy, and blood disorders. Vitamin B_6 deficiency may be responsible for the depression that often accompanies the administration of estrogen and/or oral contraceptives.

The requirement for riboflavin (vitamin B_2) is also increased by oral contraceptive use. Theoretically, when increased amounts of pyridoxine are required for normal tryptophan metabolism, the need for riboflavin is also elevated. The most characteristic overt signs of riboflavin deficiency are cheilitis or angular stomatitis, sometimes accompanied by conjunctivitis, photophobia, and seborrheic dermatitis.

The concentration of plasma ascorbic acid (vitamin C) is also decreased with ingestion of oral contraceptives, which may either increase the catabolism of ascorbic acid or change its tissue distribution. Overt deficiency symptoms include joint pain, increased susceptibility to infection, poor wound healing, easy bruising, bleeding gums, and pinpoint hemorrhages in the skin.

Overall, the effect of oral contraceptives (estrogen) on vitamin nutriture seems to be either an increase or no change in serum levels of the fat-soluble vitamins (A, E and K) and a decrease in serum levels of the water-soluble C and B vitamins. For this reason, it is recommended that a patient receiving any form of estrogen should take a B-complex plus C vitamin supplement if not otherwise contraindicated. The amounts should be within recommended dietary ranges. Large doses of any vitamins should be highly discouraged because their possible pharmacological effects may interfere with drug efficacy.

Iron deficiency—After absorption from the gastrointestinal tract, iron is transported in the plasma bound to the protein transferrin. Plasma transferrin levels are increased by administration of estrogens or contraceptive steroids. Serum iron levels may or may not be elevated in women on contraceptive steroids. Elevated serum iron levels can be deceptive because breakthrough bleeding in premenopausal women on contraceptive steroids may contribute to iron loss. Thus, subclinical iron deficiency might go undetected. Because of the idiopathic increase in the serum transferrin levels, it is recommended that serum transferrin not be used as an indicator of visceral protein production of iron nutriture in the patient receiving estrogen therapy.

Gallstones and glucose intolerance—Additional nutritional or metabolic effects reported with estrogen and oral contraceptive usage include cholelithiasis, or gallstones. Should gallstones occur, a cholesterol-restricted diet may be indicated. Impaired carbohydrate metabolism and glucose tolerance resembling Type II diabetes (noninsulin dependent) may also occur, requiring a special diet.

Sodium retention and hypercalcemia—Sodium retention is common with estrogen use and necessitates a sodium-restricted diet if hypertension and/or edema develops. Symptoms of hypercalcemia may include polyuria, polydipsia, weakness, constipation, and mental sluggishness or disorientation. Hypercalcemia is very serious and could lead to coma and death if not detected and treated appropriately. Withholding dietary calcium alone is not an effective treatment for hypercalcemia, which should be treated medically.

Constipation—Constipation is a possible side effect of this drug. Commercial laxatives may cause nutritional depletion and are habit forming. Mineral oil is discouraged because it solubilizes the fat-soluble vitamins in the gut, preventing absorption. Constipation is best treated prophylactically with dietary fiber when not contraindicated and with stool softners as needed.

Nausea and vomiting—Nausea and vomiting resembling morning sickness may occur. In some instances, these effects can be prevented by the prophylactic administration of antiemetic agents. Dietary manipulations cannot prevent this type of nausea and vomiting, but starchy foods taken with the drug may minimize nausea. Other dietary measures can mitigate the aftereffects of vomiting and lessen residual nausea.

If nausea and vomiting are a problem, favorite foods should not be ingested prior to the administration of estrogen because a conditioned aversion to foods taken immediately beforehand may result.

Refer patients, as needed, to:

Chapter One: How to Deal with Specific Problems
Problem 1—Loss of Appetite, page 4
Problem 2—Nausea and Vomiting, page 8
Problem 3—Constipation, page 24

Chapter Two: General Dietary Guidelines
Guideline 2—A High-Protein/High-Calorie Diet, page 38
Guideline 3—Food Sources of Minerals, page 45
Guideline 4—Food Sources of Vitamins, page 52
Guideline 5—The Fiber and Residue Content of Foods, page 58
Guideline 6—A Lactose-Free/Lactose-Restricted Diet, page 61
Guideline 9—A Cholesterol and Fat-Restricted Diet, page 71
Guideline 11—Transient Glucose Intolerance/Diabetic Diet, page 76
Guideline 12—A Sodium Restricted Diet, page 79

- **Etoposide** (VP-16, BP-16-213)
- **VePesid®** (Bristol)

Nutritionally Significant Side Effects

Anorexia
Altered taste and smell
Nausea and vomiting
Stomatitis and mucositis
Diarrhea
Protein loss
Loss of fluids and electrolytes

Properties and Use in Treatment

Etoposide is a semisynthetic derivative of podophyllotoxin. Its predominant macromolecular effect is the inhibition of DNA synthesis by an enzyme-mediated strand scission mechanism. Etoposide also binds DNA topoisomerase II, producing strand breakage. To a lesser degree, RNA and protein synthesis are depressed.

Etoposide is used in combination therapies with other chemotherapeutic agents and is administered intravenously in the treatment of refractory testicular tumors and orally or intravenously in the treatment of small cell lung cancer, acute non-lymphocytic leukemia, lymphomas, bladder, prostate, uterine cancers and neuroblastoma.

General Toxicities

Myelosuppression, especially leukopenia and thrombocytopenia are seen. Occasional bronchospasm is seen, which can be relieved by antihistamines. Alopecia and peripheral neuropathy are also seen occasionally. Non-nutritional side effects include fever, chills, sore throat, mouth and lip sores, unusual bleeding and bruising, numbness and tingling in the fingers and toes, rapid heart rate, shortness of breath, wheezing and weakness. Patients with hypoalbuminemia, especially post-surgery, may have an increased risk of toxicity with etoposide.

Interactions with Other Drugs

Since etoposide is highly protein bound, displacement of other agents from binding sites may occur. One report of enhanced warfarin effect has been observed after the addition of etoposide.

Food-Drug Interactions

Full meals may reduce the absorption of an orally administered drug with respect to both the rate of absorption and peak serum concentrations. Complete absorption by the oral route is a special concern if the patient is concurrently receiving drugs toxic to the gastrointestinal tract.

To promote maximal absorption, etoposide should not be taken with full meals or fatty foods that delay absorption. It is recommended that the drug be administered one hour before or two to three hours after a full meal. Because the drug on an empty stomach may engender nausea or other stomach disturbances, it should be taken along with a starchy snack such as bread or crackers that will clear the stomach quickly and not interfere with drug absorption. The drug should preferably be taken at the same time(s) each day.

Notes on Nutritional Side Effects

Anorexia—Unexplained anorexia has been noted as a side effect of this drug. It is not known whether the problem is diminished appetite, resulting from nausea and vomiting, or misperception of hunger, the body's physiological signal that it needs energy input. Whatever the cause, the result is reduced food intake. Dietary measures are available to help increase appetite.

Altered taste and smell—Altered taste and smell, or dysgeusia, has been reported with this drug and can lead to decreased appetite. The most common taste complaints are a lowered taste threshold to bitterness and sweetness. Dietary means are available to help cope with this problem.

Nausea and vomiting—Nausea and vomiting have been noted with oral preparations of etoposide. In this instance, the problem may be due to the direct stimulation of the stomach and its acid by the physical presence of the drug. Starchy foods taken with the drug may minimize nausea, and other dietary measures can mitigate the aftereffects of vomiting and lessen residual nausea.

Nausea and vomiting are mild to moderate at conventional doses and moderate at higher IV doses (> 1 gm/m2). Prophylactic use of antiemetics is recommended prior to therapy.

If nausea and vomiting are a problem, favorite foods should not be ingested prior to the administration of etoposide because a conditioned aversion to foods taken immediately beforehand may result.

Stomatitis and mucositis—This drug can be directly toxic to the rapidly replicating mucosal cells in and around the mouth and throughout the digestive tract. Standard doses of etoposide produce mild mucositis in about 30 percent of patients. With high doses used for bone marrow transplant, severe mucositis occurs in most patients. Prophylactic administration of enhanced nutrition, with an emphasis on the B vitamins, may mitigate or prevent this problem. Once the problem exists, however, certain dietary restrictions, such as a soft diet, may be needed to keep the patient eating. A prescribed mouth care program may reduce toxic symptoms.

Diarrhea—Diarrhea results from the direct toxicity of etoposide to the mucosa of the gut. The villi and microvilli become flattened, reducing the absorptive surface area, resulting in a "slick gut." Intestinal contents move rapidly through the gut, reducing absorption. Much of the water poured into the gut for digestion is not reabsorbed, and many water-soluble vitamins and minerals are lost. It is possible to mitigate some of the effects of diarrhea by dietary means.

Loss of protein, fluid and electrolytes—Etoposide may cause destruction of white blood cells and fever. Of nutritional concern is the fact that the fever can destroy lean body mass, so care should be taken to replace any protein, fluid and electrolyte losses.

Refer patients, as needed, to:

Chapter One: How to Deal with Specific Problems

Problem 1—Loss of Appetite, page 4

Problem 2—Nausea and Vomiting, page 8

Problem 3—Taste Changes, page 12

Problem 4—Sore or Ulcerated Mouth or Throat (Stomatitis/Mucositis), page 14

Problem 6—Diarrhea, page 20

Problem 9—Dehydration, page 26

Chapter Two: General Dietary Guidelines

Guideline 1—Basic Nutrition for the Cancer Patient, page 30
Guideline 2—A High-Protein/High-Calorie Diet, page 38
Guideline 3—Food Sources of Minerals, page 45
Guideline 4—Food Sources of Vitamins, page 52
Guideline 5—The Fiber and Residue Contents of Foods, page 58
Guideline 6—A Lactose-Free/Lactose-Restricted Diet, page 61
Guideline 14—A Soft-Food/Pureed-Food Diet, page 86

- **Fluorouracil** (5-FU)
- **Adrucil®** (Adria)
- **Fluorouracil** (Roche)
- **Floxuridine** (FUdR)
- **FUdR®** (Roche)

Nutritionally Significant Side Effects

Anorexia
Nausea and vomiting
Xerostomia
Dysphagia
Stomatitis and mucositis
Bleeding and ulceration of the GI tract
Bile salt losses
Diarrhea
Niacin deficiency
Thiamine deficiency
Alopecia

Properties and Use in Treatment

Fluorouracil (5-FU) and floxuridine (FUdR) interfere with DNA amount of fraudulent RNA by being incorporated into RNA and is cell-cycle specific.

5-FU must be activated to the deoxynucleotide (FdUMP) by thymidine phosphorylase and thymidine kinase as well as through other pathways. FUdR is converted rapidly to 5-FU in vivo. 5-FU is active orally but is erratically absorbed. FUdR is poorly absorbed by the oral route. It can also enter cerebrospinal fluid and malignant effusions. Continuous infusions of 5-FU and FUdR may produce dose-limiting GI toxicity manifested as stomatitis and diarrhea. In contrast, of 5-FU and FUdR, myelosuppression is dose limiting after IV bolus therapy. Both drugs may be administered by the intraperitoneal and intraarterial route.

It is primarily used for cancers of the breast, stomach, colon, liver, pancreas, ovary, bladder, and prostate. It is used topically on skin for basal cell cancer.

General Toxicities

The most significant clinical toxicities of fluorouracil and FUdR pertain to the GI tract and bone marrow. These side effects are related to how the 5-fluorouracil is administered. Hair loss is a frequent occurrence, but mild in severity, and skin hyperpigmentation and a maculopapular rash may be seen. Tingling of the palms and soles is rare. Cerebellar ataxia with headache and visual disturbances are also seen. Anterior chest wall pain has been reported, especially with infusional 5-FU as well as transient coronary vasospasm. Other non-nutritional side effects include cough, shortness of breath, difficulty in balance, fever, chills, sore throat, and unusual bleeding or bruising and in addition, watery eyes, nasal and skin dryness. The skin may also be more sensitive to sun and may burn and tan more easily.

Floxuridine (FUdR) has the same toxicity. Additionally, liver toxicity with sclerosing cholangitis and changes in the biliary tract and surrounding hepatic parenchyma have been reported after intra-arterial administration.

Notes on Nutritional Side Effects

Anorexia—Unexplained anorexia has been noted as a side effect of these drugs, resulting in decreased food intake. Dietary measures are available to help increase appetite.

Nausea and vomiting—Nausea and vomiting are common and, in some instances can be prevented by the prophylactic administration of antiemetic drugs. Diet cannot prevent this type of nausea and vomiting, but starchy snacks such as bread or crackers taken with the drug may minimize nausea. Other dietary measures can mitigate the aftereffects of vomiting and lessen residual nausea.

If nausea and vomiting are a problem, favorite foods should not be ingested prior to the administration of fluorouracil or floxuridine because a conditioned aversion to foods taken immediately beforehand may result.

Xerostomia and dysphagia—5-FU may cause xerostomia or dry mouth through its effects on the salivary glands. It inhibits the parasympathetic nervous system, causing a decrease in the usual watery secretions. However, the thick salivary secretions from the sympathetically controlled glands remain, leaving a feeling of "cotton mouth." Certain dietary practices may be needed to keep up nutritional intake. Dysphagia, difficulty in chewing and/or swallowing, has also been described with this drug. Some dietary restrictions may be necessary regarding the consistency of foods.

Stomatitis and mucositis—5-FU can be directly toxic to the rapidly replicating mucosal cells in and around the mouth and throughout the digestive tract. With continuous 5-FU infusions, stomatitis can be dose limiting. The toxicity typically begins three to five days after the initiation of the infusion course. Initial signs include a diffuse erythema (reddening) of the mucosa with mild pain, progressing to complete ulceration and occasional bleeding with moderate pain after one week. The ulcers commonly become inflamed with bacteria and fungi. In some instances, prophylactic administration of enhanced nutrition, with an emphasis on the B vitamins, may mitigate or prevent this problem. Once the problem exists, however, certain dietary restrictions, such as a soft diet, may be needed to keep the patient eating.

Bleeding and ulceration of the GI tract and bile salt losses—The enteritis caused by this drug may be severe enough to result in bleeding and ulceration of the gut. This can lead to a blood loss of iron, loss of many nutrients, and nonreabsorption of the bile salts. Dietary means can mitigate these side effects.

Diarrhea—5-FU GI toxicity is known to produce significant diarrhea, especially in patients receiving continuous infusions of the drug, due to its direct toxicity of this drug to the mucosa lining of the gut. The villi and microvilli become flattened, reducing the absorptive surface area and resulting in a "slick gut." As a result, intestinal contents move rapidly through the gut, reducing absorption. Much of the water poured into the gut for digestion is not reabsorbed, and many water-soluble vitamins and minerals are lost. It is possible to mitigate some of the effects of diarrhea with dietary means.

Niacin deficiency—An antimetabolite such as 5-FU may cause pellagra as a consequence of niacin (and/or tryptophan) deficiency. The cardinal signs of severe, advanced pellagra are dermatitis, diarrhea, dementia, and ultimately death.Pellagra is correctable by the administration of 100 to 300 mg of niacin a day given in divided doses of 50 to 150 milligrams.

Thiamine deficiency—A significant number of patients given 5-FU have been reported to develop thiamine (vitamin B_1) deficiency. 5-FU competes with thiamine for phosphorylation, resulting in reduced thiamine-dependent transketolase activity. 5-FU-mediated thiamine deficiency can be further aggravated by a number of factors, including an initial marginal dietary intake; a low caloric intake (especially low in whole grains); folic acid deficiency; intravenous glucose given without vitamin B_1; chronic alcohol intake; and chemical stresses such as anorexia, vomiting, and hypermetabolism.

Clinical signs of chronic adult thiamine deficiency include loss of appetite, tiredness, nausea, vomiting, constipation, irritability, weak and heavy extremities, depression, and disordered thinking. Thiamine deficiency that develops during treatment with 5-FU has been shown to be correctable by the administration of 100 mg of thiamine per day in two divided doses. In order not to interfere with the chemotherapy and possibly inactivate some of the drug, vitamin supplementation is best done during drug-free intervals.

Alopecia—Alopecia is frequent due to transient effects on hair follicles. No nutritional means exist to prevent hair loss, but general good nutrition will promote maximal normal regrowth. New hair growth begins almost immediately, but its color and texture may be slightly different than before.

Refer patients, as needed to:

Chapter One: How to Deal with Specific Problems

Problem 1—Loss of Appetite, page 4

Problem 2—Nausea and Vomiting, page 8

Problem 4—Sore or Ulcerated Mouth or Throat (Stomatitis/Mucositis), page 14

Problem 5—Difficulties in Chewing and Swallowing (Dysphagia) and Dry Mouth (Xerostomia), page 18

Problem 6—Diarrhea, page 20

Problem 7—Protecting the Gastrointestinal Tract (Enteritis), page 22

Problem 9—Dehydration, page 26

Chapter Two: General Dietary Guidelines

- **Flutamide**
- **Eulexin®** (Schering)

Nutritionally Significant Side Effects

Anorexia
Nausea and vomiting
Diarrhea

Properties and Use in Treatment

Flutamide (Eulexin®) is a nonsteroidal, orally active antiandrogen used in combination with LHRH agonistic analogues (such as leuprolide acetate) for the treatment of metastatic prostatic carcinoma (stage D_2).

Flutamide exerts its antiandrogenic action by inhibiting androgen uptake and/or by inhibiting nuclear binding of androgen in target tissues or both. Flutamide interferes with testosterone at the cellular level and complements medical castration achieved with leuprolide, which suppresses testicular androgen production by inhibiting luteinizing hormone secretion. To achieve the benefit of the adjunctive therapy, treatment must be started simultaneously with both drugs.

General Toxicities

Frequently reported (in more than 5 percent of patients) toxicities unrelated to nutritional status include hot flashes, loss of libido, impotence, and gynecomastia. (Some adverse experiences reported where there was no apparent relation to drug treatment are those that are common in elderly patients). The following adverse reactions were reported during treatment with flutamide plus LHRH-agonist: hypertension (1 percent); central nervous system reactions (1 percent); drowsiness, confusion, depression, anxiety, and nervousness; elevation of serum enzymes and clinically evident hepatitis (causal relationship reported with flutamide monotherapy); pulmonary symptoms (fewer than 1 percent); skin irritation at the injection site and rash (3 percent); photosensitivity reactions; edema and hematopoietic (WBC/platelets) symptoms (4 percent); neuromuscular, hepatic, and genitourinary symptoms (2 percent). Laboratory abnormalities may include elevated SGOT, SGPT, bilirubin and creatinine values.

Notes on Nutritional Side Effects

Anorexia—Unexplained anorexia is a side effect of this drug in 4 percent of patients, resulting in diminished appetite and reduced food intake. Dietary measures can help increase appetite.

Nausea and vomiting—Nausea and vomiting is reported in about 10 percent of patients and may be ameliorated by antiemetic agents. Starchy foods taken with the drug may reduce nausea, and other dietary measures can mitigate the aftereffects of vomiting and lessen residual nausea.

If nausea and vomiting are a problem, favorite foods should not be ingested prior to flutamide because a conditioned food aversion may result.

Diarrhea—Diarrhea has occurred in 12 percent of patients and may be associated with lactose intolerance. The oral formulation of flutamide contains 360.5 mg per 125 mg capsule or 210 mg of lactose per 250 mg tablet. Thus, patients with lactase deficiency may be at risk for diarrhea complications. It is recommended that the tablet form may be used in such patients (if available), along with lactase supplementation (1 to 2 tablets of generic lactaid [galactosidase]) with each dose of flutamide to help control diarrhea.

Refer patients, as needed, to:

Chapter One: How to Deal with Specific Problems
Problem 1—Loss of Appetite, page 4
Problem 2—Nausea and Vomiting, page 8
Problem 6—Diarrhea, page 20

Chapter Two: General Dietary Guidelines
Guideline 1—Basic Nutrition for the Cancer Patient, page 30
Guideline 2—A High-Protein/High-Calorie Diet, page 38
Guideline 3—Food Sources of Minerals, page 45
Guideline 4—Food Sources of Vitamins, page 52
Guideline 6—A Lactose-Free/Lactose-Restricted Diet, page 61

• Hydroxyurea (HU, HUR)
• Hydrea® (Squibb)

Nutritionally Significant Side Effects

Iron loss
Anorexia
Nausea and vomiting
Stomatitis and mucositis
Diarrhea
Constipation
Hyperuricemia

Properties and Use in Treatment

Hydroxyurea is an orally administered antimetabolite used in the treatment of resistant chronic myelogenous leukemias, especially in the blast crisis of chronic myelogenous leukemia. Hydroxyurea has been also used in the treatment of: melanoma; recurrent, metastatic, or inoperable carcinoma of the ovary; and local control of primary squamous cell (epidermoid) carcinomas of the head, neck (excluding the lip) (when used concomitantly with radiation therapy) and brain cancer.

The mechanism of action is believed to involve inhibition of ribonucleotide reductase, causing an immediate inhibition of DNA synthesis without interfering with RNA or protein synthesis. Its action is cell-cycle S-phase specific.

HU is usually well absorbed orally and given in three to four divided doses.

General Toxicities

The most significant clinical toxicity is myelosuppression with dose-limiting leukopenia. Other non-nutritional side effects include fever, chills, sore throat, unusual bleeding, bruising, dizziness, hallucinations, headache, joint pains, and swelling of the feet and lower legs.

Food-Drug Interactions

Full meals may delay and change the absorption of an orally administered drug with respect to both the rate of absorption and peak serum concentrations. Complete absorption by the oral route is a special concern if the patient is concurrently receiving drugs toxic to the gastrointestinal tract.

To promote maximal absorption, oral drugs should not be taken with full meals or fatty foods that delay absorption. It is recommended that the drug be administered one hour before or two to three hours after a full meal. Taking the drug on an empty stomach may engender nausea or other stomach disturbances. It should be taken along with a starchy snack such as bread or crackers, in order to clear the stomach quickly and not interfere with drug absorption.

Notes on Nutritional Side Effects

Iron loss—Self-limiting megaloblastic erythropoiesis is often seen early in therapy. The morphological changes resemble pernicious anemia but are not related to a deficiency of vitamin B_{12} or folic acid. Hydroxyurea may reduce the rate of iron utilization by erythrocytes, but iron supplementation will not correct the problem. If clinically indicated, transfusions may be required to correct hemoglobin and erythrocyte level. After chronic effects of the drug have worn off, the patient should be checked for inadequate iron status; supplementation may be necessary at that time.

Anorexia—Anorexia is an uncommon side effect of this drug. The mechanism is unlcear but may be related to appetite suppression. Dietary measures may help increase appetite.

Nausea and vomiting—Nausea and vomiting are uncommon side effects and may be prevented by antiemetic agents. Starchy foods, such as bread, crackers, or rice, taken with the drug may minimize nausea. Other dietary measures can mitigate the aftereffects of vomiting and lessen residual nausea.

If nausea and vomiting are a problem, favorite foods should not be ingested prior to the administration of hydroxyurea because a conditioned aversion to foods taken immediately beforehand may result.

Stomatitis and mucositis—Although stomatitis and mucositis are uncommon with hydroxyurea, toxicity to the rapidly replicating mucosal cells in and around the mouth and throughout the digestive tract may occasionally occur. Enhanced nutrition, emphasizing the B vitamins, may prevent this problem. A soft diet may be necessary to maintain adequate nutrition. A prescribed mouth care program will help reduce toxic symptoms.

Diarrhea—Diarrhea results from the direct toxicity of this drug to the mucosa lining of the gut. The villi and microvilli become flattened, reducing the absorptive surface area and resulting in a "slick gut." As a result, intestinal contents move rapidly through the gut, reducing absorption. Much of the water poured into the gut for digestion is not reabsorbed, and many water-soluble vitamins and minerals are lost. It is possible to mitigate some of the effects of diarrhea with dietary means. The patient's ability to synthesize lactose may be lost, and a lactose-restricted diet may become temporarily necessary.

Constipation—Constipation is also a noted side effect of this drug. It may not readily be relieved by an enema or suppository. Commercial laxatives can cause nutritional depletion and may also be habit forming, and thus are discouraged. Mineral oil is also discouraged because it solublizes the fat-soluble vitamins in the gut, preventing absorption. Constipation is best treated prophylactically with dietary fiber when not contraindicated.

Hyperuricemia—Hydroxyurea can cause rapid cellular destruction in leukemic patients in blast crisis, resulting in extensive purine catabolism and hyperuricemia. Renal and joint damage may result from the precipitation of urates. Hyperuricemia is best treated by medical means—that is, by the administration of a xanthine oxidase inhibitor drug such as allopurinol* without an accompanying low-protein diet. Supportive dietary measures should include increased hydration (ten to twelve 8-ounce glasses of fluid per day) and an alkaline-ash diet to alkalinize the urine and prevent the precipitation of uric acid stones in the kidney.

*Note: Allopurinol is not without its own nutritional side effects. See the discussion of this drug earlier in this chapter.

Refer patients, as needed, to:

Chapter One: How to Deal with Specific Problems
Problem 1—Loss of Appetite, page 4
Problem 2—Nausea and Vomiting, page 8
Problem 4—Sore or Ulcerated Mouth or Throat (Stomatitis/Mucositis), page 14
Problem 6—Diarrhea, page 20
Problem 8—Constipation, page 24
Problem 9—Dehydration, page 26

Chapter Two: General Dietary Guidelines
Guideline 1—Basic Nutrition for the Cancer Patient, page 30
Guideline 2—A High-Protein/High-Calorie Diet, page 38
Guideline 3—Food Sources of Minerals, page 45
Guideline 4—Food Sources of Vitamins, page 52
Guideline 5—The Fiber and Residue Contents of Foods, page 58
Guideline 6—A Lactose-Free/Lactose-Restricted Diet, page 61
Guideline 10—How to Prevent Kidney Stone Formation (Acid Ash/Alkaline Ash Diet), page 74
Guideline 14—A Soft-Food/Pureed Food Diet, page 86

- **Ifosfamide**
- **Ifex®** (Mead Johnson)

Nutritionally Significant Side Effects

Nausea and vomiting

Properties and Use in Treatment

Ifosfamide is a chemotherapeutic agent chemically related to nitrogen mustard and a synthetic analog of cyclophosphamide. It is administered intravenously and often used in combination with other antineoplastic agents for third-line chemotherapy of germ cell testicular cancer, sarcomas, lung and ovarian cancer and lymphomas. A prophylactic agent for hemorrhagic cystitis, such as mesna, should be used concomitantly.

Ifosfamide should be given cautiously to patients with impaired renal function or compromised bone marrow reserve.

General Toxicities

Ifosfamide given in combination with other chemotherapeutic agents may produce severe myelosuppression and requires cessation of therapy.

Various adverse reactions have been observed in patients receiving ifosfamide as a single agent. Dose-limiting toxicities are myelosuppression and urotoxicity. Hematuria has been reported in 6 to 92 percent of patients and renal toxicity in 6 percent. Other significant side effects included alopecia, nausea, vomiting, and central nervous system toxicities. Dose fractionation, vigorous hydration, and uroprotection with mesna can significantly reduce the incidence of hematuria, especially gross hematuria, associated with hemorrhagic cystitis. Urotoxicity consists of hemorrhagic cystitis, dysuria, urinary frequency, and other symptoms of bladder irritation.

Central nervous system side effects have been reported in 12 percent of patients, most commonly somnolence, confusion, depressive psychosis, and hallucinations. Less frequent symptoms included dizziness, disorientation, and cranial nerve dysfunction. Seizures and coma have been occasionally reported. The incidence of central nervous system toxicity may be higher in patients with altered renal function and after very high bolus disease.

Alopecia is common, occurring in approximately 83 percent of patients treated with ifosfamide as a single agent. Other less frequent side effects included phlebitis, pulmonary symptoms, fever of unknown origin, allergic reactions, stomatitis, cardiotoxicity, and polyneuropathy. Diarrhea or constipation are rare and can be prevented with proper nutrition.

Interactions with Other Drugs

Like cyclophosphamide, ifosfamide is activated in the liver by hepatic microsomal enzymes. Thus, drugs such as phenobarbital, chloramphenicol, and corticosteroids may inhibit the conversion of ifosfamide to active metabolites. Concurrent use of these drugs should be avoided.

Notes on Nutritional Side Effects

Anorexia, stomatitis, diarrhea and constipation have been reported in less than 1 percent of patients.

Nausea and vomiting—Nausea and vomiting has been reported in 58 percent of patients receiving ifosfamide as a single agent and were usually controlled by standard antiemetic therapy. Starchy foods taken with the drug may reduce nausea, and other dietary measures can mitigate the aftereffects of vomiting and lessen residual nausea.

If nausea and vomiting are a problem, favorite foods should not be ingested prior to estramustine because a conditioned food aversion may result.

Refer patients, as needed, to:

Chapter One: How to Deal with Specific Problems
Problem 2—Nausea and Vomiting, page 8

Chapter Two: General Dietary Guidelines
Guideline 1—Basic Nutrition for the Cancer Patient, page 30
Guideline 2—A High-Protein/High-Calorie Diet, page 38
Guideline 3—Food Sources of Minerals, page 45
Guideline 4—Food Sources of Vitamins, page 52

- **Interferon ALFA**
- **Intron-A** (Schering-Plough)
- **Roferon-A®** (Roche)

Nutritionally Significant Side Effects

Flu syndrome
Anorexia and weight loss
Nausea and vomiting
Diarrhea
Dry mouth
Altered taste and smell

Properties and use in Treatment

Interferon recombinant is a biologic drug used in the treatment of hairy cell leukemia, renal cancer, Kaposi's sarcoma and other cancers. The drug is administered subcutaneously or intramuscularly.

It is used primarily for melanma, renal cell cancer, myeloma, chronic myelogenius leukemia, Kaposi's sarcoma and lymphomas.

General Toxicities

The following data on adverse reactions are based on the subcutaneous or intramuscular administration of interferon as a single agent utilizing higher doses. A rapid-onset flu-like syndrome consisting of fatigue (89 percent), fever (8 percent), chills (64 percent), myalgias (73 percent), and headache (71 percent) occurred in the majority of patients. These side effects diminish with continued therapy. Toxicities occurring with moderate frequency included dizziness (21 percent), rash (18 percent) and dry skin or pruritus (13 percent).

Less common side effects included diaphoresis (8 percent), paraesthesias (6 percent), numbness (6 percent), and arthralgias (5 percent). Central nervous system side effects have been reported as vertigo (19 percent), confusion (10 percent), and depression (6 percent). These symptoms rapidly abate or discontinue. Rarely reported adverse reactions (incidence of less than 3 percent) include central nervous system effects (decreased mental status, visual disturbances, sleep disturbances, and nervousness), adverse cardiac effects (hypertension, chest pain, arrhythmias, and palpitation), epistaxis; bleeding gums, ecchymosis, petechiae, night sweats, urticaria; conjunctivitis, and inflammation at the site of injection.

Several laboratory test changes have been observed after interferon therapy. Elevated liver function tests aspartic serum transaminase, alkaline phosphatase and bilirubin. Mild proteinuria, elevated serum creatinine and uric acid may also occur. These improve after discontinuation of the drug.

Interactions with Other Drugs

Drug interactions have not yet been fully evaluated.

Notes on Nutritional Deficiencies

Flu syndrome—The fever and chills of this syndrome can cause excess losses of proteins, fluids, and electrolytes. A supportive high-protein, high-calorie diet may be indicated, and fluid and electrolyte losses should be replaced.

Anorexia and weight loss—Unexplained anorexia has been reported in 46 percent of patients, with weight loss occurring in 14 percent. The result is reduced food intake. Dietary measures can help increase appetite.

Nausea and vomiting—Nausea has occurred in 32 percent of patients and vomiting in 10 percent. These side effects may be ameliorated by antiemetic agents. Starchy foods taken with the drug may minimize nausea, and other dietary measures can mitigate the aftereffects of vomiting and lessen residual nausea.

If nausea and vomiting are a problem, favorite foods should not be ingested prior to taking the drug because a conditioned food aversion may result.

Diarrhea—Diarrhea results from the direct toxicity of this drug to the mucosa of the gut. The villi and microvilli become flattened, reducing the absorptive surface area, resulting in a "slick gut." Intestinal contents move rapidly through the gut, further decreasing absorption. Much of the water poured into the gut for digestion is not reabsorbed, and many water-soluble vitamins and minerals are lost. Some of these effects may be mitigated by dietary means.

Dry mouth—This drug has been noted to cause dry mouth, or xerostomia. The actual toxicity is to the parasympathetic nervous system, which controls salivary secretions. The thick salivary secretions from the sympathetically controlled glands remain, leaving a feeling of "cotton mouth." Certain dietary practices may be needed to keep up nutritional intake.

Altered taste and smell—Altered taste and smell, or dysgeusia, have been reported with this drug and can lead to decreased appetite. The most common taste complaints are a lowered taste threshold to bitterness and sweetness. Dietary measures can help cope with this problem.

Refer patients, as needed, to:

Chapter One: How to Deal with Specific Problems
Problem 1—Loss of Appetite, page 4
Problem 2—Nausea and Vomiting, page 8
Problem 3—Taste Changes, page 12
Problem 5—Difficulties in Chewing and Swallowing (Dysphagia) and Dry Mouth (Xerostomia), page 18
Problem 6—Diarrhea, page 20
Problem 9—Dehydration, page 26

Chapter Two: General Dietary Guidelines
Guideline 1—Basic Nutrition for the Cancer Patient, page 30
Guideline 2—A High-Protein/High-Calorie Diet, page 38
Guideline 3—Food Sources of Minerals, page 45
Guideline 4—Food Sources of Vitamins, page 52
Guideline 6—A Lactose-Free/Lactose-Restricted Diet, page 61

- **Leucovorin Calcium**
- **Wellcovorin®** (Burroughs Wellcome)
- **Leucovorin Calcium** (Lederle)

Nutritionally Significant Side Effects

Nausea and vomiting

Properties and Use in Treatment

Leucovorin calcium is an activated form of folic acid. It is indicated for the prophylaxis and treatment of undesired hematopoietic effects of folic acid antagonists, particularly methotrexate. The drug is available in both tablet and injection forms. Following chemotherapy with folic acid antagonists, initial parenteral administration is preferable due to the possibility of chemotherapy-induced vomiting and drug malabsorption.

In the treatment of accidental overdosage of folic acid antagonists, leucovorin should be administered as promptly as possible. As the time interval between antifolate administration and leucovorin rescue increases, leucovorin's effectiveness in counteracting hematologic toxicity diminishes.

It is primarily used to reverse methotrexate toxicity and potentiate and modulate action of 5-FU.

General Toxicities

Allergic sensitization has been reported following both oral and parenteral administration of folic acid. Mild nausea has been reported after intravenous administration.

Interactions with Other Drugs

Folic acid in large amounts may counteract the anti-epileptic effect of phenobarbital, phenytoin, and primidone and increase the frequency of seizures in susceptible children. Leucovorin may enhance the toxicity of fluorouracil.

Notes on Nutritional Side Effects

Nausea and vomiting—Nausea and vomiting has occurred with intravenous use.

Refer patients, as needed, to:

Chapter One: How to Deal with Specific Problems
Problem 2—Nausea and Vomiting, page 8

• Leuprolide Acetate
• Leupron® (TAP)

Nutritionally Significant Side Effects

Anorexia
Dysphagia
Taste changes

Properties and Use in Treatment

Leuprolide acetate is a synthetic nonapeptide analog of gonadotropin releasing hormone (GRH or LH-RH), which possesses greater potency than the naturally occurring hormone, somatostatin. It acts as a potent inhibitor of gonadotropin secretion when given continuously in therapeutic dosages. The metabolism, distribution, and excretion of leuprolide acetate in humans have not yet been described.

Following an initial stimulation, chronic administration of leuprolide acetate results in the reversible suppression of ovarian and testicular steroidogenesis. In males, testosterone is reduced to castrate levels within two to four weeks after initiation of treatment, which has been shown to last for periods up to five years. Leuprolide acetate is used in the palliative treatment of advanced prostatic cancer when orchiectomy or estrogen administration are either not indicated or are unacceptable to the patient. Leuprolide acetate is administered either as a single daily subcutaneous injection or as a depot suspension in a single monthly intramuscular injection.

General Toxicities

The following non-nutritionally related side effects have been reported in more than five percent of study participants given leuprolide acetate: cardiovascular system effects (congestive heart failure, ECG changes/ischemia, hypertension, murmur, peripheral edema, phlebitis/thrombosis); endocrine system (decreased testicular size, gynecomastia/breast tenderness or pain); hot flashes; impotence; anemia; bone pain, myalgia; nervous system (dizziness/lightheadedness, general pain, headache, insomnia/sleep disorders); respiratory system (dyspnea, sinus congestion); dermatitis; urogenital system (frequency/urgency, hematuria, urinary tract infection); asthenia.

Notes on Nutritional Side Effects

It should be noted that nausea, vomiting, diarrhea and peripheral edema are gastrointestinal side effects occur in less five percent of patients receiving leuprolide—it is very uncommon.

Anorexia—Anorexia or loss of appetite, has been reported in approximately five percent of patients receiving leuprolide. The source of the anorexia is unknown but may be related to nausea and vomiting. Chronic anorexia causes reduced food intake, possibly resulting in a host of nutritional deficiencies, including protein or calorie malnutrition.

A number of dietary approaches can stimulate the appetite, including an attractive, peaceful meal setting, a glass of wine before meals (if not contraindicated), mild exercise one-half hour before a meal, and smaller more frequent meals, among other things. Since appetite is generally greater in the morning, a nutritionally balanced breakfast is important. Dietary zinc supplements (Zinc Sulfate 100 mg twice daily) may also help.

Nausea and vomiting—Nausea and vomiting occur in approximately five percent of the patients, which is considerably less than with DES administration. Much of the nausea and vomiting can be prevented by the prophylactic administration of antiemetics. There are no nutritional means to prevent vomiting, but the after effects can be mitigated by dietary manipulation. If vomiting has been prolonged, the stomach will be alkalotic and can be neutralized by drinking carbonated beverages. Ginger ale and colas often work best. If there has been loss of electrolytes, electrolyte replacement drinks, such as GatoradeR, QuirshR, or ERGR, may help to stabilize the patient and eliminate some of the exhaustion and cramping. These products should be diluted one to one with water first because they tend to be very concentrated. They are often tolerated very well when given in popsicle form. Starchy foods will help quell any residual nausea. Soda crackers should be kept at the bedside for the patient who is nauseous upon waking in the morning. (NOTE: a glass of water should be kept at the bedside as well.)

Constipation—Constipation occurs in approximately 7 percent of the patients who receive leuprolide and is prevented with a prophylactic high fiber diet containing both soluble (e.g., oat bran) and insoluble fibers (e.g., cellulose,wheat bran). The chronic use of laxatives is discouraged because of potential dependency. The use of mineral oil is also contraindicated because it will solubilize out the fat soluble vitamins that may be present in the gut, rendering them unavailable for absorption.

Peripheral edema—Peripheral edema is a cardiovascular system side effect that is the retention of fluid in the tissues. A low-sodium diet may be indicated in certain patients if this occurs. A low-sodium diet will help to mitigate the condition, but it will not correct it, as it is not caused by a nutritional imbalance.

Diarrhea—Diarrhea is an infrequent, but nonetheless bothersome, side effect of leuprolide. Chronic diarrhea will result in the flattening of the microvilli, or absorptive surfaces, in the gut. Fewer nutrients are absorbed, and many, particularly those that are water soluble, are lost. Dehydration and loss of electrolytes will also occur, and a transient lactose intolerance may develop in those patients who previously had no problems consuming dairy products. The water-soluble vitamins and minerals and electrolytes will need to be replaced along with fluids.

Dysphagia—Dysphagia or difficulty in swallowing, may sometimes occur with the administration of leuprolide. It may become necessary to alter the consistency to a softer diet if this side effect occurs.

Taste changes—Taste disorders have been reported to occur occasionally, especially with foods tasting too sweet or bitter. Dietary means can disguise foods that taste too sweet or bitter. Sour or spicy foods are preferred (unless contraindicated for other reasons).

Refer patients, as needed, to:

Chapter One: How to Deal with Specific Problems
Problem 1—Loss of Appetite, page 4
Problem 2—Taste Changes, page 12
Problem 5—Difficulties in Chewing and Swallowing (Dysphagia) and Dry Mouth (Xerostomia), page 18

Chapter Two: General Dietary Guidelines

Guideline 1—Basic Nutrition for the Cancer Patient, page 30
Guideline 2—A High-Protein/High-Calorie Diet, page 38
Guideline 3—Food Sources of Minerals, page 45
Guideline 4—Food Sources of Vitamins, page 52

• Levamisole
• Ergamisol® (Janssen Pharmaceutica)

Nutritionally Significant Side Effects

Nausea and vomiting
Altered taste and smell
Abdominal discomfort
Diarrhea
Loss of appetite

Properties and Use in Treatment

It is an imidiazothiazole derivative which has been used in clinical investigational trials to help restore toward normal an impairment of the immune system. It appears to improve macrophage and T lymphocyte function and helps augment cellular immune function. It enhances antibody formation to a variety of antigens.

It is primarily used for melanoma, colon, ovary and lung cancer and myelogenous leukemia.

General Toxicities

In general, toxic reactions to levamisole when used alone are infrequent and consist of mild diarrhea, nausea, or leukopenia. Occasionally a flu-like syndrome may be seen including fever, chills, and malaise. Agranulocytosis has been reported in about 3 percent of patients treated with levamisole 150 mg/day on 2 consecutive days every week.

It produces a small incidence of stomatitis and hair loss. Rarely, it has been known to cause fever, malaise, bone marrow depression, skin rashes, blurred vision, headaches, irritability and nervousness.

Central nervous system side effects have been reported in patients receiving long-term therapy and have included: fatigue, headache, confusion, insomnia, dizziness, excitation, and convulsions.

A transient granulocytopenia (WBC depression) occurs in about 20% of patients which disappears when drug is discontinued. Fatigue, weakness and flu-like symptoms occur.

Ergamisol® has been reported to produce "antabuse-like" effects when given concomitantly with alcohol. Patients should be instructed to avoid alcohol on the days they take Ergamisol® and for a few days afterward.

Notes on Nutritional Side Effects

Nausea and vomiting—Nausea and vomiting is mild and easily managed with antiemetics.

Altered taste and smell—Altered taste and smell along with a bad taste in the mouth is occasionally seen. A metallic taste is associated with long-term therapy and may lead to decreased appetite. Breath sweetners may be helpful in improving the altered taste.

Abdominal discomfort—Cramping and abdominal pain have been reported, usually after high single doses. The drug should be subdivided into three daily doses to minimize gastric upset.

Diarrhea—Diarrhea is relatively uncommon when the drug is used alone. When combined with 5-fluorouracil, diarrhea is common, probably due to the cytotoxic effect of the pyrimidine antagonist.

Refer patients, as needed, to:

Chapter One: How to Deal with Specific Problems

Problem 1—Loss of Appetite, page 4
Problem 2—Nausea and Vomiting, page 8
Problem 3—Taste Changes, page 12
Problem 6—Diarrhea, page 20
Problem 7—Protecting the Gastrointestinal Tract (Enteritis), page 22

Chapter Two: General Dietary Guidelines

Guideline 1—Basic Nutrition for the Cancer Patient, page 30
Guideline 2—A High-Protein/High-Calorie Diet, page 38
Guideline 3—Food Sources of Minerals, page 45
Guideline 14—A Soft-Food/Pureed-Food Diet, page 86

- **Lomustine** (CCNU)
- **CeeNU®** (Bristol-Myers)

Nutritionally Significant Side Effects

Anorexia
Nausea and vomiting
Diarrhea
Stomatitis and mucositis

Properties and Use in Treatment

Lomustine is an alkylating agent used primarily in the treatment of Hodgkin's disease, brain tumors, bronchogenic carcinoma, melanoma and colorectal adenocarcinoma. The cytotoxic effect of lomustine involves both alkylation of DNA and carbamolyation of protein by isocyanate metabolites, thus inhibiting both DNA and RNA synthesis. Its action is cell-cycle nonspecific. Lomustine is active orally with prompt and rapid absorption.

General Toxicities

Hematologic toxicities are dose limiting and include leukopenia (delayed to about four to six weeks after a dose and persisting less than twenty-four hours); thrombocytopenia (occurring about three to five weeks after a dose and lasting one to two weeks); and anemia.

Other side effects unrelated to nutritional status include alopecia, awkwardness, confusion, cough, fever, chills, sore throat, shortness of breath, slurred speech, swelling of feet or lower legs, unusual bleeding or bruising, unusual reduction in urination, tiredness, weakness, yellowing of eyes and skin, darkening of skin, skin rash, and itching. Lung and kidney toxicity occur infrequently and are related to cumulative dosing for 12 to 18 months.

Interactions with Other Drugs

Cimetidine (Tagamet®) may enhance the bone marrow depression of carmustine and possibly lomustine.

Notes on Nutritional Side Effects

Anorexia—nausea and vomiting. It results in reduced food intake. Dietary measures can help increase appetite.

Nausea and vomiting—Nausea and vomiting can be quite severe, usually occurring four to six hours after drug administration, persisting less than twenty-four hours. Antiemetic agents may provide some relief. Starchy foods taken with the drug may minimize some nausea, and other dietary measures can mitigate the aftereffects of vomiting and lessen residual nausea.

If nausea and vomiting are a problem, favorite foods should not be ingested prior to lomustine because a conditioned food aversion may result.

Diarrhea—Diarrhea results from the direct toxicity of this drug to the mucosa of the gut. The villi and microvilli become flattened, reducing the absorptive surface area, resulting in a "slick gut." Intestinal contents move rapidly through the gut, further decreasing absorption. Much of the water poured into the gut for digestion is not reabsorbed, and many water-soluble vitamins and minerals are lost. Some of these effects may be mitigated by dietary means.

Stomatitis and mucositis—Rarely, lomustine can also be directly toxic to the mucosal cells in and around the mouth and throughout the digestive tract. Enhanced nutrition, with an emphasis on the B vitamins, may prevent this problem. Certain dietary restrictions such as a soft diet, may be necessary to maintain nutrition. A prescribed mouth care program can be helpful in reducing discomfort.

Refer patients, as needed, to:

Chapter One: How to Deal with Specific Problems
Problem 1—Loss of Appetite, page 4
Problem 2—Nausea and Vomiting, page 8
Problem 4—Sore or Ulcerated Mouth or Throat (Stomatitis/ Mucositis), page 14
Problem 9—Dehydration, page 26

Chapter Two: General Dietary Guidelines

Guideline 1—Basic Nutrition for the Cancer Patient, page 30
Guideline 2—A High-Protein/High-Calorie Diet, page 38
Guideline 3—Food Sources of Minerals, paage 45
Guideline 4—Food Sources of Vitamins, page 52
Guideline 14—A Soft-Food/Pureed-Food Diet, page 86

- **Mercaptopurine** (6-Mercaptopurine, 6-MP)
- **Purinethol®** (Burroughs Wellcome)

Nutritionally Significant Side Effects

Anorexia
Nausea and vomiting
Diarrhea
Stomatitis and mucositis
Abdominal discomfort
Hyperuricemia
Pellagra

Properties and Use in Treatment

Mercaptopurine is an antimetabolite used primarily in the consolidation treatment of acute lymphocytic and lymphoblastic leukemia. (This drug is also used as an immunosuppressant to prevent graft rejection in renal or cardiac transplant patients.)

Mercaptopurine is metabolized to a ribose-phosphate species that competes with hypoxanthine and guanine for the enzyme hypoxanthine-guanine phosphoribosyltranferase, ultimately halting DNA and RNA synthesis. Its action is cell-cycle S-phase specific and self-limiting. Mercaptopurine is well absorbed orally and is extensively metabolized to active and inactive forms in the liver.

General Toxicities

The most consistent, dose-related toxicity of mercaptopurine is bone marrow suppression, manifested by anemia, leukopenia, thrombocytopenia, or any combination of these. Cholestatic jaundice occurs in about one-third of patients, less commonly in children, and is usually reversible with cessation of therapy. As mentioned, mercaptopurine is an immunosuppressant; immunity to infectious agents or vaccines will be subnormal in patients receiving this drug. Mercaptopurine's immunosuppressive effect should be carefully considered with regard to intercurrent infections and risk of subsequent neoplasia.

Interactions with Other Drugs

The pharmacologic effects of mercaptopurine are increased by allopurinol. Bone marrow depression (leukopenia, thrombocytopenia, and anemia) may occur. When allopurinol and mercaptopurine are administered concurrently, the dose of mercaptopurine must be reduced to one-third to one-quarter of the usual dose. Failure to observe this dosage reduction will result in delayed catabolism of mercaptopurine and the strong likelihood of severe toxicity.

Usually complete cross-resistance occurs between mercaptopurine and thioguanine. The hypoprothrombinemic effect of oral anticoagulants may possibly be decreased by mercaptopurine. The onset of this reaction is delayed and its severity moderate. It is also suspected that the neuromuscular blocking effects of nondepolarizing muscle relaxants may be decreased by mercaptopurine. The onset of this reaction is rapid and severity is moderate.

Notes on Nutritional Effects

Anorexia—Anorexia has been noted in about 25 percent of patients, with a resultant decrease in food intake. Dietary measures can help increase appetite.

Nausea and vomiting—Nausea and vomiting occur in about 25 percent of patients and may be ameliorated by antiemetic agents. Starchy foods taken with the drug may minimize nausea, and other dietary measures can mitigate the aftereffects of vomiting and lessen residual nausea.

If nausea and vomiting are a problem, favorite foods should not be ingested prior to the administration of mercaptopurine because a conditioned food aversion to foods taken immediately beforehand may result.

Diarrhea—Diarrhea occurs in about 25 percent of patients and results from direct toxicity to the mucosa of the gut. The villi and microvilli become flattened, reducing the absorptive surface area, resulting in a "slick gut." The intestinal contents move rapidly through the gut, further decreasing absorption. Much of the water poured into the gut for digestion is not reabsorbed, and many water-soluble vitamins and minerals are lost. Some of these effects may be mitigated by dietary means.

Abdominal discomfort—Mercaptopurine can cause vague abdominal discomfort, which may be aggravated by a full or distended gut. A fiber- and residue-restricted diet may be necessary in severe cases.

Hyperuricemia—Mercaptopurine may cause rapid cellular destruction resulting in extensive purine catabolism and hyperuricemia. Renal and joint damage may result from the precipitation of urates. A low-purine, low-protein diet may be contraindicated in most cancer patients. Thus hyperuricemia is usually treated by medical means, that is, by the administration of a xanthine oxidase inhibitor drug such as allopurinol.* Supportive dietary measures should include increased hydration (ten to twelve 8-ounce glasses of water per day) and an alkaline ash diet to alkalinize the urine and prevent the precipitation of uric acid stones in the kidney.

In high doses, mercaptopurine crystals can precipitate in the renal tubules, leading to hematuria and crystalluria. Allopurinol significantly reduces the rate of inactivation of mercaptopurine by xanthine oxidase. Thus, patients receiving oral 6-MP concurrently with allopurinol must have doses reduced to one-third or one-quarter in order to prevent severe myelosuppression.

Pellagra—An antimetabolite such as mercaptopurine may cause pellagra due to deficiency of niacin and/or tryptophan. The cardinal signs of advanced pellagra are dermatitis, diarrhea, dementia, and ultimately death. Symptoms occurring with both pellagra and with antimetabolite administration include anorexia, malaise, weakness, irritability, anxiety, depression, photosensitivity of light-exposed skin, digestive gastritis, diarrhea (aggravated by highly seasoned or acidic foods), and wasting. Pellagra is correctable by the administration of 100 to 300 mg of niacin a day given in divided doses of 50 to 150 mg.

Refer patients, as needed, to:

Chapter One: How to Deal with Specific Problems

Problem 1—Loss of Appetite, page 4

Problem 4—Sore or Ulcerated Mouth or Throat (Stomatitis/Mucositis), page 14

*Note: Allopurinol also has nutritional side effects. See the discussion of this drug earlier in this chapter.

Problem 6—Diarrhea, page 20
Problem 9—Dehydration, page 26

Chapter Two: General Dietary Guidelines
Guideline 1—Basic Nutrition for the Cancer Patient, page 30
Guideline 2—A High-Protein/High-Calorie Diet, page 38
Guideline 3—Food Sources of Minerals, page 45
Guideline 4—Food Sources of Vitamins, page 52
Guideline 5—The Fiber and Residue Contents of Foods, page 58
Guideline 6—A Lactose-Free/Lactose-Restricted Diet, page 61
Guideline 10—How to Prevent Kidney Stone Formation (Acid Ash/Alkaline Ash Diet), page 74
Guideline 14—A Soft-Food/Pureed-Food Diet, page 86

- **Melphalan** (L-PAM)
- **Alkeran®** (Burroughs Wellcome)

Nutritionally Significant Side Effects

Nausea and vomiting
Stomatitis and mucositis
Hyperuricemia

Properties and Use in Treatment

Melphalan is the L-phenylalanine derivative of nitrogen mustard. It is a bifunctional DNA alkylating agent administered orally to treat multiple myeloma, ovarian cancer, and occasionally chronic leukemia. Activity is cell-cycle phase nonspecific.

General Toxicities

Melphalan primarily causes myelosuppression, which can be delayed and prolonged after chronic dosing.The major toxicity of melphalan is leukopenia, thrombocytopenia, and occasionally anemia, which is dose-limiting. Long-term administration predisposes patients to increased risk of developing secondary cancers, especially acute myelogenous leukemias.Other non-nutritional side effects include fever, chills, unusual bleeding or bruising, stomach pains, joint pains, and swelling of the feet and lower extremities.

Food-Drug Interactions

Full meals may delay and change the absorption of an orally administered drug with respect to both the rate of absorption and peak serum concentrations. Complete absorption by the oral route may be questionable if the patient is concurrently receiving drugs toxic to the gastrointestinal tract.

To promote maximal absorption, oral drugs should not be taken with full meals or fatty foods that delay absorption. It is recommended that the drug be administered one hour before or two to three hours after a full meal. Taking the drug on an empty stomach may engender nausea or other stomach disturbances. It should be taken along with a starchy food such as bread or crackers in order to clear the stomach quickly and not interfere with drug absorption.

Notes on Nutritional Side Effects

Nausea and vomiting—Nausea and vomiting are common and, in some instances, can be prevented by the prophylactic administration of antiemetic drugs. Diet cannot prevent this type of nausea and vomiting, but starchy foods taken with the drug may reduce nausea. Other dietary measures can mitigate the aftereffects of vomiting and lessen residual nausea.

If nausea and vomiting are a problem, favorite foods should not be ingested prior to the administration of melphalan because a conditioned aversion to foods taken immediately beforehand may result.

Stomatitis and mucositis—This drug can be directly toxic to the rapidly replicating mucosal cells in and around the mouth and throughout the digestive tract. Prophylactic administration of enhanced nutrition, with an emphasis on the B vitamins, may mitigate or prevent this problem. Once the problem exists, however, certain dietary restrictions such as, a soft diet may be necessary to maintain nutrition. Also, a prescribed mouth care program may reduce these symptoms.

Hyperuricemia—Melphalan causes rapid cellular destruction, resulting in extensive purine catabolism and hyperuricemia. Renal and joint damage may result from the precipitation of urates. A low-purine, low-protein diet may be contraindicated in many cancer patients. Thus, hyperuricemia should be treated by medical means, specifically, by the administration of a xanthine oxidase inhibitor drug such as allopurinol.* Supportive dietary measures should include increased hydration (ten to twelve 8-ounce glasses of water per day) and an alkaline-ash diet to alkalinize the urine and prevent the precipitation of uric acid stones in the kidney.

*Note: Allopurinol can also have nutritional side effects. See the discussion of this drug earlier in this chapter.

Refer patients, as needed, to:

Chapter One: How to Deal with Specific Problems
Problem 1—Loss of Appetite, page 4

Problem 2—Nausea and Vomiting, page 8

Problem 4—Sore or Ulcerated Mouth or Throat (Stomatitis/Mucositis), page 14

Problem 9—Dehydration, page 26

Chapter Two: General Dietary Guidelines
Guideline 1—Basic Nutrition for the Cancer Patient, page 30

Guideline 2—A High-Protein/High-Calorie Diet, page 38

Guideline 3—Food Sources of Minerals, page 45

Guideline 4—Food Sources of Vitamins, page 52

Guideline 10—How to Prevent Kidney Stone Formation (Acid Ash/Alkaline Ash Diet), page 74

• Mechlorethamine
• Mustargen® (Merck Sharp & Dohme)

Nutritionally Significant Side Effects

Anorexia
Nausea and vomiting
Bleeding and ulceration of the GI tract
Hyperuricemia

Properties and Use in Treatment

Mechlorethamine was the first of the nitrogen mustards to be introduced into clinical medicine and is the most rapidly acting drug of its class. It is an alkylating agent with cytotoxic, mutagenic, and radiomimetic actions that inhibit rapidly proliferating cells. Its action is cell-cycle phase nonspecific. Mechlorethamine is usually given intravenously and is predominantly used in the treatment of Hodgkin's and non-Hodgkin's lymphomas, malignant pleural effusions, lung cancer and mycosis fungoides.

General Toxicities

The major clinical toxicity of mechlorethamine is hematologic suppression, which is dose limiting and includes suppression of lymphocytes, granulocytes and platelets with approximately a three-week recovery. Alopecia is marked, and scarring and sclerosis with extravasation at the site of injection occurs. Non-nutritional side effects include fever, chills, sore throat, unusual bleeding and bruising, unusual tiredness and weakness, yellowing of the eyes, joint pain, swelling of the feet, black or tarry stools. Itching, ringing in the ears, numbness, burning and tingling of the fingers and toes, and shortness of breath and swelling of the feet and lower legs can also occur.

Notes on Nutritional Side Effects

Anorexia—Unexplained anorexia has been noted and may persist for twenty-four hours after administration of the mechlorethamine.

The result is reduced food intake. Dietary measures can help increase appetite.

Nausea and vomiting—Nausea and vomiting are common and in some instances can be prevented by the prophylactic administration of antiemetic drugs. Vomiting usually stops within eight hours, but nausea may persist for twenty-four hours. Starchy foods taken with the drug may minimize nausea. Other dietary measures can mitigate the aftereffects of vomiting and lessen residual nausea.

If nausea and vomiting are a problem, favorite foods should not be ingested prior to the administration of mechlorethamine because a conditioned aversion to foods taken immediately beforehand may result.

Bleeding and ulceration of the GI tract—The enteritis caused by this drug may be severe enough to result in bleeding and ulceration of the gut. This can lead to a blood loss of iron, loss of many nutrients, and nonreabsorption of bile salts. Dietary means can help mitigate these side effects.

Hyperuricemia—This drug causes rapid cellular destruction, in lymphoma patients, resulting in extensive purine catabolism and hyperuricemia. Renal and joint damage may result from the precipitation of urates. A low-purine, low-protein diet may be contraindicated in many cancer patients. Thus, hyperuricemia should be treated by medical means, that is, by administering a xanthine oxidase inhibitor drug such as allopurinol.* Supportive dietary measures should include increased hydration (ten to twelve 8-ounce glasses of fluid per day) and an alkaline-ash diet to alkalinize the urine and prevent the precipitation of uric acid stones in the kidney.

Refer patients, as needed, to:

Chapter One: How to Deal with Specific Problems

Problem 1—Loss of Appetite, page 4

Problem 2—Nausea and Vomiting, page 8

*Note: Allopurinol can also have nutritional side effects. See the discussion of this drug earlier in this chapter.

• Mesna
• Mesnex™ (Mead-Johnson)

Nutritionally Significant Side Effects

Nausea and vomiting

Properties and Use in Treatment

Mesna is a detoxifying agent that inhibits the hemorrhagic cystitis induced by ifosfamide. It is also effective in preventing cystitis from cyclophosphamide.

The active ingredient in mesna is a synthetic sulfhydryl compound designated as sodium 2-mercaptoethanesulfonate. Following intravenous administration, mesna is rapidly oxidized to its only metabolite, mesna disulfide (dimesna), which is inert. Mesna disulfide is subsequently reactivated in the kidney to the free thiol compound mesna, which reacts chemically with the urotoxic ifosfamide metabolites acrolein and 4-hydroxy-ifosfamide, resulting in their detoxification. Mesna also binds to other cytotoxic metabolites.

To obtain adequate protection, mesna must be administered with each dose of ifosfamide. Mesna prevents hemorrhagic cystitis in about 94 percent of patients.

General Toxicities

Because mesna is used in combination with ifosfamide and other chemotherapeutic agents with documented toxicities, it is difficult to distinguish its adverse reactions from those caused by concomitantly administered cytotoxic agents. In controlled clinical studies, however, adverse reactions were uncommon and mainly associated with nausea, vomiting, and diarrhea.

Notes on Nutritional Side Effects

Nausea and vomiting—Nausea and vomiting are common and may be ameliorated with antiemetic agents. Starchy foods taken with the drug may minimize nausea. Other dietary measures can mitigate the aftereffects of vomiting and lessen residual nausea.

If nausea and vomiting are a problem, favorite foods should not be ingested prior to the administration of mesna because a conditioned food aversion may result.

Refer patients, as needed, to:

Chapter One: How to Deal with Specific Problems
Problem 2—Nausea and Vomiting, page 8
Problem 9—Dehydration, page 26

Chapter Two: General Dietary Guidelines
Guideline 1—Basic Nutrition for the Cancer Patient, page 30
Guideline 2—A High-Protein/High-Calorie Diet, page 38
Guideline 3—Food Sources of Minerals, page 45
Guideline 4—Food Sources of Vitamins, page 52

- **Methotrexate**
- **Folex®** (Adria)
- **Mexate** (Bristol-Myers)
- **Methotrexate** (Lederle)
- **Methotrexate** (Cetus)

Nutritionally Significant Side Effects

Anorexia
Nausea and vomiting
Diarrhea
Bleeding and ulceration of the GI tract
Lactose intolerance
Protein loss
Iron loss
Fatty acid loss
Fat-soluble vitamin loss

Properties and Use in Treatment

Folic acid is an essential dietary constituent needed for the replication and maturation of both normal and tumor cells. Methotrexate interferes with the conversion of dietary folate to the active reduced folate tetrahydrofolic acid. Methotrexate binds competitively with the enzyme dihydrofolate reductase (DHFR), thus preventing formation of tetrahydrofolic acid. Without reduced folate, cells cannot form the nucleic acid thymidine from uracil, and DNA synthesis is halted. Thus, cells do not replicate and eventually die. Methotrexate also inhibits both RNA and protein synthesis. Its activity is cell-cycle S-phase specific.

Methotrexate may be administered orally, intramuscularly, or intravenously for a large variety of cancers. For patients with meningeal leukemia, it may also be administered via the intrathecal route. Fifty percent of the drug is bound to serum proteins. It is primarily excreted unchanged in the urine, about 75 percent of the dose excreted within eight hours.

The classic clinical manifestation of folic acid deficiency is megaloblastic anemia, accompanied by such clinical signs as diarrhea, weight loss, and a red, sore tongue (glossitis) with atrophic papillae. A low serum or red blood cell folate level before treatment with methotrexate may predispose the patient to greater toxicity. However, it does not affect the therapeutic antineoplastic efficacy of the drug.

When dietary folate is consumed during methotrexate therapy, it is not reduced by DHFR to tetrahydrofolate because of the competitive binding by methotrexate. Thus, folate is excreted, which results in a decrease in the reduced folate pool. In contrast, reduced folate can bypass the methotrexate block on DHFR. Since the binding is competitive, folinic acid (leucovorin), administered as a "rescue," can reverse some of the toxic effects of methotrexate.

It should be noted that the actions of methotrexate cannot be terminated by the administration of dietary folate or folic acid vitamins. The antidote *must be* the activated form of the vitamin, folinic acid (N^5N^{10}-methylenetetrahydrofolic acid), also known as citrovorum factor (calcium leucovorin). Dietary folic acid or folate from oral vitamins not only will not overcome the drug's toxicity, it may enhance it possibly by interfering with the excretion of the methotrexate.

It is primarily used for acute leukemia, sarcomas, chonocarcinoma, psroiasis, cancer of the head and neck, breast, lung, stomach, esophagus, lymphoma, testes, and mycosis fungoides.

General Toxicities

Myelosuppression is common and manifested by leukopenia, thrombocytopenia, and anemia between days seven and ten. Recovery usually occurs in twelve to twenty-one days for leukopenia. Acute hepatic dysfunction is rare and usually reversible and may be seen with elevation in liver function tests—hepatic enzymes. Hepatic fibrosis is seen with long-term therapy. Secondary nephrotoxicity is uncommon and related to high-dose methotrexate therapy. Skin rash, usually a maculous papular type may occur. Methotrexate pneumonitis is rare and characterized by fever, cough, and an interstitial infiltrate. Neurotoxic effects with arachnoiditis and meningeal irritation may be related to intrathecal therapy. Occasionally subacute motor paralysis, cranial nerve dysfunction, seizures, or coma is seen with intrathecal therapy.

Other non-nutritional side effects include sensitivity to sunlight, which may occasionally result in severe sunburn. Uncommon side effects include black, tarry stools, fevers, chills, sore throat, unusual bleeding and bruising, blood in the urine, blurred vision, confusion, convulsions, seizures, cough, dark urine, dizziness, drowsiness, headache, joint pain, shortness of breath, leg and feet swelling, tiredness, and yellowing of the eyes and skin.

Interactions with Other Drugs

Several drugs including aspirin may enhance methotrexate toxicity by displacing the drug from the serum protein binding sites or reducing renal excretion. Aspirin-containing preparations should not be used in patients receiving methotrexate. Sulfa and penicillin compounds may interfere with renal excretion of methotrexate. Additionally, nonsteroidal anti-inflammatory drugs such as indomethacin and ibuprofen may decrease the renal excretion of methotrexate. These drugs should not be given concurrently with methotrexate.

Food-Drug Interactions

Foods that contain high amounts of salicylates, either naturally or as additives, should be withheld for two days before and one day following methotrexate administration. Salicylates can be found in such foods as plums; gums; mints; jelly beans; root beer; apple, cherry, and blueberry turnovers, breakfast squares, and refrigerated cinnamon-sugar cookies. Flavoring agents containing methyl-salicylate, such as oil of wintergreen or teaberry, should also be avoided.

Evidence shows that orally administered methotrexate absorption is reduced by the concurrent presence of food in the gut and that oral methotrexate absorption averages one-third that of an intravenous or intramuscular amount. To promote maximal drug absorption, oral methotrexate should probably not be taken with food. Ingestion of the drug is recommended one hour before and two to three hours after a full meal or during fasting.

Although dietary folate occurs naturally in foods in microgram quantities, it is not likely to enhance or detract from methotrexate treatment. But patients should be cautioned not to take vitamin supplements high in folic acid for two days before and on the day of methotrexate administration. Foods high in folic acid content, such as dark green leafy vegetables, should also be deemphasized at this time. Complete avoidance of foods containing folic acid is not necessary, however.

Notes on Nutritional Side Effects

Anorexia—Unexplained anorexia has been noted as a side effect of this drug resulting in decreased food intake. Dietary measures are available to help increase appetite.

Nausea and vomiting—Nausea and vomiting are common with high dose methotrexate regimens. In some instances, this can be prevented by the prophylactic administration of antiemetic drugs. Diet cannot prevent this type of nausea and vomiting, but starchy foods taken with the drug may minimize nausea. Other dietary measures can mitigate the aftereffects of vomiting and lessen residual nausea. If nausea and vomiting are a problem, favorite foods should not be ingested prior to the administration of methotrexate because a conditioned aversion to foods taken immediately beforehand may result.

Diarrhea—Diarrhea may result from the direct toxicity of this drug to the mucosa lining of the gut. The villi and microvilli become flattened, reducing the absorptive surface area and resulting in a "slick gut." As a result, intestinal contents move rapidly through the gut, reducing absorption. Much of the water poured into the gut for digestion is not reabsorbed, and water-soluble vitamins and minerals are lost. It is possible to mitigate some of the effects of diarrhea with dietary means.

Stomatitis and mucositis—Methotrexate can be directly toxic to the rapidly replicating mucosal cells in and around the mouth and throughout the digestive tract. Prophylactic administration of enhanced nutrition, with an emphasis on the B vitamins (except folic acid) prevent this problem. Certain dietary restrictions, such as a soft diet, may be necessary to maintain adequate nutrition. A prescribed mouth care program may be helpful in reducing toxic symptoms.

Bleeding and ulceration of the GI tract—Toxicities of methotrexate are manifested in the intestinal tract and bone marrow which are areas with high rates of cellular replication. The entire intestinal tract may exhibit severe hemorrhagic desquamating enteritis. This can lead to a blood loss of iron, loss of many nutrients, and nonreabsorption of bile salts. Dietary therapy may be needed to prevent these side effects.

Lactose intolerance and loss of protein, iron, fatty acids and fat soluble vitamins—Lactose intolerance may develop due to gut damage or reduced protein synthesis, which leads to lactase deficiency. If the developing enteritis becomes hemorrhagic, losses of protein and iron ensue. Losses of essential fatty acids and fat-soluble vitamins can occur if bile salts are not reabsorbed.

Refer patients, as needed, to:

Chapter One: How to Deal with Specific Problems
Problem 1—Loss of Appetite, page 4
Problem 2—Nausea and Vomiting, page 8
Problem 4—Sore or Ulcerated Mouth or Throat (Stomatitis/ Mucositis), page 14
Problem 6—Diarrhea, page 20
Problem 7—Protecting the Gastrointestinal Tract (Enteritis), page 22
Problem 9—Dehydration, page 26

Chapter Two: General Dietary Guidelines
Guideline 1—Basic Nutrition for the Cancer Patient, page 30
Guideline 2—A High-Protein/High-Calorie Diet, page 38
Guideline 3—Food Sources of Minerals, page 45
Guideline 4—Food Sources of Vitamins, page 52
Guideline 5—The Fiber and Residue Contents of Foods, page 58
Guideline 6—A Lactose-Free/Lactose-Restricted Diet, page 61
Guideline 14—A Soft-Food/Pureed Food Diet, page 86

- **Mitomycin C**
- **Mutamycin®** (Bristol-Myers)

Nutritionally Significant Side Effects

Interference with bone marrow and protein synthesis
Anorexia
Nausea and vomiting
Diarrhea
Stomatitis and mucositis
Loss of protein, fluids and electrolytes

Properties and Use in Treatment

Mitomycin C functions as an alkylating agent, causing cross-linking of DNA chains. At high concentrations, RNA and protein synthesis are also inhibited. Mitomycin C is a cell-cycle nonspecific antibiotic.

Mitomycin is used primarily in the treatment of colorectal, gastric, and pancreatic adenocarcinomas, breast cancer, and lung cancer. The drug is administered intravenously, as it is poorly absorbed orally and is metabolized primarily in the liver. The most common and serious toxicities with mitomycin are thrombocytopenia and/or leukopenia and the hemolytic uremic syndrome.

General Toxicities

The dose-limiting toxicity of mitomycin C is myelosuppression, which manifests as leukopenia and thrombocytopenia with a nadir of thirty days and recovery of forty-two days. Nausea and vomiting are moderate and controlled with antiemetics. Stomatitis and alopecia are common. A long term effect is pulmonary toxicity, which manifests as interstitial fibrosis. Renal toxicity is uncommon and is associated with hemolysis and microangiopathy. Mitomycin C is a vesicant and may result in severe skin necrosis upon accidental extravasation. Local treatment of extravasation reactions include topical ice and sodium thiosulfate administration.

Notes on Nutritional Side Effects

Interference with bone marrow and protein synthesis—Interference with bone marrow and protein synthesis cannot be prevented nutritionally. A nutritionally adequate diet emphasizing protein, vitamins (especially the B vitamins), however, may enhance the body's ability to generate new bone marrow and protein when it is once again able to do so.

Anorexia—Mild anorexia has been noted as a side effect of this drug, possibly resulting in decreased appetite and reduced food intake. Dietary measures are available to help increase the appetite.

Nausea and vomiting—Nausea and vomiting are usually mild with this drug. In some instances, they can be prevented by the prophylactic administration of an antiemetic drug. A starchy food eaten before the drug administration may help to minimize the nausea. Other dietary measures can mitigate the aftereffects of vomiting and lessen residual nausea.

If nausea and vomiting are a problem, favorite foods should not be ingested prior to the administration of mitomycin because a conditioned aversion to foods taken immediately beforehand may result.

Diarrhea—Diarrhea results from the direct toxicity of this drug to the mucosa lining of the gut. The villi and microvilli become flattened, reducing the absorptive surface area, resulting in a "slick gut." Intestinal contents then move rapidly through the gut, reducing absorption. Much of the water poured into the gut for digestion is not reabsorbed, and many water-soluble vitamins and minerals are lost as a result. It is possible to mitigate some of the effects of diarrhea with dietary means.

If toxicity is prolonged, further dietary modifications may be necessary, such as restricting lactose, gluten, and long-chain triglycerides.

Stomatitis and mucositis—Mitomycin can be directly toxic to the rapidly dividing mucosal cells in and around the mouth and throughout the digestive tract. Prophylactic administration of enhanced nutrition, with an emphasis on the B vitamins, may prevent this problem. Once the problem exists, however, certain dietary restrictions, such as a soft diet may be necessary to maintain the patient's nutritional intake. A prescribed mouth care program is helpful in reducing toxic symptoms.

Loss of protein, fluids, and electrolytes—Mitomycin may cause fever, which can result in a loss of lean body tissue as well as fluids and electrolytes. These effects may be mitigated by a high-protein diet and nutritional replacement of fluids and electrolytes.

Refer patients, as needed, to:

Chapter One: How to Deal with Specific Problems
Problem 1—Loss of Appetite, page 4
Problem 2—Nausea and Vomiting, page 8
Problem 4—Sore or Ulcerated Mouth or Throat (Stomatitis/Mucositis), page 14
Problem 5—Difficulties in Chewing and Swallowing (Dysphagia) and Dry Mouth (Xerostomia), page 18
Problem 9—Dehydration, page 26

Chapter Two: General Dietary Guidelines
Guideline 1—Basic Nutrition for the Cancer Patient, page 30
Guideline 2—A High-Protein/High-Calorie Diet, page 38
Guideline 3—Food Sources of Minerals, page 45
Guideline 4—Food Sources of Vitamins, page 52
Guideline 5—The Fiber and Residue Contents of Foods, page 58
Guideline 6—A Lactose-Free/Lactose-Restricted Diet, page 61
Guideline 7—A Gluten-Restricted/Gliadin-Free Diet, page 65
Guideline 8—Long-Chain Triglyceride-Restricted/Medium-Chain-Triglyceride Fat Diet, page 68
Guideline 14—A Soft-Food/Pureed-Food Diet, page 86

- **Mitotane** (o,p,-DDD)
- **Lysodren®** (Bristol-Myers)

Nutritionally Significant Side Effects

Anorexia
Nausea and vomiting
Diarrhea

Properties and Use in Treatment

Mitotane is an oral adrenal cytoxic agent that causes adrenal inhibition without cellular destruction. It is used primarily in the treatment of inoperable adrenal carcinoma of both the functional and nonfunctional types. Mitotane's biological mechanism of action is unknown, but it appears to be directed at the mitochondria of adrenal cortical cells. Mitotane is chemically related to the insecticide DDT and has marked lipophilicity in humans. It is administered orally. Its action is cell-cycle nonspecific.

General Toxicities

A substantial number of patients treated with mitotane may develop signs of adrenal insufficiency. Patients should therefore be monitored for this problem and steroid (glucocorticoid and mineralocorticoid) replacement instituted when necessary.

Other toxicities include central nervous system side effects (depression, lethargy, somnolence, dizziness, and vertigo). Skin toxicity has been observed in about 15 percent of patients and consists primarily of transient skin rashes.

Infrequent side effects may involve the eye (visual blurring, diplopia, lens opacity, toxic retinopathy); the genitourinary system (hematuria, hemorrhagic cystitis, and albuminuria); cardiovascular system (hypertension, orthostatic hypotension, and flushing); and miscellaneous complaints, including aching muscles, muscle twitching, fever, and lowered protein-bound iodine (PBI).

Muscle aches and twitches may resolve upon administration of calcium and/or magnesium. Fever is of nutritional concern because it can destroy lean body mass. Care should be taken to replace lost protein, fluid, and electrolytes. With hematuria and hemorrhagic cystitis, blood loss of iron will need to be replaced, along with fluid and electrolytes.

Interactions with Other Drugs

Mitotane has been reported to accelerate the metabolism of warfarin, necessitating an increase in dosage requirements for the latter. Patients on coumarin-type anticoagulants should be closely monitored and anticoagulant dosage adjusted accordingly. In addition, mitotane should be given with caution to patients receiving other drugs susceptible to the influence of hepatic enzyme induction.

Food-Drug Interactions

Full meals may delay and change the absorption of an orally administered drug with respect to both the rate of absorption and peak serum concentrations. Complete absorption by the oral route is questionable if the patient is concurrently receiving drugs that are toxic to the gastrointestinal tract.

Because mitotane is lipophilic, it should be taken with meals or with fatty foods to lessen gastrointestinal upset. Taking the drug on an empty stomach may cause nausea or other stomach disturbances. If these are a problem, the patient may need to take the drug with a starchy snack, such as bread or crackers.

Notes on Nutritional Side Effects

Anorexia—Unexplained anorexia has been noted as a common side effect of this drug, resulting in decreased food intake. Some dietary measures can help to increase appetite.

Nausea and vomiting—Nausea and vomiting are common and may be ameliorated by antiemetic agents. Starchy foods taken with the drug may minimize nausea, and other dietary measures can mitigate the aftereffects of vomiting and lessen residual nausea.

If nausea and vomiting are a problem, favorite foods should not be ingested prior to the administration of mitotane because a conditioned food aversion may result.

Diarrhea—Diarrhea results from the direct toxicity of this drug to the mucosa of the gut. The villi and microvilli become flattened and reduce the absorptive surface area, resulting in a "slick gut." Intestinal contents will move rapidly through the gut, further reducing absorption. Much of the water poured into the gut for digestion is not reabsorbed, and many water-soluble vitamins and minerals are lost. Some of these effects may be mitigated by dietary means.

Refer patients, as needed, to:

Chapter One: How to Deal with Specific Problems
Problem 1—Loss of Appetite, page 4
Problem 2—Nausea and Vomiting, page 8
Problem 6—Diarrhea, page 20
Problem 9—Dehydration, page 26

Chapter Two: General Dietary Guidelines
Guideline 1—Basic Nutrition for the Cancer Patient, page 30
Guideline 2—A High-Protein/High-Calorie Diet, page 38
Guideline 3—Food Sources of Minerals, page 45
Guideline 4—Food Sources of Vitamins, page 52
Guideline 5—The Fiber and Residue Contents of Foods, page 58
Guideline 6—A Lactose-Free/Lactose-Restricted Diet, page 61

• Mitoxantrone HCl
• Novantrone® (Lederle)

Nutritionally Significant Side Effects

Nausea and vomiting
Diarrhea
Stomatitis and mucositis
Bleeding and ulceration of the GI tract
Hyperuricemia

Properties and Use in Treatment

Mitoxantrone hydrochloride is a synthetic antineoplastic anthracenedione. It is a DNA-reactive agent that is cell-cycle nonspecific. Mitoxantrone HCl is distinctly different chemically and structurally, from anthracycline agents such as daunorubicin and doxorubicin. Mitoxantrone HCl binds to nucleic acids in cancer cells in two different ways: by intercalation with DNA, like the anthracyclines, and by nonintercalative electrostatic binding. Mitoxantrone induced both protein-associated and nonprotein-associated DNA strand scissions. These actions may be responsible for the lack of complete cross-resistance with anthracyclines. Mitoxantrone HCl comes in an intense blue colored solution and is administered intravenously.

Mitoxantrone HCl has been combined with other drugs to induce high remission rates in patients with relapsed acute nonlymphocytic leukemia. Mitoxantrone HCl is also effective as a single agent in previously treated patients with lymphoma and can be safely integrated into combination chemotherapy for non-Hodgkin's lymphoma. In addition, mitoxantrone HCl has been shown to exert significant activity in the treatment of advanced breast cancer, both as a single agent and as a constituent of combination chemotherapy regimens.

General Toxicities

Mitoxantrone HCl causes severe myelosuppression, which is rapid in onset and recovers in about 21 days. Patients with preexisting myelosuppression as the result of prior drug therapy should not receive mitoxantrone HCl unless warranted.

Mitoxantrone is associated with a 3 percent risk of cardiac toxicities, which include congestive heart failure, tachycardia, EKG changes, arrhythmias, chest pain, and asymptomatic decreases in left ventricular ejection fraction. The danger of cardiac toxicity is increased in patients previously treated with daunorubicin or doxorubicin.

Occassional allergic reactions have occurred including hypotension, urticaria, dyspnea, and rashes. Phlebitis has been reported infrequently at the infusion site. Tissue necrosis following extravasation is rare. Other toxicities include petechiae and ecchymoses; gastrointestinal side effects, such as nausea, vomiting, diarrhea, stomatitis and mucositis, gastrointestinal bleeding, and abdominal pain (all significantly reduced in comparison to doxorubicin therapy); jaundice; infections (urinary tract, pneumonia, sepsis, fungal); renal failure; fever; alopecia (rare in comparison to doxorubicin therapy); cough; seizures; headache; and conjunctivitis.

Interactions with Other Drugs

Mitoxantrone HCl should not be mixed in the same infusion as heparin since a precipitate may form. Because specific compatibility data are not available, it is also recommended that mitoxantrone HCl not be mixed in the same infusion with other drugs. Previous treatment with doxorubicin or daunorubicin may increase myelosuppression and cardiotoxicity from mitoxantrone HCl.

Notes on Nutritional Side Effects

Nausea and vomiting—Nausea and vomiting may occur within two to four hours but are generally mild to moderate and are easily controlled by antiemetic agents. Starchy foods taken with the drug may minimize nausea. Other dietary measures can mitigate the aftereffects of vomiting and lessen residual nausea.

If nausea and vomiting are a problem, favorite foods should not be ingested prior to the administration of mitoxantrone HCl because a conditioned food aversion may result.

Diarrhea—Diarrhea results from the direct toxicity of this drug to the mucosa of the gut. The villi and microvilli become flattened, reducing the absorptive surface area, resulting in a "slick gut" and possible lactose intolerance. Intestinal contents move rapidly through the gut, further decreasing absorption. Much of the water poured into the gut for digestion is not reabsorbed, and many water-soluble vitamins and minerals are lost. Some of these effects may be mitigated by dietary means.

Stomatitis and mucositis—This drug can be directly toxic to the rapidly replicating mucosal cells in and around the mouth and throughout the digestive tract, causing stomatitis and mucositis within the first week of therapy. Enhanced nutrition, with an emphasis on the B vitamins, may mitigate or prevent this problem. Once the problem exists, however, certain dietary restrictions, such as a soft diet, may be necessary to keep the patients eating. A prescribed mouth care program may be helpful in reducing toxic symptoms.

Bleeding and ulceration of the GI tract—The enteritis caused by this drug may be severe enough to result in bleeding and ulceration of the gut. This can lead to a blood loss of iron, loss of many nutrients, and nonreabsorption of bile salts. Dietary means may mitigate these side effects.

Hyperuricemia—Hyperuricemia may occur as a result of rapid lysis of tumor cells by mitoxantrone HCl. Rapid cellular destruction results in extensive purine catabolism and hyperuricemia. Renal and joint damage may result from the precipitation of urates. A low-purine, low-protein diet may be contraindicated in cancer patients.

Serum uric acid levels should be monitored and hypouricemic therapy (that is, a xanthine oxidase inhibitor drug such as allopurinol*, without an accompanying low-protein diet) instituted prior to the initiation of mitoxantrone HCl therapy. Supportive dietary measures should include increased hydration (ten to twelve 8-ounce glasses of water per day) and an alkaline ash diet to

*Note: Allopurinol is not without its own nutritional side effects. See the discussion of this drug earlier in this chapter.

alkalinize the urine and prevent the precipitation of uric acid stones in the kidney.

Refer patients, as needed, to:

Chapter One: How to Deal with Specific Problems
Problem 2—Nausea, page 8
Problem 4—Sore or Ulcerated Mouth or Throat (Stomatisis/Mucositis), page 14
Problem 6—Diarrhea, page 20
Problem 7—Protecting the Gastrointestinal Tract (Enteritis), page 22
Problem 9—Dehydration, page 26

Chapter Two: General Dietary Guidelines
Guideline 1—Basic Nutrition for the Cancer Patient, page 30
Guideline 2—A High-Protein/High-Calorie Diet, page 38
Guideline 3—Food Sources of Minerals, page 45
Guideline 4—Food Sources of Vitamins, page 52
Guideline 6—A Lactose-Free/Lactose-Restricted Diet, page 61
Guideline 10—How to Prevent Kidney Stone Formation (Acid Ash/Alkaline Ash Diet), page 74
Guideline 14—A Soft-Food/Pureed-Food Diet, page 86

• Octreotide Acetate
• Sandostatin® (Sandoz)

Nutritionally Significant Side Effects

Nausea and vomiting
Diarrhea
Fat malabsorption
Hyperglycemia and hypoglycemia

Properties and Use in Treatment

Octreotide acetate is a cyclic octapeptide with pharmacologic actions mimicking those of the natural hormone somatostatin. It has the ability to suppress secretion of serotonin, vasoactive intestinal peptide, gastrin, insulin, glucagon, growth hormone, secretin, motilin, and pancreatic polypeptide. Octreotide acetate is used to treat the symptoms associated with metastatic carcinoid tumors and vasoactive intestinal peptide (VIP) secreting adenomas.

It is primarily used in metastatic carcinoid tumors to suppress or inhibit severe diarrhea and flushing episodes. In VIP-secreting tumors, octreotide acetate is indicated for the treatment of profuse watery diarrhea. Significant improvement has been noted in the overall condition of otherwise therapeutically unresponsive patients, including improvement in electrolyte abnormalities (for example, hypokalemia), often enabling reduction of fluid and electrolyte support.

The precise mechanism of its action has not yet been determined. The primary action of somatostatin within the cell remains unclear but may involve alterations in diffusion of potassium and calcium.

Data are insufficient to determine whether octreotide acetate decreases the size, rate of growth, or development of metastases in patients with these tumors. The drug has been used in patients ranging in age from one month to eighty-three years without any drug-limiting toxicity. Administration is by subcutaneous injection.

General Toxicities

The most frequently occurring adverse reactions include nausea, pain at the injection site, diarrhea, abdominal pain and discomfort, loose stools, vomiting, headache, fat malabsorption, dizziness or light headedness, hyperglycemia, fatigue, flushing, hypoglycemia, edema, asthenia or weakness, and injection site redness and wheal.

Interactions with Other Drugs

Adjustment of the dosage of drugs, such as insulin, affecting glucose metabolism may be required following initiation of octreotide acetate therapy in patients with diabetes. Many patients with carcinoid syndrome or VIPomas being treated with octreotide acetate have also been, or are being, treated with many other drugs to control the symptomatology or progression of the disease, generally without serious drug interaction. Included are chemotherapeutic agents, H_2 antagonists, antimotility agents, drugs affecting glycemic states, solutions for electrolyte and fluid support or hyperalimentation, antihypertensive diuretics, and antidiarrheal agents.

Since octreotide acetate has been associated with alterations in nutrient absorption, its effect on absorption of any orally administered drugs should be considered carefully.

Notes on Nutritional Side Effects

Nausea and vomiting—Nausea and vomiting is reported in four to 10 percent of patients and may be ameliorated by antiemetic agents. Starchy foods taken with the drug may minimize nausea. Other dietary measures can mitigate the aftereffects of vomiting and lessen residual nausea.

If nausea and vomiting are a problem, favorite foods should not be ingested prior to the administration of octreotide acetate because a conditioned food aversion may result.

Diarrhea—Diarrhea is reported in seven percent of patients studied and results from the direct toxicity of this drug to the mucosa of the gut. The villi and microvilli become flattened, reducing the absorptive surface area, resulting in a "slick gut" and possible lactose intolerance. Intestinal contents move rapidly through the gut, further reducing absorption. Much of the water poured into the gut for digestion is not reabsorbed, and many water-soluble vitamins and minerals are lost. Some of these effects may be mitigated by dietary means.

Fat malabsorption—In some patients, octreotide acetate therapy may lead to malabsorption of dietary fats. Like natural somatostatin, octreotide acetate therapy may also be associated with cholelithiasis. This may occur as a result of altered fat absorption and possibly decreased motility of the gallbladder.

Hyperglycemia and hypoglycemia—Occasionally mild, transient hypoglycemia or hyperglycemia may occur in response to changes in the balance of insulin, glucagon, and growth hormone. In patients with insulin-dependent diabetes mellitus, octreotide acetate therapy may be associated with reduction in insulin requirements. Prediabetes may be manifested after initiation of octreotide therapy.

A patient with diabetes should see their physician for reevaluation of their insulin requirements if they begin to show signs of hypoglycemia.

If the patient was previously nondiabetic but is showing signs of transient glucose intolerance, a modifier type II diabetic diet should be followed during treatment. The glucose intolerance should disappear once drug treatment is discontinued.

Refer patients, as needed, to:

Chapter One: How to Deal with Specific Problems
Problem 2—Nausea and Vomiting, page 8
Problem 6—Diarrhea, page 20
Problem 9—Dehydration, page 26

Chapter Two: General Dietary Guidelines
Guideline 1—Basic Nutrition for the Cancer Patient, page 30
Guideline 2—A High-Protein/High-Calorie Diet, page 38
Guideline 3—Food Sources of Minerals, page 45
Guideline 4—Food Sources of Vitamins, page 52
Guideline 6—A Lactose-Free/Lactose-Restricted Diet, page 61
Guideline 8—Long-Chain-Triglyceride-Restricted/Medium-Chain-Triglyceride Fat Diet, page 68
Guideline 9—A Cholesterol and Fat-Restricted Diet, page 71
Guideline 11—Transient Glucose Intolerance/Diabetic Diet, page 76

- **Plicamycin** (Mithramycin)
- **Mithracin®** (Miles Pharamceuticals)

Nutritionally Significant Side Effects

Iron loss
Anorexia
Nausea and vomiting
Stomatitis and mucositis
Diarrhea

Properties and Use in Treatment

Plicamycin is an antibiotic isolated from *Streptomyces plicatus.* The exact mechanism by which plicamycin causes tumor inhibition is not known, but it appears to form a noncovalent complex with DNA and to inhibit cellular RNA and enzymatic RNA synthesis.

Its action is cell-cycle nonspecific with some evidence of S-phase specificity.It is used primarily in the treatment of life-threatening hypercalcemia and hypercalciuria associated with advanced neoplasms. It is also used in the treatment of testicular carcinoma when surgery and radiation therapy are not possible. Because of the severe toxicity of this drug, patients should be monitored carefully during therapy. LDH, BUN, prothrombin time, and platelet count should be screened before each dose. Use of plicamycin is contraindicated in patients with hepatic and kidney dysfunction or coagulation disorder. Administration is by intravenous injection.

General Toxicities

Severe thrombocytopenia and hemorrhaging has resulted in death after daily use of plicamycin. The hemorrhagic syndrome usually begins with an episode of epistaxis or hematemesis and may progress to a more widespread GI hemorrhage. Hemorrhagic diathesis is most likely due to abnormalities in multiple clotting factors. This type of severe hemorrhagic toxicity does not occur after a single dose.

Other hematologic toxicities include leukopenia and anemia. The drug may cause local irritation if injected subcutaneously. Less frequently reported side effects include fever, drowsiness, weakness, lethargy, malaise, headache, depression, phlebitis, facial flushing, and skin rash.

Plicamycin is known to cause abnormalities in electrolytes, most notably a depression in serum calcium, phosphorus, and potassium. Serum minerals and electrolytes should be monitored closely and normalized through medical management.

Notes on Nutritional Side Effects

Iron loss—Iron deficiency may occur with the hemorrhagic syndrome. Iron replacement with vitamin C-containing supplements or beverages, such as orange juice, is effective prophylaxis.

Anorexia—Anorexia is a common side effect of plicamycin, often resulting from chronic nausea and vomiting. Dietary measures can help increase appetite.

Nausea and vomiting—Nausea and vomiting are common and may be prevented by antiemetic agents. Starchy foods taken with the drug may reduce nausea, and other dietary measures can mitigate the aftereffects of vomiting and lessen residual nausea.

If nausea and vomiting are a problem, favorite foods should not be ingested prior to the administration of plicamycin because a conditioned food aversion may result.

Stomatitis and mucositis—Stomatitis and mucositis are common and due to plicamycin's direct toxicity to the rapidly replicating mucosal cells in and around the mouth and throughout the digestive tract. Enhanced nutrition, with an emphasis on the B-vitamins, may mitigate or prevent this problem. However, once the problem exists, certain dietary restrictions may be necessary to keep a patient eating. A prescribed mouth care program may also be helpful in reducing toxic symptoms.

Diarrhea—Diarrhea results from the direct toxicity to the mucosa of the gut. The villi and microvilli become flattened, reducing the absorptive surface area, causing "slick gut." Intestinal contents move rapidly through the gut, further decreasing absorption. Much of the water poured into the gut for digestion is not reabsorbed, and many water-soluble vitamins and minerals are lost. Proper nutrition may minimize some of these effects.

Refer patients, as needed, to:

Chapter One: How to Deal with Specific Problems
Problem 1—Loss of Appetite, page 4
Problem 2—Nausea and Vomiting, page 8
Problem 4—Sore or Ulcerated Mouth or Throat (Stomatitis/ Mucositis), page 14
Problem 6—Diarrhea, page 20
Problem 7—Protecting the Gastrointestinal Tract (Enteritis), page 22
Problem 9—Dehydration, page 26

Chapter Two: General Dietary Guidelines
Guideline 1—Basic Nutrition for the Cancer Patient, page 30
Guideline 2—A High-Protein/High-Calorie Diet, page 38
Guideline 3—Food Sources of Minerals, page 45
Guideline 4—Food Sources of Vitamins, page 52
Guideline 5—The Fiber and Residue Contents of Foods, page 58
Guideline 6—A Lactose-Free/Lactose-Restricted Diet, page 61

• Procarbazine
• Matulane® (Roche)

Nutritionally Significant Side Effects

Anorexia
Nausea and vomiting
Diarrhea
Constipation
Altered taste and smell
Dry mouth
Dysphagia
Iron loss
Vitamin B_6 loss
Protein loss

Properties and Use in Treatment

Procarbazine is a unique cytotoxic agent of the hydrazine class of compounds. Its cytotoxic action is believed to involve methylation of DNA and subsequent cell growth. Procarbazine also inhibits DNA, RNA, and protein synthesis. The drug is a substrate for a variety of oxidation reactions mediated by microsomal P-450 enzymes. Its action is cell-cycle phase nonspecific.

Procarbazine is administered orally in the treatment of brain tumors, Hodgkin's disease, and non-Hodgkin's lymphomas and lung cancer.

General Toxicities

The major dose limiting toxicity is white blood cell and platelet suppression with nadirs occurring at four to six weeks. Other non-nutritional side effects include severe headaches, stiff neck, chest pain, rapid heart rate, abdominal or back pain, dizziness, fever, muscle and joint pain, shortness of breath, headaches, tiredness, weakness, and unusual weight loss. Additional rare side effects include black, tarry stools, convulsions, cough, chills, sore throat, hallucinations, missed menstrual periods, unusual bleeding or bruising, tingling of fingers, toes or numbness, unsteadiness or awkward gait, fainting, skin rash, hives, itching, and wheezing.

Food-Drug Interactions

Procarbazine is associated with many food-drug interactions. It was originally synthesized as an antidepressant monamine oxidase (MAO) inhibitor but was found to be too toxic for this use. MAO inhibitors elevate norepinephrine and serotonin levels in the nervous system and potentiate cardiovascular effects of the simple phenethlylamines, such as tyramine. High levels of tyramine in food can cause a "pressor effect" characterized by transient hypertension, headache, palpitations, nausea and vomiting, and even cerebral hemorrhage. Patients receiving procarbazine should be cautioned to avoid foods with a high tyramine or dopamine content, such as ripened cheeses (especially cheddar), wines (especially chianti), fermented milk products like yogurt, broad beans, and bananas.

Concurrent administration of barbiturates, antihistamines, narcotics, hypotensive agents, and phenothiazines may cause additive CNS depression with procarbazine. Patients receiving procarbazine should actively avoid alcoholic beverages since the aldehyde hydrogenase inhibition action of the drug causes a disulfuram-like reaction, which is manifested as flushing, throbbing headache, difficulty in breathing, and acute nausea and vomiting. Patients should be cautioned not only to avoid drinking alcoholic beverages but also to look for hidden sources of alcohol, such as in sauces and desserts. Even rubbing alcohol applied to the skin has been known to cause disulfuram reactions.

Notes on Nutritional Side Effects

Clinical observations have revealed considerable intestinal discomfort in patients on procarbazine who ingest oriental foods and other foods laden with monosodium glutamate (MSG). The patient should be cautioned to avoid soy sauce and packaged or canned foods that contain MSG or have the words "taste enhancers" listed in the ingredients. Canned soups are particularly high in MSG. Low-sodium canned or packaged foods are less likely to contain MSG.

Full meals may delay and change the absorption of an orally administered drug with respect to both the rate of absorption and peak serum concentrations. Absorption by the oral route may be affected by concurrently administered drugs that are toxic to the gastrointestinal tract.

To promote maximal absorption, procarbazine should not be taken with full meals or fatty foods that delay absorption. It is recommended that the drug be administered one hour before or two to three hours after a full meal. Taking the drug on an empty stomach, however, may cause nausea or other stomach disturbances. Procarbazine might be taken along with a starchy snack as bread or crackers, which will clear the stomach quickly and not interfere with drug absorption.

Anorexia—Anorexia has been noted as a side effect of this drug, which may result in reduced food intake. Dietary measures are available to help increase appetite.

Nausea and vomiting—Nausea and vomiting are frequent with procarbazine and may be dose limiting. In some instances, they can be prevented by the prophylactic administration of antiemetic drugs. Starchy foods taken with the oral drug may minimize nausea. Other dietary measures can mitigate the aftereffects of vomiting and lessen residual nausea. Tolerance to these side effects develops with continued administration of the drug.

Favorite foods should not be ingested with procarbazine because a conditioned aversion to these foods may result if nausea and vomiting occur.

Diarrhea—Diarrhea can result from the direct toxicity of this drug to the mucosa lining of the gut. The villi and microvilli become flattened, reducing the absorptive surface area and resulting in a "slick gut." As a result, intestinal contents move rapidly through the gut, reducing absorption. Much of the water poured into the gut for digestion is not reabsorbed, and water-soluble vitamins and minerals can be lost. It is possible to mitigate some of the effects of diarrhea with dietary means.

Constipation—Constipation is also a noted side effect of this drug, which may not be readily rectified by an enema or suppository. Commercial laxatives are not recommended because they may cause nutritional depletion and can be habit forming. Constipation is best treated prophylactically with dietary fiber. Mineral oil is also discouraged because it inhibits the absorbtion of fat-soluble vitamins.

Altered taste and smell—Altered taste and smell, or dysgeusia and dysosmia have been reported with this drug and can lead to decreased appetite. The most common complaints are a lowered taste threshold to bitterness and an elevated taste threshold to sweetness. Dietary means are available to help cope with these problems.

Dry mouth—Procarbazine may cause dry mouth, or xerostomia, by inhibition of salivary watery secretions, which is controlled by the parasympathetic nervous system. The thick salivary secretions controlled by sympathetic glands remain, however, leaving a feeling of "cotton mouth." Certain dietary practices may be needed to maintain nutritional intake.

Dysphagia—Difficulty in chewing and/or swallowing has been described with this drug. Some dietary alterations may be necessary regarding the consistency of foods, such as prescription of a softer diet.

Iron loss—Bleeding tendencies, such as petechia, purpura, epistaxis, hemoptysis, hematemesis, and melena have been described with procarbazine administration. Iron deficiency should be managed, with concurrent iron and vitamin C administration to enhance absorption.

Vitamin B_6—Because procarbazine is a methylhydrazine derivative, decreased plasma levels of pyridoxylphosphate (active vitamin B_6) may be responsible for the neurotoxic and depression side effects of the drug. A metabolite may be formed as pyridoxal methylhydrazine, which causes the B_6 depletion. Vitamin B_6 replacement should be postponed until two days after and extending up to two days before administration of the drug in order not to interfere with treatment efficacy.

Because of the myriad nutritional problems related to procarbazine administration, patients about to receive this drug should receive careful nutritional counseling. Nutritional support of the patient about to receive procarbazine is a particularly good example of how dietary discretion can greatly mitigate treatment side effects.

Foods Prohibited

Foods that have been fermented or aged or in which protein breakdown has occurred to increase the flavor are not permitted when taking this drug. Most cheeses are particularly high in tyramine. Broad beans, pods, avocados, and bananas contain dopamine, so they are restricted too. Although yogurt is a fermented product, it is not excluded from this diet, because no adverse side effects of yogurt have been reported in people taking MAOI drugs.

Beverages: alcoholic beverages, wines, beer, ale

Bread and bread substitutes: homemade yeast breads with substantial quantities of yeast; breads, or crackers containing cheese

Fats: sour cream

Fruits: bananas, red plums, avocados, figs, raisins

Meats: aged game, liver, canned meats, yeast extracts, commercial meat extracts, stored beef liver, chicken livers, salami, sausage, salt-dried fish such as herring, cod, pickled herring

Cheese: aged blue cheese, blue Boursault, brick, Brie, Camembert, Cheddar, Colby, Ementaler, Gouda, mozzarella, Parmesan, provolone, Romano, Roquefort, Tilton

Vegetables: Italian broad beans (pods contain tyramine), green bean pods, eggplant

Miscellaneous: yeast concentrates, soup cubes, products made with concentrated yeasts, commercial gravies or meat extracts, soups containing items that must be avoided, soy sauce, any protein-containing food that has been stored improperly or that may have become spoiled.

Foods Allowed

Beverages: all except alcoholic beverages; limit caffeinated coffee or tea to 1 to 2 cups per day

Bread and bread substitutes: all those not on "prohibited" list

Fats: all except sour cream

Fruits: limit of 1 small orange (2-1/2" diameter), which provides 1 mg tyramine, any other fruits not on "prohibited" list

Meats: cottage cheese and meats not on "prohibited" list, eggs

Vegetables: tomato (limit 1/2 cup daily); all vegetables not on prohibited list

Miscellaneous: anything not on "prohibited" list

Refer patients, as needed, to:

Chapter One: How to Deal with Specific Problems
Problem 1—Loss of Appetite, page 4
Problem 2—Nausea and Vomiting, page 8
Problem 3—Taste Changes, page 12
Problem 4—Sore or Ulcerated Mouth or Throat (Stomatitis/Mucositis), page 14
Problem 5—Difficulties in Chewing and Swallowing (Dysphagia) and Dry Mouth (Xerostomia), page 18
Problem 6—Diarrhea, page 20
Problem 8—Constipation, page 24
Problem 9—Dehydration, page 26

Chapter Two: General Dietary Guidelines
Guideline 1—Basic Nutrition for the Cancer Patient, page 30
Guideline 2—A High-Protein/High-Calorie Diet, page 38
Guideline 3—Food Sources of Minerals, page 45
Guideline 4—Food Sources of Vitamins, page 52
Guideline 5—The Fiber and Residue Contents of Foods, page 58
Guideline 6—A Lactose-Free/Lactose-Restricted Diet, page 61
Guideline 13—A Tyramine and Dopamine-Restricted Diet, page 84
Guideline 14—A Soft-Food/Pureed-Food Diet, page 86

- **Progestins**
- **Hydroxyprogesterone**
- **Hydroxyprogesterone Caproate Injection®** (Quad)
- **Prodrox 250®** (Legere)

- **Medroxyprogesterone Acetate**
- **Depo-Provera®** (Upjohn)

- **Megestrol Acetate**
- **Megace®** (Bristol-Myers)

Nutritionally Significant Side Effects

Vitamin deficiencies
Glucose intolerance
Increased sodium and chloride excretion
Sodium and fluid retention
Nausea and vomiting
Weight gain

Properties and Use in Treatment

Progestins are steroid compounds structurally related to the natural hormone progesterone. These drugs act locally on hormonally sensitive tissue, such as the breast or endometrium, and also at the level of the pituitary. They are primarily used in the treatment of prostatic, advanced endometrial, and breast cancers and renal cell carcinomas. Administration is either oral or intramuscular.

General Toxicities

The following adverse reactions have been observed in women taking progestins: breakthrough bleeding, spotting, change in menstrual flow, amenorrhea, edema, weight gain or loss, changes in cervical erosion and cervical secretions, cholestatic jaundice, rash (allergic) with and without pruritis, melasma or chloasma, and mental depression.

Progestins are contraindicated in the first four months of pregnancy and should be used with caution in patients with a history of thrombophlebitis.

Because progestins may cause some degree of fluid retention, other conditions that might be influenced by this factor—such as epilepsy, migraine, asthma, cardiac or renal dysfunction—require careful observation.

The following adverse reactions may occur when used in combination with estrogens: thrombophlebitis, pulmonary embolism, and cerebral thrombosis and embolism. Evidence is suggestive of an association between progestin-estrogen therapy and neuro-ocular lesions—for example, retinal thrombosis and optic neuritis.

Progestin-estrogen combinations have also been observed to cause a rise in blood pressure in susceptible individuals, premenstrual-like syndrome, changes in libido, changes in appetite, cystitis-like syndrome, headache, nervousness, dizziness, fatigue, backache, hirsutism, loss of scalp hair, erythema multiforme, hemorrhagic eruption, and itching.

The following laboratory results may be altered by the use of estrogen-progestin combination drugs: increased sulfobromophtalein retention and other hepatic function tests; increase in prothrombin factors VII, VIII, IX, and X in coagulation tests; metyrapone test; pregnanediol determination; and thyroid function (increase in PBI_3 and butanol extractable protein-bound iodine and decrease in thyroid uptake values).

Few untoward side effects have been ascribed to oral Megace® (megestrol acetate) therapy. However, reports have been received of patients developing carpal tunnel syndrome, deep vein thrombophlebitis, and alopecia while taking this drug.

The following adverse reactions are rare, but they have been associated with the use of Depo-Provera®: undesirable sequelae at the site of injection (residual lump, change in color of skin, or sterile abscess); breast tenderness or galactorrhea, nervousness, insomnia, somnolence, fatigue, or dizziness; thromboembolic phenomena (thrombophlebitis and pulmonary embolism); sensitivity reaction (pruritus, urticaria, angioneurotic edema, generalized rash, anaphylaxis and/or anaphylactoid reactions); acne, alopecia, or hirsutism; jaundice, headache, and fever.

Progestin's effects on the nutritional status are not as well described as those due to estrogens in oral contraceptives. However, patients given progestins should be observed for the same types of problems that occur with estrogens (see *Estrogens*). Progestins are known to increase appetite. Megace is used therapeutically for this purpose.

Food-Drug Interactions

Full meals may delay and change the absorption of an orally administered drug with respect to both the rate of absorption and peak serum concentrations. Complete absorption by the oral route is particularly questionable if the patient is concurrently receiving drugs that are toxic to the gastrointestinal tract.

To promote maximal absorption, oral drugs should not be taken with full meals or fatty foods that delay absorption. It is recommended that the drug be administered one hour before or two to three hours after a full meal. Taking progestins on an empty stomach may cause nausea or other stomach disturbances. The drug should be taken with a starchy snack, such as bread or crackers, in order to clear the stomach quickly and not interfere with the drug absorption.

Notes on Nutritional Side Effects

Vitamin deficiencies—Patients taking progestins should be monitored for possible vitamin deficiencies, for example, vitamin B_6, (see discussion under *Estrogens*).

Glucose intolerance—A decrease in glucose tolerance has been observed in a small percentage of patients on estrogen and progestin combinations. Careful observation of diabetic patients and screening for diabetes in suspected patients is recommended. Persons susceptible to breast cancer are often also susceptible to diabetes.

Increased sodium and chloride excretion—Large doses of progesterone (50-100 mg daily) result in a moderate catabolic effect and a transient increase in sodium and chloride excretion. Lost fluid and electrolytes will need to be replaced.

Sodium and fluid retention—Sodium and fluid retention have also been observed with the administration of progesterone. A sodium-restricted diet may be necessary. Fluids should be *increased* to help wash out excess sodium.

Nausea and vomiting—Progesterone, like estrogen, can cause some nausea and vomiting, which may be ameliorated by antiemetic agents. Starchy foods taken with the drug may minimize nausea, and other dietary measures can mitigate the aftereffects of vomiting and lessen residual nausea.

If nausea and vomiting are a problem, favorite foods should not be ingested prior to the administration of progestins because a conditioned food aversion may result.

Weight gain—Unlike estrogens, progestins do not cause anorexia. When the progesterone level of the body is higher than the estrogen level, appetite is stimulated and hyperphagia is not unusual. Thus, some of the weight gain seen with progestins is not due to fluid and water retention but is a true weight gain that is normally distributed throughout the body. If not contraindicated, caloric restriction may be necessary.

Refer patients, as needed, to:

Chapter One: How to Deal with Specific Problems
Problem 2—Nausea and Vomiting, page 8

Chapter Two: General Dietary Guidelines
Guideline 1—Basic Nutrition for the Cancer Patient, page 30
Guideline 2—A High-Protein/High-Calorie Diet, page 38
Guideline 3—Food Sources of Minerals, page 45
Guideline 4—Food Sources of Vitamins, page 52
Guideline 11—A Transient Glucose Intolerance/Diabetic Diet, page 76
Guideline 12—A Sodium-Restricted Diet, page 86

• Streptozocin
• Zanosar® (Upjohn)

Nutritionally Significant Side Effects

Nausea and vomiting
Glucose intolerance
Diarrhea

Properties and Use in Treatment

Streptozocin is a natural glucose-containing nitrosourea antibiotic derived from *Streptomyces achromogenes.* DNA synthesis is inhibited by an unknown biochemical mechanism—at least partially involving DNA alkylation—leading to cell death. Its action is phase cell-cycle nonspecific, but the S-phase is most sensitive. Streptozocin is administered intravenously.

It is used primarily in the treatment of insulinomas and other pancreatic islet cell tumors. It is also used with malignant carcinoid and Hodgkin's disease.

General Toxicities

Toxicities unrelated to nutritional status include hepatoxicity (transient and mild abnormalities in liver function are common but usually reversible); anemia, leukopenia, and thrombocytopenia (all uncommon); and hypoglycemia following drug infusion. Renal toxicity is common and includes renal tubular acidosis, glycosuria, aminoaciduria, and azotemia. Streptozocin is contraindicated in patients with renal disease. Liver toxicity may occur along with hypoalbuminemia.

Other side effects include anxiety, nervousness, or shakiness; chills,cold sweats, or cool, pale skin; drowsiness or unusual tiredness or weakness; headache; redness, pain or swelling at injection site; unusual hunger; unusually fast pulse; fever; sore throat; swelling of feet or lower legs; unusual bleeding or bruising; decrease in urination; yellow eyes or skin.

Interactions with Other Drugs

Other nephrotoxic drugs such as cisplatin, aminoglycoside antibiotics, and amphotericin B may potentiate the renal toxicity of streptozocin. Concurrent administered should be avoided if possible.

Notes on Nutritional Side Effects

Nausea and vomiting—Nausea and vomiting are common and may be prevented by administration of antiemetic agents. Starchy foods taken with the drug may minimize nausea. Other dietary measures can mitigate the aftereffects of vomiting and lessen residual nausea.

If nausea and vomiting are a problem, favorite foods should not be ingested prior to the administration of streptozocin because a conditioned food aversion may result.

Glucose intolerance—Mild to moderate glucose intolerance has been observed with administration of streptozocin (generally reversible), but insulin shock with hypoglycemia has occurred. A strictly controlled Type II diabetic diet may be necessary. Such a diet is beyond the scope of this book and is therefore not included here. If diabetes does occur, the patient should be referred to a physician and a nutritionist well versed in the management of diabetes mellitus.

Diarrhea—Diarrhea results from the direct toxicity to the mucosa of the gut. The villi and microvilli become flattened, reducing the absorptive surface area, resulting in a "slick gut." Intestinal contents move rapidly through the gut, further decreasing absorption. Gut absorption of fluid is diminshed which may result in malabsorption and many water-soluble vitamins and minerals. Some of these effects may be mitigated by dietary means. The patient may temporarily lose the ability to synthesize lactose and a lactose-restricted diet may be necessary.

Refer patients, as needed, to:

Chapter One: How to Deal with Specific Problems
Problem 2—Nausea and Vomiting, page 8
Problem 6—Diarrhea, page 20
Problem 9—Dehydration, page 26

Chapter Two: General Dietary Guidelines

- **Tamoxifen**
- **Nolvadex®** (Stuart)

Nutritionally Significant Side Effects

Anorexia
Altered taste and smell (dysgeusia)
Nausea and vomiting
Peripheral edema
Weight gain
Leg cramps

Properties and Use in Treatment

Tamoxifen is a nonsteroidal antiestrogenic agent that competes with estrogen for binding sites in target tissues, such as the breast. Tamoxifen is administered orally in the therapy of estrogen-dependent breast cancer. At high-dosage levels, it also has estrogenic effects. However, studies of tamoxifen used in breast cancer treatment have not confirmed whether the side effects are more estrogenic or progestagenic.

General Toxicities

General side effects include hot flashes, less common menstrual irregularity, vaginal irritation, and discharge with bleeding. Tamoxifen may cause an acute flare of breast cancer that has metastasized to the bone. This is characterized by bone pain and tenderness occurring shortly after initiation of therapy, and erythema at the site of metastatic nodules. Rare side effects include hypercalcemia, edema, thrombocytopenia, leukopenia, thrombophlebitis, dizziness, headache, and depression. Weight gain, skin rash, blurred vision, confusion, swollen legs, shortness of breath, and unusual weakness or sleepiness have also been reported.

Food-Drug Interactions

Full meals may reduce the absorption of an orally administered drug, affecting both the rate of absorption and peak serum concentrations.

Complete absorption by the oral route is particularly questionable if the patient is concurrently receiving drugs toxic to the gastrointestinal tract.

To promote maximal absorption, oral drugs should not be taken with full meals or fatty foods that delay absorption. It is recommended that tamoxifen be administered one hour before or two to three hours after a full meal. Taking the drug on an empty stomach may engender nausea or other stomach disturbances. It should be taken along with a starchy snack such as bread or crackers, in order to clear the stomach quickly and not interfere with drug absorption. The drug should be taken at the same time each day.

Notes on Nutritional Side Effects

Anorexia—Anorexia has been reported and may result in decreased food intake. Dietary measures should be used to help increase appetite.

Altered taste and smell—Altered taste and smell perception may occur with this drug and can lead to decreased appetite. The most common complaints are a lowered threshold to bitterness and sweetness. Dietary means are available to help cope with this problem.

Nausea and vomiting—Nausea and vomiting are usually absent or mild. If present, they may be prevented by the prophylactic administration of antiemetic agents. Dietary means cannot prevent this type of nausea and vomiting, but dietary measures can mitigate the aftereffects of vomiting and lessen residual nausea. Specifically, starchy foods may help minimize nausea.

Favorite foods should not be ingested prior to the administration of a drug that causes nausea and vomiting because vomiting may create a conditioned aversion to foods taken immediately beforehand.

Peripheral edema and weight gain—Peripheral edema and weight gain have been noted, but are uncommon. These symptoms may be related to sodium retention, and a sodium-restricted diet may be indicated.

Leg cramps—Leg cramps may be experienced and may be treated with calcium supplementation if not contraindicated. Potassium or magnesium may also reduce leg cramping if calcium is ineffective.

Refer patients, as needed, to:

Chapter One: How to Deal with Specific Problems
Problem 1—Loss of Appetite, page 4
Problem 2—Nausea and Vomiting, page 8
Problem 3—Taste Changes, page 12
Problem 9—Dehydration, page 26

Chapter Two: General Dietary Guidelines
Guideline 1—Basic Nutrition for the Cancer Patient, page 30
Guideline 2—A High-Protein/High-Calorie Diet, page 38
Guideline 3—Food Sources of Minerals, page 45
Guideline 4—Food Sources of Vitamins, page 52
Guideline 10—How to Prevent Kidney Stone Formation (Acid Ash/Alkaline Ash Diet), page 74
Guideline 12—A Sodium-Restricted Diet, page 79

• Thioguanine (6-TG)
• Tabloid® Thioguanine (Burroughs Wellcome)

Nutritionally Significant Side Effects

Anorexia
Nausea and vomiting
Diarrhea
Pellagra
Hyperuricemia

Properties and Use in Treatment

Thioguanine is a purine analogue used in the treatment of acute nonlymphocytic leukemias. It acts as an antimetabolite to block DNA, RNA, and protein synthesis, and is ribosylated to active metabolites, some of which are actually incorporated into DNA. Its action is cell cycle S-phase specific. It is orally administrated. Lower doses should be used in patients with impaired renal or hepatic function.

General Toxicities

The most consistent, dose-related toxicity with thioguanine is bone-marrow suppression. The hematologic toxicities include leukopenia, thrombocytopenia and anemia and usually appear 7 to 14 days after drug administration.

Other side effects unrelated to nutritional status include fever, sore throat, jaundice, local infection, unusual bleeding, and anemia.

Interactions with Other Drugs

There is usually complete resistance between mercaptopurine and thioguanine. Allopurinol, however, does not interfere with the metabolism of thioguanine.

Food-Drug Interactions

Full meals may delay and change the absorption of an orally administered drug with respect to both the rate of absorption and peak serum concentrations. Complete absorption by the oral route is particularly questionable if the patient is concurrently receiving drugs that are toxic to the gastrointestinal tract.

To promote maximal absorption, oral drugs should not be taken with full meals or fatty foods that delay absorption. It is recommended that the drug be administered one hour before or two to three hours after a full meal. Taking the drug on an empty stomach may engender nausea or other stomach disturbances. The drug should be taken along with a starchy snack, such as bread or crackers, in order to clear the stomach quickly and not interfere with the drug absorption.

Notes on Nutritional Side Effects

Anorexia—Unexplained anorexia is an uncommon side effect and may be due to nausea and vomiting. Dietary measures can help increase appetite.

Nausea and vomiting—Nausea and vomiting are uncommon and may be ameliorated by antiemetic agents. Starchy foods taken with the drug may minimize nausea, and other dietary measures can mitigate the aftereffects of vomiting and lessen residual nausea.

If nausea and vomiting are a problem, favorite foods should not be ingested prior to the administration of thioguanine because a conditioned aversion to foods taken immediately beforehand may result.

Diarrhea—Diarrhea results from the direct toxicity to the mucosa of the gut. The villi and microvilli become flattened, reducing the absorptive surface area, resulting in a "slick gut." Intestinal contents move rapidly through the gut, further decreasing absorption. Much of the water poured into the gut for digestion is not reabsorbed, and many water-soluble vitamins and minerals are lost. Some of these effects may be mitigated by dietary means.

Pellagra—Thioguanine may cause pellagra, a deficiency of niacin and/or the amino acid tryptophan. The cardinal signs of advanced pellagra are dermatitis, diarrhea, dementia, and ultimately death. Symptoms occurring with both pellagra and antimetabolite administration include anorexia, malaise, weakness, irritability, anxiety, depression, photosensitivity of light-exposed skin, digestive gastritis, diarrhea (aggravated by highly seasoned or acidic foods), and wasting. Pellagra is correctable by the administration of 100-300 mg of niacin a day given in two divided doses.

Hyperuricemia—Thioguanine causes rapid cellular destruction resulting in extensive purine catabolism and hyperuricemia. Renal and joint damage may result from the precipitation of urates. A low-purine, low-protein diet may be contraindicated in a cancer patient. Thus hyperuricemia should be treated by medical means, that is, by the administration of a xanthine oxidase inhibitor drug such as allopurinol,* without an accompanying low-protein diet. Allopurinol does not alter the metabolism of thioguanine and therefore no dose adjustments of thioguanine are required with concurrent allopurinol administration. Supportive dietary measures should include increased hydration (ten to twelve 8-ounce glasses of water per day) and an alkaline-ash diet to alkalinize the urine and prevent the precipitation of uric acid stones in the kidney.

Refer patients, as needed, to:

Chapter One: How to Deal with Specific Problems
Problem 1—Loss of Appetite, page 4
Problem 2—Nausea and Vomiting, page 8
Problem 4—Sore or Ulcerated Mouth or Throat (Stomatitis/Mucositis), page 14
Problem 6—Diarrhea, page 20
Problem 9—Dehydration, page 26

Chapter Two: General Dietary Guidelines
Guideline 1—Basic Nutrition for the Cancer Patient, page 30
Guideline 2—A High-Protein/High-Calorie Diet, page 38
Guideline 3—Food Sources of Minerals, page 45
Guideline 4—Food Sources of Vitamins, page 52
Guideline 5—The Fiber and Residue Contents of Foods, page 58
Guideline 6—A Lactose-Free/Lactose-Restricted Diet, page 61
Guideline 10—How to Prevent Kidney Stone Formation (Acid Ash/Alkaline Ash Diet), page 74

*Note: Allopurinol has its own nutritional side effects. See the discussion of this drug earlier in this chapter.

• Triethylenethiophosphoramide (TEPA)
• Thiotepa® (Lederle)

Nutritionally Significant Side Effects

Anorexia

Nausea and vomiting

Properties and Use in Treatment

TEPA is a nonvesicant alkylating agent whose mechanism of action is believed to be through the release of ethylenimine radicals that covalently attach to DNA (PDR). Its action is cell-cycle phase nonspecific.

Thiotepa® is administered intravenously and is used primarily in the treatment of bladder, breast, and ovarian cancers and in Hodgkin's disease.

General Toxicities

Leukopenia is dose-limiting with the nadir at ten to fourteen days and recovery by twenty-one to twenty-eight days. Dizziness, headaches, hives, bronchoconstriction are less and common side effects. Amenorrhea, loss of fertility, abdominal discomfort, bladder irritability and hemorrhagic cystitis have rarely been reported.

Food-Drug Interactions

Succinylcholine inhibits psuedocholinesterase activity. Succinylcholine should be administered cautiously in patients receiving thiotepa.

Notes on Nutritional Side Effects

Anorexia—Unexplained anorexia has been noted, which may result in reduced food intake. Dietary measures are available to help increase appetite.

Nausea and vomiting—Nausea and vomiting are usually minimal and, in some instances, can be prevented by the prophylactic administration of antiemetic agents. Starchy foods taken prior to drug administration may minimize nausea. Other dietary measures can mitigate the aftereffects of vomiting and lessen residual nausea.

If nausea and vomiting are a problem, favorite foods should not be ingested prior to the administration of TEPA because a conditioned aversion to foods taken immediately beforehand may result.

Refer patients, as needed, to:

Chapter One: How to Deal with Specific Problems
Problem 1—Loss of Appetite, page 4
Problem 2—Nausea and Vomiting, page 8
Problem 9—Dehydration, page 26

Chapter Two: General Dietary Guidelines
Guideline 1—Basic Nutrition for the Cancer Patient, page 30
Guideline 2—A High-Protein/High-Calorie Diet, page 38
Guideline 3—Food Sources of Minerals, page 45
Guideline 4—Food Sources of Vitamins, page 52

• Vinblastine Sulfate
• Velban® (Lilly)

Nutritionally Significant Side Effects

Anorexia
Nausea and vomiting
Dysphagia
Stomatitis and mucositis
Abdominal discomfort
Constipation

Properties and Use in Treatment

Vinblastine sulfate is an alkaloid extract of Vinca rosea (periwinkle). The primary mechanism of action is believed to involve binding to tubulin elements of microtubules, facilitating disruption of microtubules, especially in the mitotic spindle. Vinblastine blocks all progression out of metaphase. It also interferes with metabolic pathways of amino acids leading from glutamic acid to the citric acid cycle and urea. Its action is cell-cycle specific for the M phase. At high concentrations, vinblastine sulfate also inhibits S and G1 phases.

Vinblastine is used primarily in the treatment of Hodgkin's disease, choriocarcinoma, testicular carcinoma, non-Hodgkin's lymphomas, breast cancer, lung cancer, and Kaposi's sarcoma. The drug is administered intravenously.

General Toxicities

The dose-limiting toxicity of vinblastine is myelosuppression. Leukopenia and thrombocytopenia nadir between seven and ten days with recovery by day fourteen to seventeen. Nausea and vomiting are common but mild in severity and easily controlled with phenothiazine antiemetics. Neurotoxicity occurs less frequently than with vincristine and is manifested as peripheral neuropathy, autonomic nervous system and central nervous system toxicity. Peripheral neuropathy presents as paresthesias, foot drop, and decreased lower extremity strength. Autonomic toxicity presents as constipation, ileus, abdominal pain, or urinary retention. Central nervous toxicity is manifested by jaw pain or blurred vision. Rare side effects include orthostatic hypotension, depression, headache, and convulsions. Extravasation should be avoided since it is a vesicant agent.

Interaction with Other Drugs

Reversal of the anti-tumor effect by current glutamic acid or tryptophan, has been described, but its clincal significance is not known.

Notes on Nutritional Side Effects

Anorexia—Unexplained anorexia has been noted as a side effect of this drug, possibly resulting in reduced food intake. Dietary measures are available to help increase the appetite.

Nausea and vomiting—Nausea and vomiting are common, but can usually be readily controlled by antiemetic agents. Starchy foods taken prior to drug administration may minimize the nausea. Other dietary measures may mitigate the aftereffects of vomiting and lessen residual nausea.

If nausea and vomiting are a problem, favorite foods should not be ingested prior to the administration of vinblastine because a conditioned aversion to foods taken immediately beforehand may result.

Dysphagia—On rare occasions, difficulty in chewing and/or swallowing has been described with this drug. Some dietary restrictions may be necessary regarding the consistency of foods, such as a soft diet.

Stomatitis and mucositis—Vinblastine may be directly toxic to the rapidly replicating mucosal cells in and around the mouth and throughout the digestive tract. Enhanced nutrition, with an emphasis on the B vitamins, may mitigate or prevent this problem. Once the problem exists, however, certain dietary restrictions may be necessary to keep the patient eating. A prescribed mouth care program may be helpful in reducing toxic symptoms.

Abdominal discomfort—Vinblastine can cause vague abdominal discomfort, which may be aggravated by a distended or full gut. Temporary restriction of fiber and residue contents of the diet may be necessary.

Constipation—Constipation is a side effect of vinblastine and is not usually managed effectively readily rectified by an enema or suppository. Use of commercial laxatives is discouraged because they may cause nutritional depletion and are habit forming, but may be necessary. Senna derivatives such as SenokotR or Dulcolax plus a stool softener are recommended in mild cases. Use of mineral oil is also discouraged because it solublizes the fat-soluble vitamins in the gut, preventing their absorption. Constipation is best treated prophylactically with dietary fiber, where not contraindicated.

Refer patients, as needed, to:

Chapter One: How to Deal with Specific Problems
Problem 1—Loss of Appetite, page 4
Problem 2—Nausea and Vomiting, page 8
Problem 4—Sore or Ulcerated Mouth or Throat (Stomatisis/ Mucositis), page 14
Problem 5—Difficulties in Chewing and Swallowing (Dysphagia) and Dry Mouth (Xerostomia), page 18
Problem 9—Dehydration, page 26

Chapter Two: General Dietary Guidelines
Guideline 1—Basic Nutrition for the Cancer Patient, page 30
Guideline 2—A High-Protein/High-Calorie Diet, page 38
Guideline 3—Food Sources of Minerals, page 45
Guideline 4—Food Sources of Vitamins, page 52
Guideline 5—The Fiber and Residue Contents of Foods, page 58
Guideline 14—A Soft-Food/Pureed-Food Diet, page 86

• Vincristine Sulfate
• Oncovin® (Lilly)
• Vincasar® (Adria)

Nutritionally Significant Side Effects

Nausea and vomiting
Constipation
Abdominal discomfort
Stomatitis and mucositis
Dysphagia
Dry mouth
Altered taste and smell
Hyperuricemia
Inappropriate antidiuretic hormone secretion

Properties and Use in Treatment

Vincristine sulfate is an alkaloid derivative of *Vinca rosea* (periwinkle). The antineoplastic effects of the vinca alkaloids are related to an interference with intracellular tubulin function, with prevention of mitotic spindle formation. The action is cell-cycle specific for the M phase. At high concentrations, this drug also inhibits the S phase and is capable of killing G_1 or plateau phase cells.

Vincristine is used in the treatment of many cancers, including acute lymphocytic leukemia, breast cancer, Hodgkin's disease, non-Hodgkin's lymphomas, testicular cancer, small-cell lung cancer, brain cancer, Ewing's sarcoma, neuroblastoma, rhabdomyosarcoma, general sarcomas, and Wilms' tumor. The drug is poorly absorbed orally and is given only intravenously.

General Toxicity

The dose-limiting toxicity is neuropathy which is manifested by sensory impairment and loss of deep tendon reflexes and paresthesia. This reflects a generally mild neuropathy but may be progressive with painful paresthesia, foot drop, ataxia, and cranial nerve palsies. Autonomic toxicity, including abdominal pain, severe constipation, and ileus may occur. Hematologic myelosuppression is uncommon. Alopecia occurs in 20 percent of patients. Rare non-nutritional side effects include agitation, blurred vision, confusion, convulsions, dizziness, or light-headedness, drooping lids, fever, chills, sore throat, jaw pain, joint pain, lack of sweating, mental depression, pain in fingers, toes and testicles, difficulty and painful urination, swelling of the legs and feet, problems sleeping, unusual bleeding and bruising, weakness, and increase in urination. Extravasation should be avoided since it is a potent vesicant agent.

Notes on Nutritional Side Effects

Nausea and vomiting—Nausea and vomiting occasionally occur and may be prevented by antiemetic agents. Starchy foods taken before administration of vincristine may minimize nausea. Other dietary measures may mitigate the aftereffects of vomiting and lessen residual nausea.

If nausea and vomiting are a problem, favorite foods should not be ingested prior to the administration of vincristine because a conditioned aversion to foods taken immediately beforehand may result.

Constipation—Constipation from an adynamic ileus is a serious, painful problem and is due to cumulative autonomic neurotoxicity. This symptom resolves very slowly after drug discontinuance, and is not effectively treated by an enema or suppository. Commercial laxatives may cause nutritional depletion and can be habit forming, but may be necessary. Senna derivatives such as Senokot® or Dulcolax plus a stool softener are recommended in mild cases. Their use is discouraged. Mineral oil is also discouraged because it solublizes the fat-soluble vitamins in the gut and prevents their absorption. Constipation can be successfully treated prophylactically with dietary fiber, where not contraindicated.

Abdominal discomfort—Vincristine can cause vague abdominal discomfort, which may be aggravated by a distended or full gut. Restriction of fiber and residue contents in the diet may be necessary in some instances. Dose reduction and/or the use of stool softeners, such as dioctyl sodium sulfosuccinate, may also be indicated where high fiber diet is contraindicated.

Stomatitis and mucositis—Vincristine can be directly toxic to the rapidly dividing mucosal cells in and around the mouth and throughout the digestive tract. Enhanced nutrition, with an emphasis the B vitamins, may prevent this problem. Once the problem exists, however, certain dietary restrictions may be necessary to maintain the patient's nutritional intake. A prescribed mouth care program can also be helpful in reducing toxic symptoms.

Dysphagia—Difficulty in chewing and/or swallowing has been described with this drug. Some dietary restrictions may be necessary regarding the consistency of foods, such as a soft diet.

Dry mouth—Vincristine may cause dry mouth, or xerostomia, due to its inhibition of the parasympathetic nervous system, which decreases salivary secretions. The thick salivary secretions from the sympathetically controlled glands are not affected by vincristine, leading to a feeling of dry or "cotton mouth." If dry mouth does occur, certain dietary practices may be needed to maintain nutritional intake.

Altered taste and smell—Altered taste and smell (dysgeusia and dysosmia) have been reported and can lead to decreased appetite. The most common taste complaints are a lowered taste threshold for bitterness and a raised threshold to sweetness. Dietary measures can help cope with this problem.

Hyperuricemia—Vincristine can cause rapid cellular destruction, resulting in extensive purine catabolism and hyperuricemia. Renal and joint damage may result from the precipitation of urates. A low-purine diet, low-protein diet may be contraindicated in cancer patients. The hyperuricemia should be treated primarily by medical means, that is, by the administration of a xanthine oxidase inhibitor drug such as allopurinol* without an accompanying low-protein diet if control is achieved. Supportive dietary measures should include increased hydration (ten to twelve 8-ounce glasses of fluid per day) and an alkaline-ash diet to alkalinize the urine and prevent the precipitation of uric acid stones in the kidney.

Inappropriate antidiuretic hormone secretion—Occasionally, the syndrome of inappropriate antidiuretic hormone secretion, including high urinary sodium excretion, may occur in the presence of hyponatremia. With fluid deprivation, hyponatremia and renal

*Note: Allopurinol can also have nutritional side effects. See the discussion of this drug earlier in this chapter.

sodium loss improve. Restriction of fluid intake and the administration of a potent diuretic are indicated. If fluid restriction is inadvisable because of concurrent administration of other drugs or hyperuricemia, dietary sodium or parenteral saline may be given.

Refer patients, as needed, to:

Chapter One: How to Deal with Specific Problems
Problem 2—Nausea and Vomiting, page 8
Problem 3—Taste Changes, page 12
Problem 4—Sore or Ulcerated Mouth or Throat (Stomatitis/Mucositis), page 14
Problem 5—Difficulties in Chewing and Swallowing (Dysphagia) and Dry Mouth (Xerostomia), page 18
Problem 8—Constipation, page 24
Problem 9—Dehydration, page 26

Chapter Two: General Dietary Guidelines
Guideline 1—Basic Nutrition for the Cancer Patient, page 30
Guideline 2—A High-Protein/High-Calorie Diet, page 38
Guideline 3—Food Sources of Minerals, page 45
Guideline 4—Food Sources of Vitamins, page 52
Guideline 5—The Fiber and Residue Contents of Foods, page 58
Guideline 10—How to Prevent Kidney Stone Formation (Acid Ash/Alkaline Ash Diet), page 74
Guideline 14—A Soft-Food/Pureed Food Diet, page 86

Chapter 5

Nutrition and Radiation Therapy

Lawrence W. Margolis, M.D.*
Janet L. Ramstack, Dr.P.H.
Ernest H. Rosenbaum, M.D.

*Lawrence W. Margolis, M.D., Clinical Professor and Vice-Chairman of Radiation Oncology at University of California/San Francisco; Chief of Radiation Oncology of the Claire Zellerbach Saroni Institute at Mount Zion Hospital.

Radiation Therapy in Cancer Treatment

Approximately 50% of all patients with cancer will require radiation therapy at some time during their illness—either alone or in conjunction with either surgery or chemotherapy.

Special care must be taken with patients who also receive chemotherapy or surgery, as the side effects of radiation may be enhanced. The radiation oncologist must select the most effective tumor dose, with maximum protection of normal tissue.

The radiation is usually delivered over several weeks, spread out to allow repair of normal tissues. A balance is attempted, aiming for necessary therapeutic effectiveness with minimal damage to normal tissue, based on the overall situation and the region treated. Nonetheless, there are often acute effects during the treatment, and possibly chronic effects later. Acute radiation effects are primarily on rapidly dividing tissues such as skin, esophageal mucosa, bladder, small intestine, and rectum.

Healing usually occurs within a few weeks after completion of radiation. Chronic radiation side effects may result in fibrosis, necrosis, ulceration and damage to a specific organ, depending on the region of radiation.

The principles of basic good nutrition recommended for the cancer patient on chemotherapy are applicable to the cancer patient receiving radiotherapy. In addition, specific nutritional problems may be anticipated in relation to the region irradiated.

Oral Cavity

Irradiation in the mouth and throat may result in painful mucositis, altered or loss of taste, dry mouth or dental problems. A complete dental evaluation is mandatory for any patient receiving radiation to the oral cavity or pharynx. This requires x-ray examination of teeth and repair or removal of any decayed teeth.

If it is necessary to remove teeth, the extraction site must be completely healed before the radiotherapy, to avoid late and irreversible bone damage. Radiation treatment generally should not start until about 14 days after the extraction. The remaining intact teeth should be treated daily with topical fluoride to help prevent dental caries.

Radiation mucositis frequently occurs with radiation to the head and neck. The patient may need a nourishing, soft diet. (See Chapter

One, page 18, Chapter Two, page 86.) Foods that tend to form sharp edges should be avoided. Extremely hot or cold foods also may irritate the mucosa. The drinking of alcoholic beverages and the smoking or chewing of all forms of tobacco must be avoided completely, because they are irritating to the mouth and throat.

If mucositis causes a patient to curtail intake of nourishing foods, a protein supplement may be needed to meet daily requirements. (See Chapter Three, Table 2, page 187, for a list of protein supplements.) A consultation with a dietitian can help the patient plan an adequate diet. Occasionally, when swallowing becomes too painful, tube-feeding may be necessary until the mucosa heals.

The maintenance of good oral hygiene is crucial. Frequent use of a gentle mouthwash may help reduce the discomfort or pain from mucositis. A solution of baking soda and salt dissolved in warm water should be used instead of commercial mouthwashes which may be irritating to the oral mucosa. In severe cases of mucositis, where eating or drinking may be difficult, viscous xylocaine, a topical anesthetic may be used (one tablespoon gargled) before meals. Also, slurry of sucralsulfate (Carafate®), prepared by dissolving sucralfate in water and sorbitol, will coat the oral mucosa and sooth the discomfort. (It is minimally absorbed from the GI tract, and on rare occasions there are systemic side effects; it may cause constipation.)

The radiation oncologist must carefully evaluate the patient with mucositis on a regular basis to rule out monilia infection. Existing infections may be treated locally or systemically, either with Nystatis® (oral suspension or tablets) or ketoconazola (Nizoral®).

Patients should work closely with their physician, dietitian, and nurse to ensure a continued nutritionally sound diet. Often a nutritional supplement, such as Ensure®, will be needed to ensure adequate nutrient intake. In severe cases, feeding through a nasogastric tube may be required.

A common problem of radiation of the oral cavity and pharynx is xerostomia, or dry mouth, caused by reduction in saliva following irradiation of the salivary glands. This may be temporary, but if doses exceed 4,000 rads, the patient may be left with some degree of permanent dryness of the oral cavity. The use of artificial saliva, such as Salivart®, moisturizing gels such as Oral Balance®, and a special dry mouth toothpaste such as Biotene®, will help minimize symptoms. (See Chapter One, Problem 5 on page 18.)

Patients should also increase their intake of fluids, particularly with meals, to ease swallowing and help moisten their mouths. They should avoid dry, hard food, using instead creams, gravies and sauces to moisten their food.

Patients will often suffer loss of taste with oral cavity radiation. This is usually self-limiting, and taste will commonly return within two months after completion of radiation. This symptom is secondary to the irradiation of the taste buds. It is also associated with the decrease and thickening of the saliva, as a result of radiation of the salivary glands. Emphasizing foods with distinctive flavors and odors, or adding spices may help combat the problem. (See Chapter One, Problem 3, page 12.)

Thorax

Radiation is frequently delivered to the thorax in the treatment of lung cancer, esophageal cancer, and lymphoma. This necessitates inclusion of the esophagus within the radiation area. Doses in excess of 3,000 rads may, within three weeks, result in an esophageal mucosal reaction, with symptoms of pain on swallowing. The reaction of the mucosa is usually self-limited, and reduction in the daily dose of radiation or a short interruption in the treatment will usually allow rapid healing.

A soft, bland diet, antacids, and a topical anesthetic such as viscous 2% xylocaine (Lidocaine®) solution will often minimize symptoms. Slurry of sucralfate will coat the esophagus and soothe the discomfort as it does in the oral cavity. If symptoms persist, a candida infection may be present, which is effectively treated with ketoconazole (Nizoral®, Nystatin® or Mycostatin®).

Abdomen and Pelvis

Radiation is often delivered to the upper abdomen or pelvis, potentially causing radiation enteritis. However, only 5 to 15% of patients treated with radiation to the abdomen will develop chronic problems.

Because of their rapidly dividing cells, the mucosa of both the large and small bowel, including the rectum, are quite sensitive to even modest doses of radiation. The severity of symptoms depends on several factors, including the extent of the irradiated area, the daily dose, the total dose required, and the possible concomitant use of chemotherapy. In addition, patients with a previous history of abdominal surgery, pelvic inflammatory disease, atherosclerosis, diabetes or hypertension, are predisposed to radiation injury.

The type and size of the tumor determines the treatment area and the size of the dose required. Patients treated to the upper abdomen are more likely to develop nausea and vomiting, while pelvic irradiation is more likely to result in rectal irritation, frequent bowel movements, or even water diarrhea. This disturbance of the intestinal mucosa may alter the absorptive functions of the gastrointestinal tract with resultant malabsorption of fat, bile salts, and vitamin B_{12}.

It is of utmost important to fully evaluate the extent of the enteritis by assessing the frequency of diarrhea, the character of the stools, the presence of rectal bleeding, or abdominal distention. The physician must evaluate the patient with regard to possible dehydration or electrolyte imbalance resulting from diarrhea and/or malabsorption.

The medical management of radiation enteritis includes dietary manipulation, medication and, in severe cases, the interruption of radiation treatment. Patients receiving abdominal or pelvic radiation should use a low-fat, low-fiber/residue diet (see Chapter Two, General Guidelines 5 and 9, pages 58 and 71), beginning with the first radiation treatments. They should limit their intake of milk products, except for buttermilk, yogurt and/or acidophilus or lactose-free milk (see General Guidelines 6, page 61).

Greasy foods, fried foods or fatty foods, also tend to be difficult to digest. Vegetables should be cooked. Whole-grain and high-bran products, such as whole wheat bread, and also nuts, popcorn, potato chips and beans should be avoided. Patients can drink fruit juices (except prune juice), but they should not eat raw fruits. They should also reduce their alcohol consumption.

If radiation enteritis persists despite dietary changes, medications will be needed. A 5-ASA ( ) 250mg suppository every night has helped reduce or control colitis and proctitis during and after radiation therapy. Oral medications include:

1. Kaopectate® (dose: 30 cc to 60 cc after each loose bowel movement.
2. Lomotil® (dose: one or two tablets orally every four to six hours as needed to a maximum of eight tablets a day—most patients will find they require only two or three tablets per day after the diarrhea has been initially controlled).

3. Immodium® (dose: two tablets initially followed by one tablet after each loose stool, but not to exceed 16 tablets per day); Immodium® is also now available in liquid form without a prescription.
4. Donnatol® (dose: one or two tablets every four hours for abdominal cramping).
5. Paregoric® (dose: one teaspoon orally every four hours for diarrhea).

Nausea can usually be controlled with Compazine® (10mg every four hours) or Reglan®, tablets or liquid (dose: 10mg four times daily 30 minutes before each meal and at bedtime). The severity of the side-effects may, at times, make it necessary to reduce the radiation dose.

In addition, relief from abdominal pain may be obtained with narcotics. If proctitis is present, a steroid foam given rectally may offer relief. Finally, if patients with pancreatic cancer are experiencing diarrhea during radiation therapy, they should be evaluated for potential administration of oral pancreatic enzyme replacement, to cure deficiencies which alone can cause diarrhea.

Medication Summary

1. Kaopectate®, an antidiarrheal agent. Dose: 30cc to 60cc po after each loose bowel movement.
2. Lomotil® (diphenoxylate hydrochloride with atropine sulfate). Usual dose: one to two tablets po every four hours as needed, adjusted for the individual pattern of diarrhea—but not to exceed eight tablets within a 24-hour period.
3. Paregoric®, an antidiarrheal agent. Usual dose: one teaspoon po qid as needed for diarrhea. Can be used alternatively with Lomotil®.
4. Cholestyramine®, a bile salt sequestering agent. Dose: one package po after each meal and at bedtime.
5. Donnatal®, an anticholinergic, antispasmodic agent used to alleviate bowel cramping. Dose: one to two tablets every four hours as needed.
6. Imodium® (loperamide hydrochloride), a synthetic antidiarrheal agent. Recommended initial dose: two capsules (4mg) po every four hours, followed by one capsule (2mg) po after each unformed stool. Daily dose should not exceed 16 capsules.

Dietary Summary

See *Chapter Two: General Dietary Guidelines*:
Guideline 1—Basic Nutrition for the Cancer Patient, page 30
Guideline 2—A High-Protein/High-Calorie Diet, page 38

Foods to avoid:

- Milk and milk products, because of potential lactose intolerance. Exceptions are buttermilk and yogurt (often tolerated because the lactose is altered by lactobacillus), and processed cheese (because the lactose is removed with the whey when it is separated from the cheese curd). Milkshake supplements such as Ensure[R] are lactose-free and may be used.
- Whole bran bread and cereal
- Nuts, seeds, coconuts
- Fried, greasy or fatty foods
- Fresh and dried fruit and some fruit juices such as prune juice
- Raw vegetables
- Rich pastries
- Popcorn, potato chips, and pretzels
- Strong spices and herbs
- Chocolate, coffee, tea, and soft drinks with caffeine
- Alcohol and tobacco

Foods to encourage:

- Fish, poultry, and meat that is cooked, broiled or roasted
- Bananas, apple sauce, peeled apples, apple and grape juices
- White bread and toast
- Macaroni and noodles
- Baked, boiled or mashed potatoes
- Cooked vegetables that are mild, such as asparagus tips, green and waxed beans, carrots, spinach, and squash
- Mild processed cheese, eggs, smooth peanut butter, buttermilk, and yogurt

Helpful hints:

- Ingest foods at room temperature.
- Drink 10-12 cups of fluid per day. Carbonated beverages should be allowed to lose their carbonation prior to drinking. (Stir drink until bubbles have disappeared.)
- Add nutmeg to food, which will help reduce motility of the GI tract.
- Start a low-residue diet on day one of radiation therapy treatment.

References

1. Fajardo, L. "Pathology of Radiology Injury." Chapter 5: Alimentary Tract, New York: Mason Publishers, pp. 47-76, 1982.
2. Stryker, J.A., Bartholomew, M. "Failure of lactose-restricted diets to prevent radiation-induced diarrhea in patients undergoing whole pelvis irradiation." *International Journal of Radiation Oncology, Biology, Physics* 12(5):789-792, 1986.
3. Yasco, J.M. "Care of the Client Receiving External Radiation Therapy." Reston Publishing Company, Inc., Reston, Virginia, p. 258, 1982.
4. PDQ. *Physician Data Query,* 1990.

Appendices

Appendix A

Drug Companies

For further information about some nutritional products mentioned, please refer to these companies.

CARNATION COMPANY
800 N. Brand Blvd.
Glendale, CA 91203
(818) 549-6000
Carnation Instant Breakfast®

LACTAID, INC.
P.O. Box 111
Pleasantville, NJ 08232
1(800) 257-8650
LactAid®

MEAD JOHNSON
Nutritional Division
2400 Pennsylvania Street
Evansville, IN 47721
(812) 429-5000
Sustacal®, Isocal®

NATIONAL LIVE STOCK AND MEAT BOARD
Attn: Nutrition Information Dept.
444 N. Michigan Avenue
Chicago, IL 60611
(312) 467-5520

NORWICH EATON PHARMACEUTICALS, INC.
17 Eaton Avenue
Norwich, NY 13815-0231
(607) 335-2111
Vivonex T.E.N.®, Standard Vivonex®

ROSS LABORATORIES
625 Cleveland Avenue
Columbus, OH 43216
(614) 227-3333
Ensure®, Ensure Plus®, Osmolite®, Vital HN®, Polycose®)

SANDOZ NUTRITION
Clinical Products Division
5320 W. 23 St.
P.O. Box 370
Minneapolis, MN 55440
1(800) 369-3000
Resource®, Resource Plus®

SHERWOOD MEDICAL
Cheesebrough-Ponds, Inc.
Hospital Products Division
33 Benedict Place
Greenwich, CT 06830
(203) 661-2000
Magnacal®

For information on the diet supplements, write to:

ROSS LABORTORIES
Columbus, OH 43216

SANDOZ NUTRITION
5320 West 23 Street
Minneapolis, MN 55440

EATON LABORATORIES
Morton-Norwich Products, Inc
Norwich, NY 13814

MEAD JOHNSON LABORATORIES
Evansville, IN 47721

Products

*LACTAID®—for information on LactAid®, write:

LACTAID, INC.
P.O. Box 111
Pleasantville, NJ 08232

Self-Help Companies

The following self-help companies deal directly with the consumer and provide catalogs of their products:

FRED SAMMONS, INC.
Be O/K Sales Company
Box 32
Brookfield, IL 60513
(708) 325-1700

CLEO LIVING AIDS
3957 Mayfield Rd.
Cleveland, OH 44121
(216) 382-9700

*Acidophilus Products—acidophilus milk is available at most grocery stores. Health Food stores also carry high potency acidophilus tablets or liquid.

Appendix B

Mouth and Dental Care

To help prevent mouth ulcerations, mucositis and esophagitis, patients who are prone to develop or who are developing mouth or esophageal problems (or changes in taste or swallowing) should conscientiously follow an oral hygiene program—a half hour after eating, and after each course of chemotherapy, and at least every four to six hours (four times a day).

In April, 1989, NIH Consensus Conference made several recommendations after concluding that pre-chemotherapy and radiation therapy dental care would reduce oral complications. It was recommended that patients obtain a dental hygienic evaluation, including prior dental history and an assessment of current periodontal, oral and nutritional status.

Patients should be scheduled for regular dental cleaning and scaling, and taught oral hygienic care, with daily brushing and flossing to reduce plaque. Extractions should be completed at least two weeks prior to cancer therapy. Ill fitting dentures should be fixed or replaced.

Oral problems including stomatitis, complicate chemotherapy and radiation treatments, and can be detrimental (and very aggravating) to the patient. When oral complications become severe, oncologic therapy has to be suspended, and the risk of a major systemic infection may necessitate hospitalization. Thus, appropriate dental risk assessment and treatment of pre-existing problems will help reduce the potential of oral complications related to cancer therapy.

General Recommendations:

1. Use a soft bristle or nylon toothbrush, soaked in warm water; brush teeth at a 45-degree angle between the gums and the teeth in a vertical motion.

2. Swish the mouth with a neutral, nonirritating dentifrice such as a baking soda solution. Obtain your dentist's recommendation for other solutions.
3. Floss twice a day with unwaxed dental floss, avoid when the white count or platelet counts are low.
4. Clean your dentures on a daily basis. Dentures should be removed about a half hour after eating, at least four times a day, and cleaned to help reduce mouth irritation after chemotherapy. If mouth ulcers or sores are present—dentures should not be worn until they are healed.
5. Use a mouthwash after each meal and at bedtime. Frequency may be increased if a problem develops. NOTE: Many commercial mouthwashes contain higher amounts of salt or alcohol, and in general, are not recommended.

   Mouthwash Solutions:

   Baking soda—One teaspoon with one cup warm water, rinse mouth for about one minute.

   Saline (salt water)—One level teaspoon of salt per pint of water.

   Chloroseptic® containing benzocaine, an anesthetic, used as a spray or as a liquid, full strength or diluted 1 : 1 with water.

   Hydrogen peroxide—Must be mixed right before use. Dilute with 3 or 4 parts water. Swish and spit. Rinse mouth afterward with normal saline solution or water. Hydrogen perioxide can be irritating and should be discontinued in patients with concurrent oral candida (monilia).

   Chlorhexicine (Peridex®)

6. Lips—Use of Chapstick®, lip balm or cocoa butter, or a water-based lubricant can help.
7. Gum massaging with finger or a rubber tip on a toothbrush may help.
8. Avoid drinking alcohol, smoking, and chewing tobacco as they are often very irritating to the oral mucosa.
9. Lukewarm tea may help healing, as it may form a base for antacids of Gelusil® to settle, these may be applied with a cotton-tipped applicator to areas of irritation,and the mouth can be rinsed with saline solution about 15 minutes later.

Treatments for Xerostomia, Mouth Lesions, Infections and Mouth Pain

I. Xerostomia (Dry Mouth)

Patients with chronic dry mouth, xerostomia, are best treated with an active oral hygiene program to reduce oral pathogens; frequent use of water or artificial saliva substitutes to prevent mouth dryness also may help stimulation of the salivary glands for the production of saliva. Diluted solutions of Pilocarpine may also be of help.

1. Mouth Cote™: Dry Mouth—A natural oral saliva. Contains: Water, xylitol, sorbitol, mucoprotective factor (MPF) extract yerba santa, citric acid, flavor, ascorbic acid, sodium benzoate, sodium saccharin. Available from: Parnell Pharmaceuticals, 1111 Francisco Boulevard, San Rafael, CA 94901, (415) 459-7600

2. Biotene™: Dry mouth toothpaste produces hydrogen peroxide and hypothicyanate during brushing. Used daily, the active enzyme in Biotene™ can be effective in helping the defense system normally found in saliva. Biotene dental chewing gum can be used for protection between brushings. Helps reduce plaque and gum diseases due to dry mouth. Contains: glucose oxidase, lactoperoxidase, sodium monofluorophosphate; sorbitol, calcium pyrophosphate, hydrated silica, PEG-8 isoceteth, cellulose gum, flavor, sodium benzoate, beta-d-glucose potassium, thiocynate. (Laclede Lab.)

3. MOI-STIR™: Oral swab stick, used as an aid to mouth care and oral hygiene. Contains a moisturing solution using a solution of chemicals and water similar to natural saliva; an aqueous solution of sorbitol. (Kingswood Lab.)

4. Saliva Substitutes: Saliva substitute (Roxane Laboratories, Inc.), Salavart® (Westport Pharmaceuticals).

5. Topical fluoride: Topical fluoride has become very important in preventing dry mouth in conjunction with an intense program of oral hygiene. Sodium fluoride topical solutions: Kari-Rinse (Lorvic), Karidium Liquid (Lorvic), Flura Dropt® (Kirkman).

II. Mouth Lesions (Stomatitis, Mucositis)

It is important to examine the mouth daily for changes. Examine mouth with flashlight and mirror. Look under tongue and on all sides of mouth. Changes must be reported and evaluated. Infections in the mouth must be treated promptly to prevent more serious systemic infections.

When mucosal infections or lesions occur, appropriate cultures for bacteria, fungi, and viruses are important so that appropriate antibiotic therapy can be initiated.

If platelets are low or mouth is sore, don't use a toothbrush. Toothettes® are recommended (Hallbrand, 4413 Industrial Parkway, Willoughby, OH 44094).

Medications and Mouthwashes

1. Allopurinol Mouthwash
   Indications: 5FU stomatitis prophylaxis
   Ingredients: Allopurinol 600 mg in 60 ml of 5% methylcellulose. Store in amber glass bottle. Refrigerate. Shake well before using.
   Dose: Rinse and spit 10–15 cc (5 cc = 1 tsp.; 15 cc = 1 Tbl.) 1 hr. 2 hr., and 3 hr. every morning after treatment, on days of treatment.
2. Carafate® Slurry
   Indications: Stomatitis-esophagitis
   Ingredients: Sucralfate 1 gm per 15 cc of 1 : 1 water and sorbitol (70%).
   Dose: 15 CC qid; swish and swallow.
3. Kaopectate®: one to three teaspoons applied to the areas of mucositis as needed.
4. MOM—milk of magnesia (1/2-full strength): swish but don't swallow.
5. 1-2-3: (Viscous Xylocaine, Benadryl® elixir, antacid) 2 tsp (10 cc), swish and spit for mouth soreness, swallow for inflammation in esophagus.
6. Orabase® (with or without Kenalog®): To coat local mouth sores. Apply directly or with cotton swab.

7. Oral Balance: Moisturing Gel™ (Laclede Professional Products. 15011 Staff Court, Gardena, CA 90248 (213) 770-0463). Protective, non-drying, clear gel for mucositis and to protect or coat tissue.
8. UC Swish
   Indications: Stomatitis phophylaxis, mouth soreness (use with Xylocaine and narcotics) Benadryl® 25 mg/10 cc; Nystatin® 60,000 U/10 cc; Hydrocortisone 2.3 mg/10 cc
   Dose: 10 cc q4H swish/spit for mouth lesion, swallow for inflammation in esophagus. Hold in mouth for 15 seconds.
9. Dyclone® Dyclonine HCL-0.5 or 1% (Astra Pharmaceuticals)

III. Infections

1. Herpes Simplex Virus
   Patients with recurrent or reactivated HSV infections (including patients who are seropositive) are at high risk. Oral acyclovir, 400 to 600 mg per day for a period of up to a year and a half may be very helpful. For those at a lower risk, early acyclovir therapy may reduce the chance for recurrent infection.
2. Monila—Candida Mucositis
3. a. Clotrimazole (Mycelex®) 10 mg troches after meals and hs (4–5 times a day).
   b. Nystatin suspension 1–3 tsp (5–15 cc) q4–6 hrs. The suspension can be frozen in medicine cups. The patient then is allowed to melt one popsicle in mouth qid.
   c. Mycostatin (Nystatin®) Pastilles® 200,000 U 1–2 Pastille 4–5 times daily oral to suck and swallow—dissolution in mouth (refrigerate between 2° and 8°C, 36°–46°F).
   d. Ketoconazole used orally (200–600 mg per day)check liver functions with blood chemistries periodically.

IV. Mouth Pain

Pain from mouth sores can be significant and may be aggravated by eating. Avoid acidic foods (e.g., orange juice), spicy, and extremely hot or cold foods. Practice meticulous mouth care and paint lesions with any of the following topical solutions before eating and as required. Narcotics may be required while stomatitis is severe to allow eating and mouth care.

1. Often adding Chloriseptic® or Hurricaine® solution may be of help.
2. For local pain, Hurricaine® spray which is benzyl benzocaine or Dyclone®, 1% applied with a cotton swab for painful lesions.
3. Xylocaine Viscous®, 10–15 ml every four hours, and especially before meals for swish and swallow. (Limit 125 ml/24 hrs.)
4. 1-2-3 solution: mixing viscous Xylocaine, Benadryl elixer and antacids; using two teaspoons swish and swallow; Benadryl elixer can also be used on local lesions.
5. Zilactin™—forms a tenacious and long lasting film over ulcers. For intraoral lesions—helps decrease pain so you can eat and drink normally with comfort. Provides up to six hours of pain relief from a broad range of oral ulcers.

Appendix C

Drugs to Treat Nausea and Vomiting

Patients report nausea and vomiting as the most disturbing side effects of chemotherapy. A combination of antiemetic drug protocols and attention to psychological effects can often alleviate nausea and vomiting and control its disturbing outcomes.

There is a strong physchological component present with many people who have had problems with nausea and vomiting with chemotherapy. They develop a conditioned response that will cause nausea and vomiting before chemotherapy is given. When the chemotherapy is given, the nausea and vomiting may be more severe. This becomes a very set pattern for some people and can limit the extent of chemotherapy treatment.

Food aversions can develop when people associate them with chemotherapy and vomiting. A smell, taste or a particular food can elicit a patterned Pavolvian response (anticipating nausea and vomiting).

Anticipatory nausea and vomiting occurs in about 25% of patients. The stimulus can be the room in which the chemotherapy is given, colors, odors, or seeing a physician or nurse. Such conditioned responses often are experienced after two to four sessions of chemotherapy. The symptoms may be relieved with psychological anti-aversion therapy such as relaxation or special tape-recorded self-hypnotic techniques.

Along with the food suggestions and relaxation, a quiet, often darkened environment, avoiding hot foods or temperatures, and eating slowly may be of help. If cooking odors are a problem, have friends or family cook the meals.

Sometimes the time of day the treatment is received makes a difference; it may have to be adjusted accordingly. Avoid foods which obviously upset the stomach or gastrointestinal tract and employ diversions such as art, television, or socializing to reduce the stress of a physician chemotherapy visit.

Common Antimetics for Nausea

1. Phenothiazines (Compazine®) 5 and 10 mg tablets every 4–6 hrs; or 15 or 30 mg spansules (tablets) every 10–12 hrs. Thiethylperazine (Torecan®) 10 mg, IMor PO q 6 hr. Start Compazine® or Torecan® one day before chemotherapy, and continue one day after chemotherapy if there is no nausea or vomiting.
2. Benzodiazepines (Lorazepam®, Ativan®) 1–2 mg IM, IV, PO or sublingual q 4–6h.
3. Metaclopramide (Reglan®) 20–30 mg PO q 8 h. For cisplatin 1–2 mg per kilogram IV q 3–4 hours × 4 doses. Give concurrent diphenhydramine (Benadryl®) to prevent dystonic reactions (trismus—muscle spasms of the mouh; or torticolis—muscle spasms of the shoulder).
4. Butyrophenones (droperidol®) 1–2 mg q 4–6H or 5 mg IV push 30 minutes before chemotherapy, then infusion (1–1.5 mg) q 9–12 hrs.
5. Haloperidol (Haldon®) 1–2 mg orally at bedtime (1–2 mg q 3–6 h IV, IM or oral).
6. Corticosteroids (Dexamethasone (Decadron®) 10–20 mg IV 30 min prior to chemotherapy then Q 6 hrs × 4 for highly emetogenic regimen.
7. Antihistamines (Benadryl®) 25 mg IM or IV or PO q 6 hr × 4.
8. Delta-9-tetrahydrocannabinol (THC) (Marinol®) 2.5 mg tid or qid.
9. A new investigational antiemetic drug—Ondanstetron® (Glaxo, Ltd) is scheduled to be released in late 1990 or early 1991, as well as other anti-serotonin analogues (Granisetron®) which are currently under investigation. Ondanstetron® is a $5/HT_3$ brain receptor blocker which binds serontonin to decrease or stop the initiation of nausea and vomiting in the lower brain (chemotherapy trigger zone). Vomiting is suppressed 60–80% of the time. Combining Ondanstetron® with corticosteroids may increase the vomiting suppression to approximately 90%. Side effects are minimal—headaches and transient elevation of liver enzymes (SGOT-transaminase).

   Common antiemetic combinations: Haldon, Decadron® and Compozine® or other combinations including Ativan®, Decadron® and Compozine®.

Appendix D

Antidiarrheal Medications

1. Lomotil® (diphenoxylate hydrochloride with atropine sulfate). Usual dose: 1 to 2 tablets po every 4 hours as needed. Dose should be adjusted to the individual patient and his or her pattern of diarrhea. Do not exceed 8 tablets within a 24 hour period.
2. Immodium® (loperamide hydrochloride), a synthetic antidiarrheal agent. Recommended initial dose: 2 capsules (4 mg) po every 4 hours, followed by one capsule (2 mg) po after each unformed stool. Daily total dose should not exceed 16 capsules.
3. Kaopectate®, an antidiarrheal agent. Dose: 30–60 cc po after each loose bowel movement.
4. Paregoric, an antidiarrheal agent. Usual dose: 1 teaspoon po qid as needed for diarrhea. Paregoric may also be used alternating with Lomotil.
5. Donnatal®, an anticholinergic, antispasmodic agent used to alleviate bowel cramping. Dose: 1 to 2 tablets every 4 hours as needed.

In addition to the above, relief from abdominal pain may be obtained by the use of narcotics. If proctitis is present, a steroid form, (Anusol-HCR) given rectally may offer relief of symptoms.

Finally, if patients with pancreatic cancer are experiencing diarrhea during radiation therapy, they should be evaluated for needed oral pancreatic enzyme replacement, as deficiencies in these enzymes alone can cause diarrhea. (Pancrease® or Cotazyme®)

Radiation colitis and proctitis may be helped by 5-ASA (5-aminosalicylic acid) 250 mg suppository—one qd in rectum.

Narcotics for Diarrhea:

1. Codeine 30–60 mg q 3–4 hr P.O. or IM
2. Tincture of opium 0.6–0.8 ml po q 4 hr prn diarrhea

GLOSSARY

Albumin—the main protein found in the blood.

Antiemetic—medications that prevent vomiting.

Appetite—psychologic desire to eat.

Anorexia—loss of appetite leading to decreased food intake.

Aspiration—inhalation of liquid or solid food materials into the nose, throat or lungs.

Cheilosis—reddened and cracked lips and mouth, frequently seen in riboflavin (a B vitamin) deficiency.

Dysphagia—difficulty swallowing.

Edema—swelling, condition resulting from excessive amounts of fluids in the body tissues.

Enteral administration routes—feeding via gastrointestinal tract either via mouth (P.O.) or through a feeding tube (nasogastric).

Epidemiologial evidence—appearance of an infectious disease or condition that attacks many people at the same time in the same geographical area.

Glossitis—inflammation of the tongue, often causing difficulty in swallowing and mouth pain.

Hemorrhagic cystitis—bleeding, inflamed or infected bladder.

Hunger—physiologic desire for food.

Hyperkeratosis—an overgrowth of cells on the cornea of the eye.

Lactose intolerance—inability to fully digest milk sugar (lactose) resulting in bloating, flatulence, and/or diarrhea.

LCT—long-chain triglycerides

MAOI—monamine oxidase inhibitors

MCT—medium-chain triglycerides

µg—microgram; 1/10 of a milligram

mg—milligram

MSG—monosodium glutamate

Mucositis—ulceration in the throat.

Parenteral administration routes—feeding nutrients directly to bloodstream for utilization by the body—used when enteral feeding route not functioning.

RDA—Recommended Dietary Allowance—safe and adequate levels of vitamins and minerals for a general, healthy population group.

Renal lithiasis—formation of kidney stone or calculus.

Steatorrhea—fat in the stool.

Stomatitis—ulceration in and around the mouth.

Transferrin—a protein in the blood that binds and transports iron.

Xerostoma—dryness of the mouth.

Recipe Index

Index

Nutrition Prescription Form

Nutrition Prescription for: ______________________________

This prescription will help you use *Nutrition for the Chemotherapy Patient*, your personal guide to food selection and eating. Nutrition is very important for you now—to help minimize side effects from your drug therapy, and to keep you as strong and healthy as possible to help your treatment.

Nutrition for the Chemotherapy Patient is designed to help lay out a specific nutritional strategy for the particular drugs you are receiving. To develop your strategy, use the following sections in Part I.

Chapter One—How to Deal with Specific Problems
Consult problem numbers:

- ❑ 1—Loss of Appetite
- ❑ 2—Nausea and Vomiting
- ❑ 3—Taste Changes
- ❑ 4—Sore or Ulcerated Mouth or Throat (Stomatitis/Mucositis)
- ❑ 5—Difficulties in Chewing and Swallowing (Dysphagia) and Dry Mouth (Xerostomia)
- ❑ 6—Diarrhea
- ❑ 7—Protecting the Gastrointestinal Tract (Enteritis)
- ❑ 8—Constipation
- ❑ 9—Dehydration

Chapter Two—General Dietary Guidelines
Consult guideline numbers:

- ❑ 1—Basic Nutrition for the Cancer Patient
- ❑ 2—A High-Protein/High-Calorie Diet
- ❑ 3—Food Sources of Minerals
- ❑ 4—Food Sources of Vitamins
- ❑ 5—The Fiber and Residue Contents of Foods
- ❑ 6—A Lactose-Free/Lactose-Restricted Diet
- ❑ 7—A Gluten-Restricted/Gliadin-Free Diet
- ❑ 8—A Long-Chain-Triglyceride-Restricted Medium-Chain-Triglyceride Fat Diet
- ❑ 9—A Cholesterol and Fat-Restricted Diet
- ❑ 10—To Prevent Kidney Stone Formation (Acid Ash/Alkaline Ash Diet)
- ❑ 11—To Control Transient Glucose Intolerance
- ❑ 12—A Sodium-Restricted Diet
- ❑ 13—A Tyramine and Dopamine-Restricted Diet
- ❑ 14—A Soft-Food/Pureed-Food Diet

In addition, the sections prescribed for you in Chapters One and Two will refer you to helpful recipes and tables in Chapter Three. If you have questions or need more information at any time, contact:

______________________________ at ____________________
name telephone number

Prescription Date: ____________________

Physician's Signature: ____________________ Phy. # ____________